DISEASE FREE

AT 60 PLUS

Hundreds of Life-Preserving Tips and Techniques to
Defy Heart Trouble, Cancer, and Stroke

By Doug Dollemore, Cathy Raymond,
and the Editors of
PREVENTION Magazine Health Books

Rodale Press, Inc.
Emmaus, Pennsylvania

The two-for-one recipe for chili and spaghetti sauce by Constance Pittman Linder on page 50 is reprinted by permission of the *Tufts University Diet and Nutrition Letter.*

The "Do You Use Food to Quell Emotions?" test on page 188 is adapted from *Thin Tastes Better* by Stephen P. Gullo, Ph.D. Copyright © 1995 by Stephen Gullo Food Control Center. Reprinted by permission of Crown Publishers, Inc.

The chart on page 16 was reprinted by permission of *The M-Fit Grocery Shopping Guide:* Your Guide to Healthier Choices by Nelda Mercer, M.S., R.D.; Lori Mosca, M.P.H., M.D.; and Melvyn Rubenfire, M.D. Copyright © 1995 by Regents of the University of Michigan.

Library of Congress Cataloging-in-Publication Data

Dollemore, Doug.
    Disease free at 60-plus : hundreds of life-preserving tips and techniques to defy heart trouble, cancer, and stroke / by Doug Dollemore, Cathy Raymond, and the Editors of Prevention Magazine Health Books.
        p.   cm.
    Includes index.
    ISBN 0–87596–342–0 hardcover
    1. Aged—Health and hygiene. 2. Longevity. I. Raymond, Cathy.
II. Prevention Magazine Health Books. III. Title.
RA777.6.D65   1997
613'.0438—dc21   96-46765

Distributed in the book trade by St. Martin's Press

2 4 6 8 10 9 7 5 3   hardcover

Contents

PART 1
A LIFESTYLE OF LONGEVITY

Introduction

More Life to Enjoy—As We Defy Heart Disease,
Cancer, and Stroke

By virtually every measure we are living longer, healthier, and more productive lives than any generation in history.

Every year fewer Americans in their sixties, seventies, eighties, and even nineties are disabled or are unable to care for themselves, according to the National Long-Term Care Surveys, a federally funded study that regularly polls nearly 20,000 people over age 65 about their health and lifestyles.

That means more of us are enjoying life—robustly facing joys and challenges every day. It means that even though we are getting older, we're staying young in both mind and body, says John Weisburger, M.D., Ph.D., a 75-year-old senior member at the American Health Foundation in Valhalla, New York. "In good part the improvement in longevity without being ill is due to changes in lifestyle. People at any age, but especially over 60, are making more of an effort to stay healthy."

But getting older would be even better if we could banish heart disease, stroke, and cancer from our lives. In fact, if all major forms of heart disease could be eliminated, the average American could add nearly a decade to his life expectancy, according to the American Heart Association. And if all forms of cancer were eradicated, the gain would be three years—years that you could use to give hundreds more hugs to your grandchildren and marvel at a thousand more sunrises.

The unfortunate truth is that these diseases disable thousands of people over age 60 each year and are the top three killers in this age group, claiming more than 1.1 million lives annually. Nearly 87 percent of the deaths caused by stroke and heart disease and 70 percent of deaths caused by cancer occur after age 65, according to the National Center for Health Statistics.

Overall, one in three men and one in four women will develop cancer after age 60. For each decade after age 55, the risk of stroke doubles, and for a person over age 65, the risk of dying of a stroke is seven times greater than for those who are younger. Then there is heart disease, the number one cause of hospitalization and death for people over age 65. More than 619,000 people in this age group are killed by heart disease annually.

But as you'll discover in this book, these diseases don't have to happen to you. It's never too late to make lifestyle changes that will greatly reduce your chances of getting these diseases. And if you do develop one of these disorders, lifestyle changes may even help you slow or reverse its progress.

"If you assume a lower-risk lifestyle—eat less fat and more fruits and vegetables, exercise, and quit smoking—all of this will put you on the track to good health at any age," Dr. Weisburger says. "In fact, it is entirely possible to die healthy at an old age. There is no need to have long, debilitating diseases like stroke, heart disease, or cancer. You actually can rearrange your lifestyle so that you stay healthy until your time comes. At age 89, 99, or 100, you can just go to sleep one night and not wake up. That's the way I want to die. And by eating right, exercising, and doing other things, I'm working to make sure that's how it happens."

In these pages you'll learn life-preserving strategies from many of the nation's leading doctors and researchers and meet average people over 60 doing their best to combat these dreaded diseases and add years to their lives.

In part 1, "A Lifestyle of Longevity," we discuss all of the important ways that you can take control of your health and minimize the odds that you'll get one of these three diseases. In part 2, "Crucial Answers for a Longer Life," we tackle some of the most asked—and most controversial—questions surrounding these diseases. Finally, in part 3, "Don't Let It Happen Again," we speak to those of you who have already been diagnosed with heart disease, stroke, or cancer, and we suggest ways to prevent a recurrence. At the end of each chapter, we have summarized the core advice in a "Prescription for Prevention."

Our wish is that you find a new vision of healthy aging in our words. "Tell me and I'll forget; show me and I may not remember," advises an old Native American proverb. "Involve me and I'll understand."

We hope these pages involve and inspire you to make changes that will oust the threat of these killers from your life.

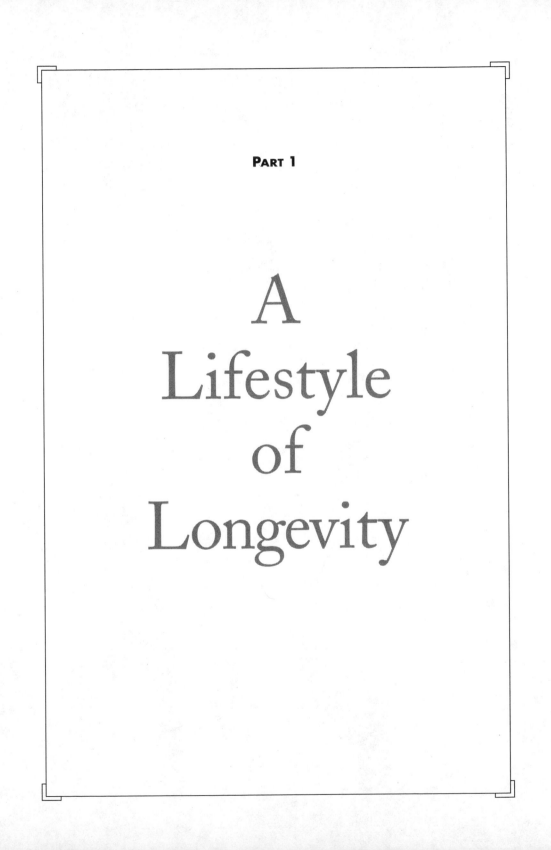

PART 1

A
Lifestyle
of
Longevity

Chapter 1

Low-Fat Eating

A Luscious, Rejuvenating Approach to Food

After a two-year, 24,000-mile voyage aboard a 71-foot sailboat, Graham Kerr was stunned by a mutiny in his own kitchen. Kerr, who gained fame as television's "Galloping Gourmet" in the 1960s, his wife, Treena, and their three children had willingly forsaken his delectable but high-fat meals after they discovered that rich foods aggravated seasickness. But they revolted against the famed chef's improvised low-fat cuisine as soon as they docked for the final time in 1974.

So while Kerr clung to his newly found low-fat lifestyle, his family eagerly returned to typical high-fat favorites like cheese, eggs, and sausages. The result? Seven years later, Treena suffered a stroke and a heart attack.

"When the family rebelled, I think if I had said, 'Look, we'll recreate the table so that we eat healthy food but get it in a way that you'll like it,' what happened to Treena wouldn't necessarily have occurred," says Kerr, now in his sixties and the author of *Graham Kerr's Best*.

Although she fully recovered, Treena was still at high risk for recurrent strokes and heart attacks because she was overweight and her total cholesterol hovered near 350 milligrams per deciliter (mg/dl). So in 1982, she agreed to change her diet. Since then, the couple has stuck to a low-fat lifestyle that consists mainly of fruits, vegetables, and grains. Treena eats no more than 2 ounces of fish, poultry, or red meat daily. Graham's diet allows him to have slightly more, but never more than 6 ounces. By 1995, when she was in her early sixties, Treena had lost 15 pounds; dropped her total cholesterol to 220 mg/dl raised her high-density lipoproteins (HDLs), the so-called good cholesterol; and slashed her low-density lipoproteins (LDLs), the "bad cholesterol."

"She's done very well," Kerr says. "I think there is no question that you can do wonderful things if you adopt low-fat eating."

In fact, more and more doctors are convinced that eating excessive amounts of fat is second only to smoking as a health threat. A growing arsenal of powerful evidence is also proving that cutting way back on dietary fat at any age can prevent or reverse heart disease, short-circuit strokes, and stifle the growth of many cancers, says Michael Klaper, M.D., director of the Institute of Nutrition Education and Research in Manhattan Beach, California.

How Bad Can Fat Be?

Americans love fat. So much that we eat the fat equivalent of six sticks of butter each week. But doing that month after month, year after year, takes its toll.

Of the estimated 13.5 million Americans alive today with a history of heart attack, angina, or both, about 50 percent are age 60 and older. Overall, heart disease and strokes annually kill more than 40 percent of all people who die in the United States. Of the eight controllable risk factors for those two diseases, five—elevated cholesterol and triglycerides, high blood pressure, diabetes, and excessive weight—have been linked to high-fat eating, says Hans Diehl, Dr.H.Sc., director of the Coronary Health Improvement Project, a lifestyle intervention program based in Loma Linda, California, that has helped more than 15,000 people worldwide reduce their risk of heart disease.

Eighty-three percent of the people who die of heart attack, which can be attributed in part to diet, are age 65 or older.

Heart disease, particularly due to atherosclerosis—hardening of the arteries caused by fatty buildups in the circulatory system—can at least double your risk of stroke, says Ralph L. Sacco, M.D., director of the North Manhattan Stroke Study at Columbia-Presbyterian Medical Center, an ongoing project examining stroke incidence among 260,000 people living in racially diverse neighborhoods in New York City.

The risk of ischemic stroke, the most common type caused by blood clots that block arteries supplying blood to the brain, may be even higher if you also have heart disease. French researchers who examined 250 men and women in their sixties and seventies found that those who had deposits of fatty plaque narrowing their aortic arches, the main artery leading out of the heart, were up to nine times more likely to have ischemic strokes than those who didn't have such buildups.

"If you have plaque there, more than likely you're going to have it in the arteries leading to or inside the brain, too," Dr. Sacco says.

...And Then There's Cancer

Dietary fat also may have a role in up to 40 percent of cancers in men and 60 percent of those that affect women, says Moshe Shike, M.D., director of clinical nutrition at Memorial Sloan-Kettering Cancer Center in New York City and co-author of *Cancer Free.*

Research shows that men in their sixties and seventies who continue to eat lots of red meat are at 2 to 3 times greater risk for colon cancer. They also are more likely to develop rectal cancer and 2.6 times more likely to have prostate cancer than men who limit dietary animal fats. Women older than age 60 who load up on red meat are 2.5 times more likely to develop colon cancer.

Scientists also are learning more about the role of fat in the development of breast cancer. Researchers at the University of Hawaii, for instance, compared the eating habits of 272 postmenopausal women who were being treated for breast cancer with 296 women who lived in the same area but who were cancer-free. They found that overweight women who ate a lot of foods high in saturated fat like sausage, processed cold cuts, beef, lamb, and whole-milk dairy food were at greater risk for breast cancer.

"We know that saturated fats have an impact on hormone levels in the body, and we think that has a role in promoting breast cancer," says Cheryl Ritenbaugh, Ph.D., head of nutrition research at the Arizona Cancer Center in Tucson.

Eating fat also might increase your risk of lung cancer even if you don't smoke, says Michael Alavanja, Ph.D., senior scientist at the National

Cancer Institute in Rockville, Maryland. In his study of 429 female non-smokers ranging up to age 84, Dr. Alavanja concluded that those who ate the most saturated fat were six times more likely to have lung cancer than those who consumed the least amount of that fat.

"At least seven studies worldwide have shown an effect of saturated fat on lung cancer," Dr. Alavanja says. "It's not conclusive, but the evidence is pointing toward the fact that fat increases the risk of lung cancer among smokers and nonsmokers."

But the truth is that none of these things need to happen to you. You could help prevent and possibly subdue almost every one of these diseases if you did just one thing: Slash the fat.

"It's very clear that our diet is totally devastating us," Dr. Diehl says. "We know that if we cut the fat content and ate a more plant food–centered diet, we could drastically cut our risk for most cancers, heart disease, and stroke."

So Why Do We Still Eat It?

A surprising number of people—particularly among those of us over age 60—haven't gotten the word yet.

In fact, one-third of 4,480 people who cook household meals told University of Nebraska researchers that they had never heard that fat was a problem.

"I was very surprised by that finding. The information about fat has been around for a long time. You'd think that by the 1990s everyone would be aware of it, especially the people who are taking care of food preparation for an entire household," says Nancy Betts, R.D., Ph.D., associate professor of nutritional science at the university in Lincoln, who conducted the survey.

Why are we so perplexed?

Well, you probably can guess that fat exists for a reason. Eating it provides us with essential fatty acids that we need to regulate body temperature, maintain healthy skin and hair, and insulate and protect nerves and vital organs like the heart and kidneys.

The problem is that all fats are not created equal. Monounsaturated fats like olive and canola oils and polyunsaturated fats, like corn and safflower oils are considered healthier than saturated fats, which are found mainly in meats, eggs, and dairy products. Trans-fatty acids, another type of harmful fat, are unsaturated fats that have been artificially solidified by food manu-

The Skinny on Fat

This table lists the percentage of saturated fat and unsaturated fat in some common cooking oils and fats. (The percentages do not add up to 100 percent because these fats have small amounts of other fatty substances.)

Oil/Fat	Saturated (%)	Monounsaturated (%)	Polyunsaturated (%)
11 superb choices...			
Canola oil	7	60	30
Safflower	9	13	76
Walnut oil	9	23	65
Sunflower oil	11	20	67
Corn oil	13	25	59
Olive oil	14	76	9
Soybean oil	15	24	59
Peanut oil	17	47	32
Rice oil	19	42	38
Wheat-germ oil	19	15	63
Margarine	20	48	32
...And 7 ugly ones			
Coconut oil	89	6	2
Butter	64	29	4
Palm oil	50	36	9
Lard	39	45	11
Chicken fat	30	45	20
Cottonseed oil	26	18	53
Vegetable shortening	25	45	20

Sorting Out Lean, Light, and Everything in Between

For some of us, telling the difference between Minnesota Fats and monounsaturated fats is a challenge. (Here's a hint: Monos don't play pool.) Here are some of the key words and phrases that you should look for on food labels and what they really mean.

Saturated fats are loaded (saturated) with hydrogen atoms. Saturated fats are found primarily in animal foods like meat, poultry, and dairy products such as butter. These fats tend to raise levels of the "bad" low-density lipoprotein (LDL) cholesterol in the blood and increase the risk of heart disease and stroke. Saturated fat has also been linked to several cancers including colon, prostate, lung, and breast.

Monounsaturated fats like olive and canola oils lower levels of LDL cholesterol in the blood and may reduce the risk of heart disease, stroke, and cancer. They are called monounsaturated because they are missing one pair of hydrogen atoms and, therefore, are unsaturated.

Polyunsaturated fats such as corn, safflower, sesame, and sunflower oils are missing more than one pair of hydrogen atoms. Although they aren't as harmful as saturated fats, polyunsaturated fats should be used cautiously because they do lower both LDL and "good" high-density lipoprotein (HDL) cholesterol levels and may increase your risk of cardiovascular disease. Polyunsaturated fats also promote cell division and that can increase your cancer risk.

facturers to make products like margarines and vegetable shortenings.

Unfortunately, many foods aren't purely unsaturated or saturated. So when you eat a typical American meal, you're likely consuming a mixture of these good and bad fats. Therefore, it is possible to unwittingly load up on bad fats even if you chop obvious fats like butter out of your life.

Why Cut Back Now?

The average American eats about 34 percent of calories from fat—down from 43 percent just a few years ago. But many people in their six-

Hydrogenated fats are created when food manufacturers add hydrogen atoms to unsaturated fats so that they solidify and transform into saturated fats like vegetable shortenings and margarine.

Trans-fatty acids are solidified polyunsaturated fats created during hydrogenation and raise LDL cholesterol levels about as much as saturated fat. To be safe, avoid foods with ingredient lists that include hydrogenated or partially hydrogenated fat.

Cholesterol, a fatty chemical compound manufactured by the body, also is found in many meats, dairy products, and other animal foods. It helps make important hormones and cell membranes. But excessive amounts of LDL cholesterol narrows artery walls. HDL cholesterol helps sweep LDL out of the body.

Fat-free. A product carrying this label has less than 0.5 gram of it.

Low-fat. This food has 3 grams of fat or less per serving.

Lean. Less than 10 grams of total fat, 4 grams of saturated fat, and 95 milligrams of cholesterol per serving are in this food.

Light. Contains one-third fewer calories or no more than half the fat of the regular product.

Cholesterol-free. Fewer than 2 milligrams of cholesterol and 2 grams or less of saturated fat are in this product.

ties, seventies, and eighties continue to consume 40 to 50 percent of their calories from fat, says Cheryl Pingleton, R.D., a dietitian at the Grand Court Lifestyles, a retirement community in Phoenix.

"Many of the people I see are eating a lot of fried foods, creamy salad dressings, and rich desserts," Pingleton says. "They feel as if they've worked their whole lives and now literally want to enjoy the fat of the land."

But as we have seen, enjoying fat too much can lead to serious health problems. If, however, you switch to a low-fat lifestyle, you may quickly feel rejuvenated, particularly if you have a chronic ailment.

"You can lose weight, feel more energetic, have fewer digestive problems, and just feel better about yourself," Pingleton says. "No matter what your age or medical condition—diabetes, gout, high cholesterol, heart disease—low-fat eating is the way to go."

The American Heart Association (AHA) and the National Cancer Institute recommend that no more than 30 percent of total calories come from fat. The AHA says that less than 10 percent of calories should come from saturated fat. Many researchers believe that fat should have an even smaller role on our dinner plates—down to 20 percent or possibly as low as 10 percent of total calories.

"Cutting back on fat will help, and the more drastically you can cut back, the better off you'll be, with the lower limit being around 7 percent of calories from fat for nutritional adequacy. If you have angina, you'll certainly have less angina. You'll also have less risk of stroke, heart attack, and cancer. And every study that I've ever looked at says it's never too late to make these important changes in your diet," says Lee Lipsenthal, M.D., medical director of Preventive Medicine Research Institute in Sausalito, California, where Dean Ornish, M.D., is conducting his pioneering research on reversing heart disease.

In fact, according to Dr. Diehl, switching to a low-fat lifestyle even in your later years can help quash the big three killers—heart disease, stroke, and cancer. Here's a look at how dietary fat does its harm and how you can stop or even reverse some of this damage.

The Heart of the Matter

Within five hours of eating a fatty meal like a slice of pepperoni pizza or a bologna sandwich, which are loaded with saturated fat, radical and dangerous changes occur in your body's chemistry, Dr. Klaper says.

First, a tide of fat oozes into the bloodstream and coats red blood cells with a sticky film. "Under normal conditions, blood serum is clear. But after you eat a fatty meal, it is thick, white, and greasy. It looks like household glue," Dr. Klaper says.

Because they're more sticky, these cells begin to clump together. It is this clumping that eventually forms the blood clots in the arteries, which lead to stroke or heart attack. At the same time, saturated fat raises the harmful LDL cholesterol levels in the blood by suppressing the production of enzymes in the liver that would normally help destroy these compounds. Adding to your woes, as the body processes the fat, it produces free radicals, the same oxidizing molecules that cause metal to rust and food to spoil. Inside your body, these free radicals cause cholesterol to cling to artery walls and clog them up. Years of eating like that virtually guarantees that a person age 60-plus will have at least some atherosclerosis, the underlying disease that can lead to stroke and heart attack.

In addition, this arterial rust makes it more difficult to deliver oxygenated blood, says Dr. Diehl. This starves the tissues and leads to degenerative changes that can cause impotence, hearing loss, degenerative disk disease, memory loss, and vision problems, Dr. Diehl says.

But remember, it doesn't have to happen.

"Atherosclerosis is totally unnecessary. But it is reversible, even after age 60. All you have to do is take better care of yourself, particularly how you eat. The simpler your diet, the better your chances of reversing these narrowed arteries and increasing blood flow to more adequate levels once again," Dr. Diehl says. "In as little as three weeks, most people can eat themselves out of angina symptoms just by switching to a simpler diet that includes very low fat foods."

Going into Reverse

Several exciting studies have shown that eating a very low fat and low cholesterol diet in conjunction with other lifestyle changes like exercise, smoking cessation, and stress reduction can, as Dr. Diehl says, actually reverse heart disease.

"Our experience has shown that within days of starting a low-fat diet, patients with angina can show an immediate and dramatic decrease in their symptoms," says Monroe Rosenthal, M.D., medical director of the Pritikin Longevity Center in Santa Monica, California. In addition, studies have shown that coronary artery blockages can actually be reversed over a one- to two-year period, he says.

Pritikin researchers, for example, studied a group of 4,587 men and women that included people in their eighties and nineties. After three weeks, those who ate a diet that was less than 10 percent of calories from fat and consisted mostly of fruits, vegetables, and whole grains lowered their total cholesterol levels by 23 percent. This reduction sliced their heart attack risk in half.

"There was little difference in drop in cholesterol levels between the young people and the older people. This is clear proof that it's never too late to change your lifestyle and improve your health," says R. James Barnard, Ph.D., author of the study and professor of physiology in the Department of Physiological Science at the University of California, Los Angeles.

The Ornish Way Works

Even more dramatic results come from Dr. Ornish's landmark work. Dr. Ornish divided 43 men and 5 women—many in their fifties, sixties and seventies who had severe atherosclerosis—into two groups. The "treatment" group was instructed to go on a strict vegetarian diet deriving fewer than 10 percent of calories from fat. No meat, poultry, fish, or cheese. No nuts or seeds. No chocolate, no coffee, no cooking oils. In addition, they walked for at least 1 hour, three times a week; practiced meditation and yoga daily; and if they smoked, they quit.

Meanwhile, the other group was advised to follow the standard American Heart Association lifestyle program. That is, reduce their fat intake to less than 30 percent of calories, stop smoking, and exercise moderately.

After one year, 82 percent of those in the treatment group had shown reversal of coronary blockage. The average amount of reduction was about 5 percent. But even that modest regression can mean a 100 percent improvement in blood flow, says Dr. Lipsenthal. Those on the AHA diet didn't experience these striking results. At best, their disease appeared to progress at a slower rate.

"It's a world of difference. I'm doing things that I never imagined I could do again," says Victor Karpenko, in his seventies and a retired nuclear engineer in Danville, California. When he began the Ornish program in 1987, he had one artery almost completely blocked, had suffered from persistent angina, and could walk less than a block.

Since then, his total cholesterol has dropped from 290 to 150 mil-

Fat-Busting Starts Here

Before you can break away from high-fat living, you need some information about your dietary needs. First, you need to roughly calculate how many calories you should eat daily based on your age, says Moshe Shike, M.D., director of clinical nutrition at Memorial Sloan-Kettering Cancer Center in New York City and co-author of *Cancer Free.*

To do that, multiply your body weight by 13. (The average person needs to eat 13 calories per pound to do normal daily activities.) Next, subtract 2 percent of that total for each decade after age 30.

So if you are 70 years old and weigh 160 pounds, for example, multiply 160 by 13. That's 2,080 calories. Now deduct 10 percent to account for your age—that leaves you with 1,872 calories. That's your basic caloric need. Now you can use the following chart to figure out the maximum number of fat grams you want to eat per day based on 30, 25, 20, 15, or 10 percent of calories from fat. Tallying your fat grams each day will help you make better decisions when you're reading food labels and preparing meals.

If You Eat (in Calories)	Calories from Fat				
	30%	25%	20%	15%	10%
1,200	40 g.	33 g.	27 g.	20 g.	13 g.
1,400	47 g.	39 g.	31 g.	23 g.	16 g.
1,600	53 g.	44 g.	36 g.	27 g.	18 g.
1,800	60 g.	50 g.	40 g.	30 g.	20 g.
2,000	67 g.	56 g.	44 g.	33 g.	22 g.
2,200	73 g.	61 g.	49 g.	37 g.	24 g.
2,400	80 g.	67 g.	53 g.	40 g.	27 g.
2,600	87 g.	72 g.	58 g.	43 g.	29 g.
2,800	93 g.	78 g.	62 g.	47 g.	31 g.

ligrams per deciliter, he has lost 30 pounds, his angina is gone, and he regularly hikes in the hills surrounding his home. He also climbs the equivalent of 130 floors on his stair-climber in a half-hour and backpacked in the High Sierras at 8,000 feet with 40 pounds on his back.

"The diet is really the foundation of the whole program," Karpenko says. "I feel so much better now physically and mentally because of it. And it's a diet that really isn't hard to stick to when you consider the benefits."

Little Trims Add Up, Too

But even if you can't see yourself curbing your fat consumption as much as Dr. Ornish suggests, just shaving a modest amount of fat from the obvious sources might have some positive effects.

In the St. Thomas' Atherosclerosis Regression Study in London, for instance, 26 men up to age 66 were put on a diet that limited fat intake to 27 percent of calories and lowered saturated fat to 8 percent of calories. In a similar group, 24 men were allowed to eat their usual English diets, which typically consist of about 40 percent of calories from fat. Three years later, researchers found that 10 men in the dietary group (compared to 1 man in the usual-care group) had small regressions of artery blockages. As a result, the dietary group reported better control of angina and had three times fewer deaths and coronary surgeries and two times fewer heart attacks.

"Anything that you can do to lower your fat is better than doing nothing at all," Dr. Barnard says. "It's like a game of Russian roulette. It just depends on how many bullets you want to stick in that revolver. If it holds six bullets and you eat the typical American diet, then you have five bullets in it. If you want to eat 20 percent, you're down to four. If you go to 15 percent, you're down to three. And if you can manage to get down to less than 10 percent, you may only have one bullet in that pistol, and your risk of these diseases is dramatically reduced."

The Cancer Link: Another Reason to Lower Fat Now

Fat doesn't directly cause cancer. Instead, it promotes it—much like ice on a porch step increases the chances that you'll slip and fall, Dr.

Klaper says. Although researchers aren't certain how this happens, they do have plenty of theories. Some suspect that free radicals, produced as the body metabolizes fat, damage a cell's genetic codes and spark cancers. Others believe that fat may interfere with the body's ability to shut down cell growth or that it disrupts the immune system, which may have a protective role against cancer.

High-fat meals also may stimulate production of sexual hormones like estrogen and testosterone that can promote cancer, particularly in the breast and prostate, Dr. Klaper says.

But whatever the reason, it is becoming increasingly clear that the longer you stick to a high-fat lifestyle, the less likely it is that you will remain cancer-free in what should be the best years of your life.

"Eating high-fat foods is like throwing gasoline on a fire," Dr. Klaper says. "You're just fanning the flames of the cancer and helping it spread."

But as with heart disease and stroke, this doesn't have to be your future. In fact, slashing dietary fat might help many of us in our sixties, seventies, and eighties halt the progression of certain tumors before they become cancerous and prevent recurrences, Dr. Ritenbaugh says.

It may be too late, for instance, for dietary changes to stop a tumor from developing in the next couple of years, but "tumors that would have gotten you 4, 5, or 10 years from now, you can still do something about," Dr. Ritenbaugh says.

Derailing Tumors

Cutting back to 20 percent of calories from fat, for example, may reduce your risk of precancerous skin growths and prevent skin cancer in your sixties and beyond, according to researchers at Baylor College of Medicine in Houston. In their study, researchers found that people who continued eating the typical American diet developed three times more precancerous skin lesions, called actinic keratosis, than those who ate a low-fat diet.

Men over the age of 60 who have been cancer-free all of their lives run a 21 percent risk of being diagnosed with prostate cancer, the second leading lethal cancer among American men. But switching to low-fat eating may help stop the growth of microscopic prostate cancers before

15

Minor Metamorphosis Makes a Menu Magnificent

Small changes can make a big difference in percentage of calories from fat in your meals without sacrificing taste. Here's a pair of examples. The daily menu on the left is similar to the typical American diet—2,400 calories, 34 percent of calories from total fat and 12 percent of calories from saturated fat. The healthier menu on the right provides 2,300 calories, but only 26 percent of calories from total fat and 7 percent of calories from saturated fat. The changes are subtle, but enough to make a huge dent in the amount of fat. Both were prepared by Nelda Mercer, R.D., of the University of Michigan Medical Center and co-author of *The M-Fit Grocery Shopping Guide: Your Guide to Healthier Choices.*

Typical American Diet   **The Healthy Alternative**

Breakfast

Typical American Diet	The Healthy Alternative
8 oz. orange juice	8 oz. orange juice
12 oz. coffee	12 oz. coffee
1 Tbsp. half-and-half creamer	1 Tbsp. half-and-half creamer
1 cup puffed rice cereal	1¼ cups ready-to-eat oat cereal
¾ cup 2% milk	1 cup skim milk
	¾ cup strawberries

Midmorning Snack

Typical American Diet	The Healthy Alternative
12 oz. coffee	12 oz. coffee
1 tsp. nondairy powdered creamer	1 tsp. fat-free creamer
1 plain doughnut	1 blueberry muffin

Lunch

Typical American Diet	The Healthy Alternative
12 oz. cola	12 oz. instant tea (unsweetened)
1 cup carrot sticks	1 cup carrot sticks

they have a chance to cause major problems, says William R. Fair, M.D., chief of urologic surgery and chairman of urologic oncology at Memorial Sloan-Kettering Cancer Center in New York City. In his animal studies, Dr. Fair is finding that dipping fat consumption below 20 per-

1 oz. potato chips
Ham-and-cheese sandwich
   made with:
1 oz. regular ham
1 oz. Cheddar cheese
1 Tbsp. mayonnaise
2 slices white bread

—
Grilled chicken sandwich
   made with:
4 oz. grilled chicken breast
1 oz. Swiss cheese
2 leaves lettuce
1 slice tomato
1 Tbsp. mayonnaise
1 wheat bun

Afternoon Snack

1 chocolate bar

1 oz. pretzels
1 medium apple
12 oz. can of diet cola

Dinner

5 oz. chicken breast (fried)
3/4 cup mashed potatoes

1½ cups cooked spaghetti
3/4 cup tomato and mushroom
   sauce

3/4 cup canned peas and carrots
Salad made with:
1 cup iceberg lettuce, tomatoes,
   and carrots
2 Tbsp. ranch salad dressing
1 brown-and-serve roll
1 tsp. corn oil margarine

1 oz. meatballs
Salad made with:
1 cup romaine lettuce, tomatoes,
   and carrots
2 Tbsp. light ranch dressing
1 whole-wheat roll
1 tsp. corn oil margarine

Evening Snack

1 cup vanilla ice cream

1 cup low-fat vanilla ice cream

cent of calories can halt the progression of these tiny tumors.

    "I really don't think a low-fat diet could cure a sizable tumor, but if it can halt the progression of a microscopic tumor, then that would be tantamount to a cure," Dr. Fair says.

Cutting back on fat may also stave off colon cancer, according to Harvard University researchers who followed nearly 52,000 male health professionals for two years. Those who ate the least amount of animal fat—about 24 percent of calories—were half as likely to develop precancerous colon polyps as the men who consumed more fat.

"These studies suggest that eating a healthy diet that includes lower amounts of animal fat and higher amounts of fruits and vegetables that have lots of fiber and micronutrients is an important part of what we can do to prevent colon cancer," says Eric Rimm, Sc.D., assistant professor of epidemiology and nutrition at the Harvard School of Public Health.

Women can dramatically reduce their risk of other common types of cancer—particularly breast cancer—if they significantly ease up on fat, Dr. Klaper says.

Researchers put 13 postmenopausal women at the Pritikin Longevity Center in Santa Monica, California, on an eating plan that included less than 10 percent of calories from fat. In three weeks, their blood levels of estradiol, a form of the hormone estrogen linked to breast cancer, fell nearly 50 percent. As a result, the women were far less likely to develop breast cancer at the end of the study, Dr. Barnard estimates.

Even if a woman age 60 or older does get breast cancer, reducing fats may be a good move. Women who have breast cancer might substantially improve their chances of surviving if they are on low-fat diets, according to researchers at the University of Minnesota in Minneapolis who polled 42,000 women between the ages of 55 and 69 on their eating habits. Of the 698 women who developed breast cancer in the next five years, those who reported eating 56 grams of fat a day (almost 2 ounces) had twice the risk of death as women who ate less fat, says Aaron Folsom, M.D., professor of epidemiology at the university and co-author of the study.

"I'm not surprised that lower-fat diets are effective in the prevention of breast cancer as well as its treatment," Dr. Klaper says. "High-fat diets raise the levels of sex hormones like estrogen in the bloodstream, and many breast cancers depend on estrogen to grow."

Cutting down on fat also may help women slash their risk of ovarian cancer, a disease that becomes more common as women reach their early sixties, says Harvey A. Risch, M.D., Ph.D., associate professor of epidemiology and public health at Yale University School of Medicine.

Dr. Risch and his colleagues evaluated the eating habits of 450 women up to age 79 with ovarian cancer and 564 without the disease. They concluded that cutting 10 grams of saturated fat a day (about the same amount as in one cheeseburger with all the fixings) could trim the risk of ovarian cancer by 20 percent. And adding 10 grams of vegetable fiber a day—what you would get in about 1 cup of cooked lentils—may take the risk down by another 37 percent.

"It appears possible to cut your risk of ovarian cancer in half by assertive modification of the diet," Dr. Risch says.

How to Start Now

Really cutting back on total fat and sorting out the best low-fat foods from the worst high-fat offenders takes some adjustments, but these changes don't have to be time-consuming or costly or sap flavor from your favorite meals.

"Changing a lifetime of eating habits, particularly for people age 60-plus, can be challenging. But I don't think it's as hard to do as many people perceive. It doesn't have to be all or nothing. Over time, even small changes in your eating habits can improve your health," says Sheah Rarback, R.D., an American Dietetic Association spokesperson in Miami.

Here are some basics to get you started.

Keep score. For the next couple of days, jot down on a piece of paper or handy 3-by-5-inch cards all the foods and beverages that you eat and drink. Note the amount and type of fat listed on the nutrition labels. If you're eating in a restaurant, estimate your intake of food, Dr. Shike suggests. This will give you an idea about how much fat you're eating now and how much you'll need to cut back. Every three months or so, do this all over again so that you can see your progress.

Set a goal. Give yourself something to strive for, but make it practical, Pingleton says. Making over a lifetime of eating habits in a week probably isn't realistic. But getting your total fat intake under 25 percent of calories in the next six months is a reasonable goal.

Be bold. Most doctors and dietitians recommend that no more than 30 percent of your calories come from fat. But it seems that the more you slash the fat you eat, the more dramatic the impact on your health. So be adventurous, Dr. Klaper suggests. Experiment with lower levels of fat in your meals. To begin, pick a day of the week and on that day, make a bean dish, pasta, or salad the centerpiece of your meals. If you dine out, try low-fat ethnic foods or vegetarian dishes. Then gradually, over a month or two, increase the number of days of the week you eat like that. All of this will help your taste buds adapt to eating less fat and help you become comfortable with a new lower-fat lifestyle.

Count the grams. Figuring the percentage of fat in a meal can be tricky.

An easier way to control fat consumption is to count grams, because that's how fats are measured on nutrition labels, says William Castelli, M.D., epidemiologist, medical director of the Framingham Cardiovascular Institute and former director of the Framingham Heart Study in Massachusetts. So if you eat 2,000 calories a day and want to keep your fat intake below 20 percent, multiply 2,000 by 20 percent. That's 400 calories. Now divide 400 by 9—which is the number of fat calories in 1 gram. You get 45, the number of grams of fat you're allowing from all the foods that you eat in one day. How much is that? A beef bologna sandwich made with two pieces of meat and a 1-ounce slice of regular Cheddar cheese has about 36 grams of fat—nearly an entire day's fat allowance in one meal. So use those fat grams thoughtfully, Dr. Castelli says.

Take 20. Try to keep your consumption of saturated fat—the really bad fat—under 20 grams a day (10 grams if you have suffered a heart attack), Dr. Castelli says. Again, read the food labels carefully. What can you eat and stay under 20 grams? A lot more than wheat germ.

"You could have rolled oats, fruit, and low-fat yogurt for breakfast; a chicken, tuna, or turkey sandwich for lunch; and shrimp cocktail, a 3-ounce filet mignon, vegetables, salad, and fat-free dressing for dinner—

and you'd still be under 20 grams of saturated fat for the day," Dr. Castelli says. "Now does that sound like such a miserable experience?"

Make the switch gradually. Cravings for fat won't disappear immediately, but you can retrain your taste buds, says John Foreyt, Ph.D., director of the Nutrition Research Clinic at Baylor College of Medicine in Houston.

"You can retrain yourself at any age by making shifts gradually away from high-fat foods," he says.

Make one gradual change a week. If you use whole milk in your coffee or on cereal, for example, try a 50/50 mixture of whole milk and 2 percent milk for a week. Then switch to 2 percent for seven days. Then use a mixture that is half 2 percent and half 1 percent, and so on until you are using skim milk. If skim milk alone doesn't satisfy your taste buds, you can stir in some nonfat powdered milk to improve its texture and flavor, Dr. Foreyt says. You can use the same strategy to wean yourself off cheeses, shortenings and oils, ice cream, and other high-fat traditions.

Reinvent your favorites. The worst thing that you can do is give up your favorite dishes, because you'll feel deprived and may develop cravings that make it harder to stick to a low-fat lifestyle, Dr. Foreyt says. Instead, experiment with low-fat ingredients.

"Take your 10 favorite recipes and go into the supermarket and buy all the low-fat substitutes for the ingredients that you would normally use," says Dr. Castelli.

If you prefer not to modify your recipes, then serve the original versions less often—on holidays and special occasions, for instance—and take only half of the portion that you would normally eat, Dr. Foreyt suggests.

Eat with friends. Make your transition to low-fat living a social celebration, Rarback says. Ask a few friends to join a lunch or dinner club. On a rotating basis, one of you makes a low-fat main entrée while the others bring the bread, salad, fruit, or dessert.

"It will help all of you experiment with new low-fat recipes, and it is fun to eat together," she says.

Splurge now and then . . . Make high-fat foods like country fried
(continued on page 24)

21

Slash More Than 100 Fat Grams Painlessly

Cutting fat out of your foods can be fun and tasty. Here are some simple ways to cut more than 100 fat grams from your meals and snacks, according to Cheryl Pingleton, R.D., a dietitian at the Grand Court Lifestyles, a retirement community in Phoenix.

If You Eat:	Grams of Fat
Blueberry muffin	6
1 oz. bag of potato chips	10
3½ oz. fried chicken with skin	17
2 Tbsp. regular French dressing	13
3 store-bought chocolate chip cookies	7
½ cup rich chocolate ice cream	15
3 oz. corned beef	16
1 cup cream of mushroom soup	19
3-in. square fudge brownie	6
1 Tbsp. margarine	11
1 Tbsp. half-and-half in 2 cups of coffee = 2 Tbsp. daily	4
2 oz. whole-milk American cheese	18
TOTAL:	142

Switch To:	Grams of Fat	Fat Savings
A toasted (unbuttered) English muffin with jam	1	5
1 oz. bag of pretzels	1	9
3½ oz. roasted light meat chicken without skin	5	12
2 Tbsp. reduced-calorie French dressing	2	11
3 fig bars	3	4
½ cup peach frozen yogurt	4	11
3 oz. lean roast beef (eye of round)	4	12
1 cup minestrone soup	3	16
2-in. square angel food cake with fresh strawberries	0	6
1 Tbsp. whipped margarine	7	4
2 Tbsp. evaporated skim milk in 2 cups of coffee = 4 Tbsp. daily	0	4
2 oz. light cheese	8	10
	38	104

steak a once-a-month treat rather than daily fare, says Michele Tuttle, R.D., director of consumer affairs for the Food Marketing Institute in Washington, D.C.

"I've never met anybody who can eat perfectly. In fact, that's probably the best recipe for failure because the thought that you can never have chocolate fudge double cake again in your life will drive you crazy," Tuttle says. "So go ahead and have a little bit with some friends. One dessert split four ways is not a big deal."

. . . But make up for it later. Any one food or any one meal can have some extra fat as long as you compensate for it, Dr. Foreyt says.

"Over a week you want your fat consumption to be certainly less than 30 percent of calories and closer to 20 percent of calories if you can get there," Dr. Foreyt says. "So if you eat a hamburger or cheesecake on a Monday, that's fine. But you should adjust your eating plans so that you eat less fat during the rest of the week."

With these essentials in mind, here are some ideas for stocking your pantry, shopping for groceries, eating at home, and dining out that will help you become a savvy low-fat role model for your grandchildren.

The Pantry: Low-Fat Living Starts Here

Filling your pantry with high-fat foods is like asking a compulsive gambler to live next door to a casino.

It's too much of a temptation.

"If you don't have the right things in your pantry, you're going to pre-pare the foods you do have in the same old way, or you're going to be tempted to say 'the heck with it' and go out to eat at a high-fat restaurant," Tuttle says. "So it only makes sense to stock your pantry well."

For low-fat living, here is what should be readily at hand in the kitchen of anyone who is age 60 and over.

Remember the 75/25 rule. "Whenever you open the refrigerator, a kitchen cabinet, or the bread box, 75 percent of what you see should be plant-derived foods—pastas, breads, beans, cereals, grains, and fresh, frozen, or canned fruits and vegetables. Then the remaining 25 percent can be made up of small amounts of lean meats and low-fat dairy products like milk and cheese. If the bulk of your pantry is like that, then your plate will probably look that way, too," says Elizabeth Somer, R.D., author of *Nutrition for Women*.

Consider the pastabilities. Pastas like spaghetti, linguine, and fettucine have earned a bizarre reputation for being fattening. But in reality, these grain foods are almost devoid of fat and are a great source of complex carbohydrates—your body's best fuel.

"If you fill up on pasta, you'll be more inclined to eat less meat, and that will mean that you're eating even less fat," Rarback says. So keep several boxes of your favorite pastas within reach.

Be wary of what you put on pasta. What fattens up most pastas is what we put on it, says Rarback. A typical white sauce, for instance, is 71 percent calories from fat. And most bottled spaghetti sauces have up to 9 grams of fat in a ½-cup serving.

Instead of those, always keep in your refrigerator a jar of spaghetti sauce that has 5 grams of fat or less to pour over pasta, spread on pizza crust or even on baked potatoes, says Elaine Moquette-Magee, R.D., author of the book series *Fight Fat and Win: How to Eat a Low-Fat Diet without Changing Your Life.*

Count on beans and rice. Dried beans like pinto, navy, lima, and black beans, and grains like brown rice are virtually fat-free and are terrific sources of protein that can reduce or eliminate the need for fat-laden meats in stews, chili, salads, and other traditional dishes, Rarback says. Instead of using 10 ounces of beef in a stew, for example, use 5 ounces and round out the dish with lentils.

Be aware that beans can cause gas. To prevent it, soak your beans overnight in a bowl of water and then use new water for cooking them, suggests Rarback. Or try over-the-counter products containing enzymes such as alpha-galactosidase (Beano) that can prevent gas by breaking down sugars in the digestive system.

Get cracking. Unlike packaged bread crumbs, which have some fat, cracker meal is fat-free, Moquette-Magee says. Cracker meal can be used for coating oven-roasted chicken or fish, as a topping for low-fat fruit crisps and casseroles, or as a filler for meat loaf.

Stock up on low-fat cream soups. Be sure to have in your pantry

25

plenty of low-fat condensed cream soups, like 99 percent fat-free cream of broccoli or cream of chicken, says Evelyn Tribole, R.D., author of *Healthy Homestyle Cooking*. They're great in casseroles and as sauces on meats, poultry, and fish.

Stay away from solids. If you use cooking oils, stock up on liquid olive or canola oils that are loaded with monounsaturated fat. These oils and tub margarines are better for you than solid oils and fats like shortenings that contain lots of saturated fat, says Edith Howard Hogan, R.D., a spokesperson for the American Dietetic Association in Washington, D.C. Better yet, coat your cookware with a vegetable oil cooking spray.

Brown it in broth. Keep defatted chicken broth in your cupboard instead of vegetable oil, Moquette-Magee says.

"I use chicken broth all the time to sauté vegetables, pan-simmer meats or boil and flavor rice. All it does is keep the food moist and transfer heat. Those are the same things the oil would be doing, except the broth doesn't have all that fat," she says.

Slash fat with a splash from the vine. Alcohol is another good fat substitute to have on hand, Moquette-Magee says. You can use beer and wine to stir-fry meats and simmer mushrooms, green peppers, onions, and other vegetables.

Juice up your meals. White grape, apple, orange, and pineapple juices are all light-flavored alternatives to oil in homemade salad dressings or marinades, Tribole says.

Bring on the prunes. Pureed prunes are one of the best fat substitutes in baked chocolate favorites like brownies and cakes, Tribole says. They're chewy and contribute a naturally sweet flavor to the dessert. A ½-cup can save you more than 800 calories and almost 100 grams of fat compared to a ½-cup of butter. For convenience, Tribole suggests buying jars of baby-food prunes that have already been pureed.

Peel away calories with applesauce. "Applesauce is another great substitute," Tribole says. "You can use it in place of cooking oils or butter in brownies, muffins, and cakes. For every ½ cup of applesauce you use, you'll save about 109 grams of fat and 900 calories."

Cocoa satisfies taste buds. If you bake, keep your pantry well-stocked with unsweetened cocoa powder. It provides rich chocolate taste without the fat of unsweetened baking chocolate, Tribole says. For each ounce of unsweetened chocolate called for in a recipe, substitute 3 tablespoons of unsweetened cocoa powder, she advises.

Keep the cow in the cupboard. Cartons of skim milk that can be stored without refrigeration until opened have no fat and are convenient and cost-effective because they reduce spoilage, Hogan says. The milk contains no preservatives, but is safe because it is pasteurized at a higher temperature than other milk products. You can store it for up to five months in your pantry, she says. These products are available on most grocery shelves. Look for "UHT" (ultra-high temperature) on the label.

Make that fat evaporate. Evaporated skim milk is terrific for sauces and soups because it has the texture and flavor of cream but without the fat, Tribole says. Each cup contains 80 grams less fat and 600 fewer calories than heavy cream.

Expand yogurt's horizons. Plain nonfat or low-fat yogurt is a versatile addition to any refrigerator, Moquette-Magee says. It can be used to replace sour cream and make salad dressings, and it is a good, quick add-on to breakfast cereals and desserts.

Take a chance on butter substitutes. Butter-flavored sprinkles like Molly McButter or Butter Buds add taste to foods without the fat or calories, Rarback says.

Teach old spices new tricks. Low-fat foods may seems less flavorful when you first try them. There are a couple of reasons for that. First, fat adds flavor to some foods, and it's a taste that you're used to. Second, as we age, our taste buds become less acute. So keep plenty of herbs and spices like basil, garlic, ginger, onion powder, tarragon, and oregano in your pantry to add zip to low-fat meals, Rarback says.

"By using some different spices and herbs in your food, you're going to bring back flavor and zest to the meal and make it more enjoyable while still eliminating fat," she says. Tinker with low-fat foods and spices until you find combinations that you like.

Invigorate with vinegar. "Using a flavorful vinegar like raspberry, tarragon, or rice wine vinegar will allow you to decrease the amount of oil in homemade salad dressings. So I'd encourage you to have them in your kitchen and experiment with them," Rarback says.

Do a mayo makeover. Regular mayonnaise is 98 percent fat. "It's just egg yolks and oil," Moquette-Magee says. "I can't think of anything worse for you."

Try one of the light, low-fat or fat-free varieties. If you don't like how they taste on sandwiches, opt for mustard, cranberry sauce, barbecue sauce, or plain yogurt, says Moquette-Magee. You also might want to try creating your own mayo. Either mix ½ cup of light or low-fat mayonnaise with ½ cup of plain yogurt, or whip ½ cup of low-fat cottage cheese in a food processor or blender.

Have a "biteables" box. Put a variety of low-fat snacks like grapes, dates, celery, rice cakes, and other crunchy, chewy things into a container in your kitchen so that you can quickly satisfy yourself without being tempted to dash out for higher fat goodies between meals, Graham Kerr suggests.

Shopping: Surviving the High-Fat Maze

"If you're the cook in the family, your first line of defense against high-fat living is at the grocery store," Pingleton says.

But while most supermarkets have a tremendous variety of nonfat and low-fat options, they are also filled with prominently displayed, high-fat enticements.

Here are some ways to get through the grocery store without loading up on fat.

Make a list. This may seem like obvious advice, but some people in their sixties, seventies, and eighties still don't do it, Somer says.

Before you go to the store, sit down and plan out what you would like to eat that week. In the long run, a list will save time and reduce the risk that you'll impulsively throw a high-fat food into your cart, Somer says.

Don't shop on an empty stomach. "You want your mind working, not your stomach, as you stroll the grocery store aisles," Somer says. "If you're hungry, you're going to be reaching for all the high-fat stuff that you shouldn't be eating." Go grocery shopping after a meal or a snack like low-fat cheese and crackers, she says.

Shop outside in. Generally, the fresher, lower-fat foods like fruits and vegetables are on the perimeter of the store. So shop on the outside aisles first. That way, you'll load your cart with healthier foods and be less tempted to fill it with the more processed, higher-fat products on the inner aisles, says Jayne Newmark, R.D., a nutrition consultant in Phoenix.

Read those labels . . . Nutrition Facts labels can be your best weapon in your war against high-fat eating. Among other things, each label is now required by law to list the amount of total calories, total fat, saturated fat, and sodium per listed serving size.

When reading the Nutrition Facts label, says Kathy Pompliano, R.D., manager of the M-Fit Supermarket Program at the University of Michigan in Ann Arbor, remember the following rules of thumb: If an item contains 5 percent or less of the Daily Value for a particular nutrient, it is considered "low." On the other hand, if an item contains 20 percent or more of the Daily Value for a particular nutrient, it is considered "high." Look for foods that are low in total fat, saturated fat, and sodium and foods that are high in fiber, vitamin A, vitamin C, and calcium. Read the ingredients list, too, she suggests. Compare products and choose the one with fewer fat sources listed. Common fat sources included vegetable oil, meat fat, whole milk, butter, cream, and eggs. Check breads and cereals for fiber-rich whole grains, such as whole or rolled oats, whole wheat, cracked wheat or stone-ground.

. . . But take a few at a time. Of course, reading every label on every food every time you shop would be tedious and time-consuming. Instead, each time you shop pick out a couple of foods and read those labels very carefully, recommends Mona Sutnick, R.D., Ed.D., a nutrition consultant in Philadelphia and a spokesperson for the American Dietetic Association.

"Today, for example, you could read salad dressing labels and pick one that has little or no fat," she says. "If you like it, you don't have to read salad dressing labels anymore, because you've found one that suits you. That approach will work for virtually every food in the store."

Eat Like a Peasant, Live Like a King

It's cheap, it's easy, and it's quick. A hamburger and fries at a drive-through? Hardly. It's the traditional Mediterranean diet, and from Spain to Sicily, Corsica to Crete, and Athens to the Alps, it has been a staple of peasant life for centuries. Ranging up to 40 percent of calories from fat, it would seem to be a sure killer. Yet people in this vast region live longer than Americans do, and heart disease and cancer are far less common.

"It's one of the healthiest diets that human beings have developed in the past 2,000 years," says R. Curtis Ellison, M.D., chief of preventive medicine and epidemiology at Boston University School of Medicine.

Researchers aren't absolutely certain why this lifestyle works. But it may have a lot to do with the type of fat that Mediterraneans eat. Most foods are low-fat fresh fruits, vegetables, and grains, including oranges, apples, tomatoes, eggplant, spinach, onions, peppers, and lots of bread. Nearly 75 percent of the fat that is consumed is from heart-healthy olive oil, which is loaded with monounsaturates.

French researchers have shown that people in their sixties who begin living this lifestyle can have a 70 percent drop in heart attack risk. Preliminary evidence also suggests that monounsaturated fats may reduce your risk of breast, endometrial, and perhaps lung cancer, says Dimitrios Trichopoulos, M.D., director of the Harvard Center for Cancer Prevention at the Harvard School of Public Health.

Red meat, a prime source of worrisome saturated fat, isn't daily fare in the traditional Mediterranean diet. In fact, it is usually only eaten once or twice a month. Poultry and fish are also eaten less often than in the United States. But is it better than eating low-fat?

"I think both are excellent alternatives to the traditional American fare of meat and potatoes," Dr. Ellison says. "But low-fat is a huge change that is less acceptable to many Americans. Mediterranean eating is a less-radical change, and more Americans are trying it and liking it."

Give hydrogenated foods the heave-ho. Avoid foods like baked goods or margarines that list hydrogenated or partially hydrogenated oils as ingredients. This means hydrogen has been added to unsaturated liquid oils to make them solidify. But adding hydrogen does two things. First, it transforms unsaturated fat into saturated fat, says George Seperich, Ph.D., a food scientist and associate professor of agribusiness at Arizona State University in Tempe. Second, it creates trans-fatty acids, molecules that raise LDL cholesterol as much as saturated fat does.

"When I'm shopping and I see the word 'hydrogenated' on the label, that food goes right back on the shelf because I know it is loaded with things that I don't want in my body," Dr. Klaper says.

Water it down or whip it up. Pick a margarine that lists water as its first ingredient. It will almost certainly be low-fat, Dr. Castelli says.

Whipped margarines also are a good choice because they have more air, and that reduces the fat content, says Gerry Bates, R.D., nutritional program manager for the Florida Department of Elder Affairs in Tallahassee.

Keep veggies on ice. "For many people in this age group who live alone, buying fresh fruits and vegetables is often a problem because they rot before they're eaten," Rarback says. "Frozen vegetables packed without sauces are a very good alternative. Then a person living alone or a couple doesn't have to worry about spoilage, and they have a fresh-tasting vegetable readily available that they can take out of the freezer and microwave quickly, or use as a base in soups or stews."

Become a cereal fan. "There didn't used to be a lot of low-fat, low-sodium breakfast cereals, but now there is a multitude of very good ones," says Jeanne Jones, cookbook author and "Cook It Light" syndicated columnist in La Jolla, California. In particular, look for shredded wheat, oatmeal, and puffed rice, corn, or wheat.

Smile when you say low-fat cheese. Most regular cheeses have about 9 grams of fat per ounce. Instead look for low-fat cheeses that have about 6 grams of fat or less per ounce or part-skim varieties of ricotta and mozzarella that have about 5 grams or less, according to Moquette-Magee.

Nonfat cheeses taste fine in sandwiches but don't cook well, Kerr says.

Reach for nonfat cream cheese. Regular varieties of cream cheese are very high in fat and saturated fat. Look for the nonfat or low-fat varieties to accompany a breakfast bagel, says Pompliano.

Pass on the processing. Make foods that are naturally low-fat your first choice, says Dr. Seperich. That's because many nonfat products—particularly nonfat sweets like cakes and cookies—are highly processed, Dr. Klaper says. Instead of fat, they're packed with gums and sugars that cause the formation of free radicals and drive up triglycerides, a type of fat that increases your risk of heart disease.

People also tend to eat larger amounts of nonfat foods because they don't give the feeling of fullness that fat does. Dutch researchers also have found that fat substitutes can reduce your body's ability to absorb vitamin E and health-promoting antioxidants like carotenoids.

Some nonfat products such as fat-free sour cream, cream cheese, yogurt, and mayonnaise are fine if they are used sparingly on sandwiches or to make other foods like vegetable dips and salad dressings, Dr. Seperich says.

Find a fresh path. Instead of heading straight to the meat department, purchase a new fruit, vegetable, grain, bean, or pasta that you've never tried before, like kiwifruit, bok choy, couscous, Anasazi beans, or ziti, Pingleton says. It will awaken your taste buds and give you another way to experiment with low-fat living.

Gobble up ground turkey breast. Ground turkey or chicken breast are among the leanest meats you can buy, Pingleton says. Be wary, though, if the label doesn't indicate that it is 100 percent breast meat, because the package may include skin and other poultry fat.

If ground turkey or chicken breast isn't available, consider 15 percent–fat ground beef. It is leaner than plain ground turkey, Pingleton says.

Select the "select" meats. The more marbling a meat has, the more tender and tasty it will be. But that marbling is pure fat. Look for the U.S. Department of Agriculture grade on the package. Choose "select" grade meats, which have the least amount of marbling and may be cheaper than other meats, Tuttle says. If that isn't available, get "choice," the next highest grade. "Prime" grades have the most marbling, so save these for special occasions.

Look for loin. Leaner cuts of beef contain the words "round" or "loin," as in "top round" or "sirloin." Lean cuts of pork usually are loins or legs. For ham, choose lower-fat varieties or Canadian bacon, Pingleton says.

As always, go fish. Researchers are backing away from claims that eating five or six servings of fish a week—fish like salmon and tuna, which are rich in a polyunsaturated fat called omega-3 fatty acids—is any more beneficial to your heart than eating one or two servings a week. But those one or two servings will clearly protect your heart better than none at all.

"Fish isn't a magic bullet, but it is a fine choice in the grocery store. It's a healthy food, and from all we know, it is better for you than red meat," says Walter Willett, M.D., Dr.P.H., professor of epidemiology and nutrition and chairman of the Department of Nutrition at the Harvard School of Public Health and author of several classic fish-consumption studies.

Try eating fish like salmon, trout, or tuna once or twice a week in place of red meats like beef, Dr. Willett suggests.

Be a deli detective. While it is true that many deli meats and salads are loaded with fat and sodium, there are healthier varieties at supermarkets today, says Pompliano. Look for chicken breast, turkey breast, or other lean and extra-lean meats for a low-fat and low-saturated protein source. To reduce the amount of sodium on these meats, rinse the meat gently under cool water and pat dry before making a sandwich, suggests Pompliano.

If traditional deli items are too hard to resist, ask the deli clerk about lower-fat options. Some delis have fat-free or low-fat macaroni salads and potato salads, says Pompliano.

To really slash the fat that you carry away from the deli, ask the clerk to slice the meat as thin as possible, and instead of ordering it by the quarter- to half-pound, ask for only the number of slices that you think you'll eat that week, Tuttle says. That also may prevent overindulging or wasting food.

Send the oil packing. Tuna and other seafoods packed in oil just add unwanted fat to your meal. Pick water-packed tuna or seafood like clams canned in their own juices, Jones says.

Dump doughnuts, muzzle the muffins. Because half of the calories in a doughnut comes from fat and a third of the calories in a muffin comes from fat, a bagel is your best choice—it's nearly fat-free.

"A bagel is a great breakfast food. It is fast, convenient and readily available in most areas," Pompliano says.

Eat a few, but don't go nuts. Eating nuts, which are good sources of monounsaturated and polyunsaturated fats, may protect you from heart disease, according to researchers at Loma Linda University in California. These researchers, who studied the eating habits of 31,000 Seventh-Day Adventists in their fifties, sixties, and seventies, found that those who ate nuts four or more times a week had half the risk of fatal heart attacks than people who munched on them less than once a week.

But keep in mind that the fats in nuts still count toward your daily fat total, and most nuts are chock-full of calories. A cup of peanuts, for example, has about 800 calories.

"For the average person nuts can be dangerous because they're like potato chips. It's hard to just have one," Newmark says. If you're going to eat them, avoid doing it by the handful. Instead just use five or six nuts to add flavor or texture to foods like salads or frozen desserts, she says.

Eating at Home: Give Low-Fat a Personal Touch

By age 70, the average person who cooks for a family has made about 49,000 meals. Unfortunately, most household cooks also have a limited repertoire of about 14 entrée dishes, so they're feeding their families the same high-fat meals day after day, says Kerr. For a low-fat entrée to replace one of those 14—particularly after decades of cooking the same way—you need to personalize the effort.

"Go to some degree of trouble to find out what works well for you," Kerr says. "If you readdress how you prepare food and spice it the way you like it, then it is possible to make the change to low-fat living."

Stick with no-stick. No-stick cookware is worth the modest investment because it has a special coating that allows you to cook or bake without greasing it with fat, Rarback says.

"I know a woman in her sixties who has been using the same cooking pots and pans since her wedding years ago, and there have been a few innovations since then," Rarback says.

Don't drown the pans. If you normally use oil or butter to grease your pans, try dabbing a small spot—about the size of a quarter—onto a paper towel and swabbing it into the pan, Hogan says. That should cut back on the amount you use during cooking. Better yet, use fruit juice or defatted chicken broth instead.

Throw out the frying pan . . . Bake, roast, grill, microwave, or sauté foods that you would normally fry, Dr. Foreyt says. These cooking methods allow fats to run off the meats and be discarded.

. . . But not the chicken. Instead of frying chicken, remove the skin, coat it with a dusting of flour and egg white, dip it in bread or cornflake crumbs, and bake it. "It comes out remarkably well," Tribole says. "That keeps it moist and reduces the amount of fat you're eating significantly."

Be a poacher. Poaching fish in white wine, rather than frying it, trims fat and helps keep the fish flavorful and moist, Rarback says.

Bake those fries. If you crave french-fried potatoes, try this simple low-fat alternative: Cut four medium potatoes into strips, coat them with 1 tablespoon of oil by stirring in a bowl, and bake on a baking sheet in a 450°F oven for 30 to 40 minutes, turning frequently. Sprinkle with paprika or lightly with salt or salt substitute, Dr. Foreyt says.

Honey, I shrunk the meat . . . "Many people of this generation, especially men in their sixties and seventies, are used to eating 16-ounce steaks. But the real serving size that they should be eating is about 3 ounces, which is about the size of a man's palm," Somer says. "So if you eat a 16-ounce steak, you're eating more than three days' worth of meat in one serving."

Use a small amount of meat—2 to 3 ounces after cooking—to complement low-fat meals instead of letting it crowd fruits and vegetables off the plate, Pingleton says. In any case, try to limit your meat consumption to no more than 6 ounces a day, Tuttle says.

. . . And blew up the vegetables. For every bite of meat, take four bites of fruits, vegetables, beans, and grains, Somer says. It will help keep you on track for a low-fat lifestyle.

Freeze out TV dinners. Many frozen meals are loaded with fat and sodium, and in some cases take just as much time to prepare as fresh foods, Jones says. In the same 10 minutes that it takes to make fat-laden boil-in-the-bag Swedish meatballs, for instance, you could brown ground turkey breast in a skillet, add some low-fat spaghetti sauce, and pour it over pasta.

Do a macaroni makeover. To lower the fat content of packaged macaroni and cheese, add vegetables like broccoli, carrots, or cauliflower, and use low-fat or skim milk and half as much butter or margarine, Moquette-Magee says.

"Try using 1½ tablespoons of margarine or butter and 2 tablespoons of light sour cream instead of the 4 tablespoons of butter called for. It's wonderful and you won't notice the difference," she says.

Lighten up puddings. Evaporated skim milk adds body and richness to puddings, but unlike whole milk, it doesn't have any fat, Tribole says.

Ditch the yokes. If your recipe calls for whole eggs, use fat-free egg substitute instead (¼ cup substitute equals 1 whole egg). Since fat content of the substitutes varies, check the label before buying. For baking, however, using two egg whites in place of each whole egg is a better choice, because it reduces the fat yet maintains the flavor and texture of the original recipe, Rarback says.

Soak it in yogurt. Instead of oil-based marinades, try pleasant-tasting plain nonfat yogurt, Rarback says. Allow meat or skinless poultry to soak for several hours or overnight. Marinate fish for only an hour or so because of its delicate texture.

Lose 100,000 fat calories in 25 seconds. "Butter has gone the way of all flesh in our household," Kerr says. "In its place, I've been making fresh cheese from nonfat yogurt. That has actually saved me 100,000 calories a year in fat."

It takes about 25 seconds to prepare, Kerr says. Put a cheesecloth into a hand sieve and scoop in a tub of plain nonfat yogurt. Put a plate on top of the sieve and set it over a bowl in the refrigerator so that the whey can drip out.

After 12 hours it should look like thick, creamy, loosely packed cream cheese. If it tastes too sour, add a few drops of maple syrup to sweeten it, Kerr says.

Shred that cheese. Instead of putting a full slice of cheese on a sandwich, grate it or shred it. You'll use less cheese, yet get the same flavor and cut the fat in half, Rarback says.

Cook now, eat later. Once or twice a month make large quantities of low-fat soups, stews, waffles, and other favorites. Then divide them into one- or two-serving packets and store them in the freezer, Pingleton says. Then when you don't feel like cooking, you'll have a ready-made low-fat meal that you can reheat in minutes.

Kick the grease bucket. "A lot of people in this age group like to save the grease from bacon and other fatty foods in a bucket for use in cooking later. Get rid of it," Pingleton urges. That fat is mainly saturated and causes the most havoc in your body.

If you insist on using it, discard the oils that harden on top and use the liquid oil underneath, because it is less saturated, Pingleton says.

Squeeze the fat out of gravy. "People over 60 absolutely love their gravies," Pingleton says. "If you're going to make it, put the drippings in the freezer and let the saturated fat harden on top, then discard it. Use the broth underneath. It has very little fat and delivers all of the flavor you want in a gravy. Be sure to use skim or low-fat milk, too."

For quick low-fat gravy or sauce, take a can of condensed low-fat cream soup such as cream of chicken or mushroom out of your pantry and mix it with a half-can of water. Then pour the mixture over cooked meat, fish, or poultry and let it simmer for 5 to 10 minutes, Pingleton says.

Turn vinaigrette upside down. Traditional vinaigrette is made with two parts oil to one part vinegar. Flop that around: Double the vinegar and halve the oil, and you've created an exciting lower-fat salad dressing and marinade, Kerr says. Try this formula with a balsamic or Japanese rice wine vinegar and a tasty olive oil. Throw in a crushed garlic clove and dash of dry mustard and brown sugar for flavor. Whip in a blender and keep it in your refrigerator.

Back away from butter. "It's hard for a 60-plus person to get away from butter for some reason, probably because they were raised eating lots of it," Pingleton says. If you use butter, don't use it in cooking, but add a small amount—about the size of a postage stamp—after the dish is done

How I Did It: A Weatherman Alters His Forecast

Fred Pattle thought he was doing all he could to protect himself from heart disease. He was wrong.

Although he ran 5 miles a day and didn't smoke, Pattle drank whole milk by the gallon, ate eggs by the dozen, and eagerly sopped up every bit of fat on his dinner plate.

"When I was pre-40, my diet was absolutely atrocious. I overindulged in fats, heavy creams, cheeses, and meats . . . the works. Now when I think about what I ate, I just want to pass out. I really was a walking time bomb," says Pattle, in his seventies and a retired newspaperman and television weatherman in Eugene, Oregon.

Fortunately for Pattle, doctors defused the bomb in his arteries before it killed him—although it did take quadruple heart bypass surgery to do it. That was 20 years ago, but Pattle still remembers the lesson he learned.

"After the surgery, I knew what I had to do. Throw the fat out," Pattle says. And he did. Now he briskly walks 2 miles a day and doggedly sticks to a low-fat diet.

"I just know that I wouldn't be here if I had continued eating and drinking the junk that I used to," he says.

The first food that he abandoned was whole milk.

"When you make the switch, the message you need to put into your brain is simply this: Skim milk is a clean, cold, delicious drink that doesn't have any fat," he says. "I wouldn't be caught dead drinking anything else now."

He eats lots of fruits and vegetables, prefers poultry with all the visible fat trimmed, rarely eats red meat, uses the lowest-fat margarine he can find, and dresses his salads with oil and vinegar only.

"The funny thing is, once you get yourself off all that high-fat junk, you wonder how you ever managed to eat it," Pattle says. "I don't miss it one bit. I enjoy the good low-fat foods I eat now more than ever, and I feel like a million."

for flavoring only. On bread or toast, spread it thinly, so that you can still see the bread fiber. If you're making a sandwich, only butter one slice of bread. Better yet, use an all-fruit spread, low-fat mayonnaise, or margarine instead, Pingleton says.

"A lot of foods will surprise you by how good they taste without butter," Tribole says. "You really won't miss it in most cases."

Dining Out: Dodging the High-Fat Temptations

"The same rules you use for eating at home apply when you eat out. You just have to be more vigilant, and you can't assume anything," Somer says. "You still want to minimize the amount of meat that you eat and focus on fruits, vegetables, and grains."

Call first. Most high-quality restaurants will accommodate you if you give them sufficient notice, Dr. Lipsenthal says. Call a day or so beforehand, explain that you're eating low-fat foods, and ask if they can fulfill some specific requests.

Take a menu with you. If you eat at a restaurant frequently, ask for a copy of the menu to take home with you, Dr. Shike suggests. That way you can study your food choices without feeling pressured to order.

At fast-food restaurants—where many foods are 40 to 55 percent fat— try salads, plain hamburgers, or grilled chicken or ask for a copy of their nutritional information so that you can make wise selections, Dr. Shike says.

Ask for it any way but fried. If a fried entrée is offered on the menu, ask if the chef can bake it, broil it, grill it, or steam it to cut down on the fat, Dr. Shike says.

Ease back on the appetizers. Many appetizers, like buffalo wings, fried zucchini, and creamed soups, are high in fat. If you want something to munch on while you wait for your entrée, ask for bread sticks, grain breads, crackers, pretzels, or fresh vegetables like carrots and celery with honey-mustard dressing (not ranch), and salads with dressings on the side, Pingleton says.

Get feisty. Ask the waiter lots of questions and don't stop until you're satisfied, Somer says. How is the fish grilled? If it is in butter, ask for it dry.

Frying Isn't the Only Way to Cook

Gerry Bates has an easy time recalling her late husband's favorite dishes: fried chicken, fried catfish, fried eggs . . .

"My husband didn't think something was cooked unless it was fried," says Bates, a registered dietitian, who is the nutritional program manager for the Florida Department of Elder Affairs in Tallahassee. His eating habits contributed to his 1985 death of heart disease at age 59, she says.

But times are changing. A growing number of people in their sixties, seventies, and eighties are adopting low-fat cooking methods in hopes of avoiding a similar fate or simply to add variety to their meals, Bates says.

"It is surprising to a lot of them that they get away from the frying pan and cook something in a different way and still have it taste good," Bates says.

Here's a glimpse at some of the lean ways Bates says that you can create delicious meals without added grease, butter, or oil.

Steaming and microwaving quickly cook rice, vegetables, and other foods without added fat. These methods also help retain the nutrients, flavor, and moisture in the food. To steam vegetables, for instance, bring about 1 inch of water to a boil in a large saucepan. Place the

"It's your meal, you're paying for it, and within reason you should be able to get it the way you want it," Somer says. "If they say they can do something and they don't, send it back. You need to hold them to their promise."

Create a take-home portion. Ask your server to bring a doggie bag when your meal is served. That way you can cut the meal in half and put it in the bag for take-home before you take your first bite, Somer says. You'll not only have a meal for the next day, you'll slash the amount of fat and calories in each serving.

"Don't start eating until you do that, because once you start eating you'll be likely to finish it," Somer says.

veggies in a steamer basket and set the basket in the saucepan so that it sits above the water. Cover the saucepan with a tight-fitting lid and cook until the vegetables are crisp-tender. When microwaving vegetables, you need to add only a small amount of water before cooking.

Poaching means cooking food in a simmering liquid, often stock, broth, or water. This healthful alternative to frying works well with boned poultry and firm-fleshed fish like salmon.

Baking and roasting are excellent ways to cook meats, poultry, fish, squash, potatoes, and many other foods. To keep foods moist, be sure to cover them for at least part of the cooking time. Bake meats by using a roasting rack or meat-loaf pan to keep them from sitting in fat drippings.

Braising, also known as stewing, means slowly cooking food in a small amount of boiling water or other liquid. The longer you braise the meat, the more fat leaches into the cooking liquid. When the meat is done, strain the broth into a container and refrigerate it overnight. The next day, skim off and dispose of the fat that has congealed on top and reserve the remaining broth for soup stock. This works well for any combination meat dishes such as chicken and rice, chicken and dumplings, meat stews, or soups made with meat.

Carry a restaurant survival kit. In a small sandwich bag, carry packets of low-fat dressings, herbal teas, spices, hot-pepper sauce, and other essentials that may not be readily available at the restaurant, Newmark says.

Split a meal with a friend. Order soup or salad à la carte with one entrée. It will save you money and reduce the fat in each meal, Somer says.

Get dressings on the side. Many restaurants put more than 3 tablespoons of dressing on their salads, which can add more than 16 grams of fat to those veggies, Somer says.

Always order salad dressings on the side so that you can control the

41

portion and try to stick with oil and vinegar. It spreads more evenly than cream dressings, so you'll use less of it, she says.

Let go of the extras. Cheese, bacon, olives, eggs, and croutons add unnecessary fat to a salad. Ask your server not to add them, Bates says.

Cut back on the rich sauces. The sauce for fettuccine Alfredo is often referred to as "heart attack on a plate," Dr. Foreyt says. Avoid rich sauces on pasta, meats, or fish or ask for the sauce on the side.

Satisfy the kid within. If you want dessert, ask if you can get a child's portion, Somer says. That will cut some of the fat and still satisfy your sweet tooth.

Say *ciao* to meat toppings. Choose a pizza parlor that has a salad bar so that you can fill up on fresh fruits and vegetables while you're waiting for your pizza to cook, Somer says. Steer clear of pies that have lots of fatty meats like sausage or pepperoni. Try a vegetarian pizza—ask for extra veggies and skimp on the cheese—and limit yourself to two to three pieces.

Hold the mayo. Many delis use regular mayonnaise on their sandwiches. Ask if they have a low-fat substitute. If not, ask them to leave it off. If mayo is a must, ask the clerk to just wet the bread with it rather than slathering it on, Moquette-Magee suggests.

Sail clear of tartar sauce. Tartar sauce, which is served with many fish entrées, gets 96 percent of its calories from fat, Moquette-Magee says. So use it sparingly, if at all.

"If you order a fish fillet sandwich at a fast-food restaurant and scrape the tartar sauce off the bun, or ask that it not be put on in the first place, you're cutting the fat in that sandwich by 50 percent," she says.

Take a no-thank-you portion. "Years ago, if a child told his mother that he didn't want a particular food, she'd put a little on his plate anyway. It was called a no-thank-you helping. You can do the same thing now. If you are tempted by a high-fat food, ask for a no-thank-you helping—a tablespoon of it—so that you still get a taste and don't feel deprived," Hogan says.

Wash that veggie sauce away. In restaurants, ask for your vegetables steamed without added oils, butter, margarine, or creamed sauces. If the waiter tells you that the vegetables are already prepared with one of those ingredients, ask if your portion can be put in a colander and rinsed with boiling water to wash away the unwanted add-ons, says Francine Grabowski, R.D., at Cooper Hospital in Camden, New Jersey, and co-author of *Low-Fat Living for Real People*.

Make bacon a special treat. "People who are age 60 and up just love bacon. But just one slice of cooked bacon has approximately 3 to 5 grams of fat, and it's about 80 percent calories from fat. I tell people not to even buy it or keep it at home," Pingleton says. "If you must have it, get it at a restaurant where you're only going to be served 1 to 2 slices instead of the 10 that you would be tempted to eat at home."

Prescription for Prevention

Regularly eating foods loaded with fat can clog arteries and lead to heart disease and stroke. Excessive dietary fat also can promote the growth of cancers. Lowering the amount of fat you eat, even after age 60, can prevent or even reverse these diseases.

Do:

- *Count grams. Take the average number of calories that you eat each day and multiply that by 20 percent. Then divide the resulting number by 9 (the number of fat calories in a gram). The result is the maximum number of fat calories you should eat daily.*

- *Read labels. Almost all foods list fat grams per serving. Study these labels carefully before buying.*

- *Make a grocery list. It will discourage you from impulsively buying high-fat foods.*

- *Leave foods that contain hydrogenated or partially hydrogenated oils on the grocery shelf.*

- *Buy ground turkey or chicken breast that has been processed without the skin. These are among the leanest meats that you can get.*

- *Fill your pantry and refrigerator with plant foods—pastas, breads, beans, cereals, grains, and fresh, frozen, or canned fruits and vegetables. Only one in four items should be a lean meat or low-fat dairy product.*

- *Keep low-fat snacks like grapes, dates, celery, and rice cakes handy.*

- *Experiment with low-fat ingredients in your favorite recipes.*

Don't:

- *Use solid oils like shortening for cooking. Instead, reach for liquid canola or olive oils.*

- *Shop on an empty stomach.*

- *Automatically reach for nonfat foods. They may contain substances that drive up triglycerides, a type of fat that increases your risk of heart disease. A low-fat alternative may be a better choice.*

- *Grease your cooking pans. Use fruit juice or defatted chicken broth instead.*

- *Eat fried foods. They're loaded with fat. Grill, bake, broil, or steam food instead.*

- *Order appetizers in restaurants. Many are high in fat.*

Chapter 2

Fiber

Roughage—The Smooth Disease Fighter

I f your body had a yard sale, fiber would be the junk in the bin marked "free—take it away." It's the last vestige of the food you eat, the waste that remains after your body has wrung out all the goodness it can.

But fiber is far from being an expendable part of your diet. As it passes through your system, this throwaway stuff is actually an important fighter against cancer, heart disease, and stroke. What's more, it prevents a number of other unpleasant side effects of aging.

• Fiber stops constipation.

• It alleviates diverticulosis, the formation of little pockets in the colon that can trap bacteria, bleed, and become inflamed. This malady affects more than half of all people over age 70.

• Fiber reduces hemorrhoid flare-ups.

• And a balanced diet including fiber can make your hair and fingernails look better than they have in years.

But those benefits are, well, small potatoes compared to the big-time disease prevention that you get from fiber. Researchers note that people who do nothing more than increase fiber and cut fat see cholesterol levels plummet from over 300 milligrams per deciliter (mg/dl) to under 200. That 33 percent drop in cholesterol translates into a whopping 60 percent lower risk of heart disease and stroke.

High-fiber diets also slash your risk of some forms of cancer. On its way through your body, fiber keeps cancer-causing substances from combining forces to make trouble. And it sends them toward the exit a lot faster.

Get Rid of the Gas

Now the question you have been waiting to ask: How can high-fiber eating be, well, socially acceptable? You know that old song about beans. Along with all the benefits, fiber has two side effects that you would rather do without. It might give you that bloated feeling that makes you need to loosen your belt. And, of course, there is always gas.

Here's how to get the fiber you need without the unpleasantness.

Up your intake gradually. You can avoid most of fiber's unfortunate by-products by introducing it slowly. Each week, increase your daily intake by no more than 5 grams. That is the amount of fiber that you would get in 2 cups of sliced, unpeeled apples, says Belinda Smith, R.D., research dietitian at the Veterans Affairs Medical Center in Lexington, Kentucky. If you add fiber gradually but experience discomfort, keep your fiber intake constant for a few days until symptoms clear up. If they still persist, cut back a few grams. Wait a few days before trying to make another addition. Also, introduce high-fiber cereals or fiber supplements even more slowly and take them with low-fiber foods to help ease your system into a high-fiber routine.

Remember your fluid assets. "You need to increase the amount of water as you increase the fiber you take in, because fiber actually draws water into the bowel," says Alan Adelman, M.D., associate professor in the Department of Family and Community Medicine at the Milton S. Hershey Medical Center of Pennsylvania State University in Hershey. Nutritionists recommend 8 to 12 (8-ounce) glasses of water or juice per day. This will also help reduce the buildup of gas that leads to bloating.

Soak the beans. "Before you cook them, soak dried beans," says Dr. Adelman. Replace the soaking water with fresh water when it is time to cook. This will help get rid of the sugars that cause gas.

Add a gas preventer. Try an over-the-counter product containing enzymes such as alpha-galactosidase (Beano) to reduce gas, suggests Dr. Adelman.

Fiber doesn't travel alone. A lot of good stuff goes along for the ride. Perillyl alcohol, for instance, is concentrated in fiber. One of a group of compounds called isoprenoids, it is now being tested as an experimental treatment for people with advanced cancer.

"These compounds, isoprenoids, actually slow down the growth of tumors or stop their growth entirely," says Charles Elson, Ph.D., a researcher at the University of Wisconsin at Madison. Tumors are always trying to get started in the body, and researchers suspect that isoprenoids routinely prevent a lot of them from forming. And no one ever says thanks.

Most foods contain a combination of the two types of fiber—insoluble and soluble. Good news: Each type fights disease differently, so you get two forms of protection when you take in a mouthful of some fiber-rich foods. Wheat products and vegetables boast lots of insoluble fiber but tend to be stingy with soluble fiber. Heart-protecting soluble fiber shows up mostly in fruits, barley, oats, and beans, and these foods generally contain even more of the cancer-fighting insoluble fiber.

Now for the bad news: If you're like most older Americans, you probably get no more than 14.8 grams of fiber a day. You need 25 to 35 grams for disease protection. Luckily, you can make up the difference easily.

Keep Cancer at Bay with Insoluble Fiber

At first glance insoluble fiber doesn't seem much like a cancer fighter. It's much more like lawn mulch than food. But studies show that insoluble fiber protects you from colon cancer, and researchers believe it wards off breast, prostate, and pancreatic cancer as well.

Lots of insoluble fiber comes from the substances that form in the cell walls of plants. It's called insoluble because your body can't easily break down this type of fiber during the digestive process.

Insoluble fiber gives your stool its bulk, which helps it move more quickly through your system. That is why foods that are high in insoluble fiber—bran, for instance—are known as nature's own laxatives. In fact, one nursing home found that people who added bran cereal to their breakfasts no longer needed laxatives.

In Finland diets rich in cereals go along with low rates of breast and colon cancer. In some parts of Africa, where people eat lots of high-fiber foods, there is virtually no intestinal disease—and that includes colon cancer. In laboratory studies one component of insoluble fiber, phytic acid, actually prevents the beginning of colon cancer.

Here's how insoluble fiber works to protect you.

Dilutes the risk. Lucky you—the same stuff in insoluble fiber that keeps you from getting constipated protects you from cancer, too. Insoluble fiber soaks up water like a sponge. This makes stools bulkier. The extra bulk means that cancer-causing agents get spread out over a larger area. They can't join forces to do as much damage.

Gives a high-speed boost. On the interstate large loads move slowly. But in the intestinal highway, bulk translates into speed. Insoluble fiber gets things moving fast, so there is less time for interaction between the cells that line the colon and cancerous agents.

Creates a cancer-unfriendly environment. Fiber tinkers with the acid levels in your intestines. This changes the way bacteria do their jobs. The end result: more fermentation. While that may give you gas (okay, nothing is perfect—not even fiber), it also makes it harder for carcinogens to get into your system. Fiber also helps control levels of the intestinal bile acids that play a part in the start-up of colon cancer.

Ties up carcinogens. Substances that lead to cancer of the breast, prostate, and pancreas tend to latch onto fiber. This means that when the body says good-bye to fiber, it also waves *adios* to any carcinogens that have joined up.

Keeps breast cancer at bay. Insoluble fiber may reduce levels of the harmful estrogen that contributes to the beginnings of breast cancer.

In an Australian study women who ate 28 grams of fiber a day had half the breast cancer risk of women who ate less than 14 grams a day. In addition, when you eat a lot of fiber, you generally eat less fat. Researchers believe that dietary fat is a big player in postmenopausal breast cancer.

Laboratory experiments also suggest that doubling fiber intake and lowering the amount of fat you eat can drop the tumor rate by 50 percent.

Insoluble Fiber: How to Bulk Up

Insoluble is easy. If you're eating fiber-rich foods, chances are that you're getting an ample amount of the insoluble type. That's because virtually all fiber-rich foods contain more insoluble than soluble fiber. Here is how to make sure that you're getting enough.

With beans, you can do it. Hey, who needs more work? You get as much fiber benefit from canned beans as dried beans that you soak and cook yourself. Add a can of beans to vegetable and other soups, suggests Belinda Smith, R.D., research dietitian at the Veterans Affairs Medical Center in Lexington, Kentucky.

Sneak it in. Add fiber to the foods that you normally prepare. For instance, use oat bran instead of white bread as a filler in meat loaf. Add canned kidney beans to lasagna. Introduce beans into casseroles and salads, Smith suggests.

Try instant brown rice instead of instant white rice, says Alan Adelman, M.D., associate professor in the Department of Family and Community Medicine at the Milton S. Hershey Medical Center of Pennsylvania State University in Hershey.

Go whole grain. If you want refinement, take an art appreciation course. Refinement in food is another thing entirely. Refined bread, for instance, loses fiber in the milling process. So choose whole-grain bread products, which can provide 3 grams of fiber or more per slice—meaning you can get 6 grams from one sandwich.

"Refined, processed foods not only lose the fiber, but refining takes out a lot of the trace minerals and possibly the beneficial phytochemicals," notes Rosemary Newman, R.D., Ph.D., professor of food and nutrition at Montana State University in Bozeman.

Phyto-whats? She is talking about protective plant chemicals. In living plants these chemicals guard the plants from harsh weather and insects. In your body phytochemicals guard against a wide number of diseases, including heart disease, cancer, and stroke.

Read the fine print. Nutrition labels tell you the amount of fiber per

(continued on page 52)

Keep Fiber High and Kitchen Time Low

If you're used to buying off-the-shelf prepared products (usually made with low-fiber, highly processed ingredients), it may seem like a lot of work to switch to high-fiber. Belinda Smith, R.D., a research dietitian at the Veterans Affairs Medical Center in Lexington, Kentucky, recommends this two-in-one recipes developed by Constance Pittman Lindner for the *Tufts University Diet and Nutrition Letter.* You'll see how easy it can be. When you are finished, store individual servings in the freezer and have a home-cooked meal whenever the mood strikes.

Chili and Spaghetti Sauce: Two Recipes in One

This two-for-one recipe for high-fiber chili and low-fat spaghetti sauce gives you a lot of good eating. Start by making the basic meat mixture, then divide it and turn one portion into chili and the rest into spaghetti sauce. The whole process takes well under an hour and leaves you with several future meals.

Basic Meat Mixture

2	tablespoons olive oil	1	can (12 ounces) tomato paste
2	onions, chopped	1½	cups water
2	cloves garlic, minced		
1	pound ground turkey or chicken		
2	cans (28 ounces each) chopped tomatoes or tomato puree		

Chili

2	cans (16 ounces) kidney beans, rinsed and drained	1½–2	teaspoons chili powder
½	green pepper, seeded and chopped	1½	teaspoons ground cumin
		1	cup shredded low-fat sharp Cheddar cheese

Spaghetti Sauce

2	tablespoons honey	½	teaspoon ground black
1	teaspoon dried basil		pepper
1	teaspoon dried oregano		

To make the basic meat mixture: In a large saucepan, add the onions and garlic to the heated oil. Sauté over medium heat for 5 minutes, or until the onions are tender. Crumble the turkey or chicken into the pan. Break up the meat with a wooden spoon and cook for 5 minutes, or until it is browned. Drain off fat that has accumulated in the pan.

Add the tomatoes or tomato puree, tomato paste, and water to the meat mixture. Simmer for 20 minutes. Divide the meat mixture into two portions: Using a slotted spoon, remove two-thirds of the meat and one-third of the sauce for chili and put into another large saucepan. One-third of the meat and two-thirds of the sauce will remain in the original pan for spaghetti sauce.

To make the chili: Add the beans, green peppers, chili powder, and cumin to the chili meat and sauce mixture. Simmer for 5 minutes. Serve sprinkled with the Cheddar.

Makes 8 (1 cup) servings.

Per serving: 276 calories, 7.1 g. fat (23% of calories), 7 g. dietary fiber, 38 mg. cholesterol, 911 mg. sodium

To make the spaghetti sauce: To the meat and sauce mixture remaining in the first saucepan, add the honey, basil, oregano, and pepper. Simmer for 5 minutes.

Makes 5 (1 cup) servings.

Per serving: 325 calories, 8.4 g. fat (23% of calories), 6.6 g. dietary fiber, 53 mg. cholesterol, 1,110 mg. sodium

---

Maximize the Bean Benefit

Maybe you bring packages of beans home from the store in little plastic bags, plop them into the cupboard and forget about them. Well, here's how to bring beans out into the open and get the most out of them, says James W. Anderson, M.D., professor of medicine and clinical nutrition at the Veterans Affairs Medical Center in Lexington, Kentucky.

Put them on the shelf. Store beans in airtight containers at room temperature. They'll keep for up to a year.

Let them hang out. Store beans in glass containers where you can see them—they're attractive and you'll be more likely to use them if you see them every time you're in the kitchen.

Root out debris. Before you soak beans, get rid of pebbles and other debris that may be in the package along with the beans.

Give them a thorough soaking. Soak dried beans overnight, or boil them and then soak them for two hours before cooking.

---

serving in a food. But also look at the ingredients list. "In a bread, for instance, the first listed ingredient should be a whole grain. Better yet, the first three or four listed should be whole grains. That means there are more grains than anything else in the product," says Dr. Newman.

If you get tired of picking up and checking every loaf, concentrate on those with labels that make high-fiber claims, such as "good source of fiber."

Weigh the benefits. Not all high-fiber products are created equal. Say that you want to snack on a high-fiber granola bar. Even if the bar of your dreams has 1 or more grams of fiber, it's a good fiber deal only if the fat and calorie content are low.

"A snack bar with something like 100 calories, 2 grams of fat, and a gram of fiber is fine. But some have around 300 calories and a lot more fat. That's too much," says Dr. Newman.

Set goals. Don't try to become a fiber-gobbling machine overnight. If you think that you'll have trouble staying the course of a high-fiber diet, set small, realistic goals that you can meet, suggests Smith. Once you have accomplished those goals, set new ones. To keep yourself on track, keep a diary of what you eat.

Single out singles. Keep your fiber consumption high by lining your kitchen cabinets with easy-to-prepare, fiber-rich staples in packages that are small enough for one or two people. Even if you're an avid cook, says Smith, there will be days when you don't feel like going into the kitchen. Stock up on items such as baking potatoes, canned soup, canned beans, and cereals.

Eat with a friend. Get on the phone and flesh out your social calendar. When there are friends and family to share with, fixing a high-fiber meal seems like no effort at all, Smith notes. Other avenues for social eating: Join community groups or start your own luncheon club.

Soluble Fiber Protects the Heart

Study after study shows that soluble fiber lowers cholesterol, cutting your risk of heart disease and stroke. It may also help clear out your arteries, dropping your risk of high blood pressure.

You get soluble fiber in the outer part of some grains, the white rind in citrus fruits, and the membranes that contain each little section of grapefruit pulp. But in some plants, such as beans or barley, you find soluble fiber throughout.

One-fourth of the fiber that you take in should be soluble, says Dr. Newman. The problem is that most people don't get that much of the soluble type. A lot of foods are gold mines of insoluble fiber but contain almost no soluble materials. For example, you'll get 3 grams of fiber from 3 cups of popcorn. But a mere 0.1 gram will be soluble fiber.

In your body, soluble fiber combines with water, swelling up to create a gelatinous goo that does wonders to protect you from heart attacks and strokes. Here's how it works.

Cuts cholesterol. The higher your cholesterol levels, the greater your risk of heart disease and stroke. The soluble goo gets your cholesterol levels down. Researchers believe that once the soluble fiber reaches the small intestine, it interferes with absorption of fat. "The total amount of

53

Shoot Down Cholesterol and Cancer Risk

Imagine substances right in your food that stop or slow the growth of tumors. Substances that researchers are using—right now—to treat advanced cancers. And imagine that these same substances block the synthesis of cholesterol in your body.

You would eat such a food morning, noon and night, right? Well, that's exactly what you get when you eat foods that are rich in fiber. That's because tocotrienols, part of a powerful group of compounds called isoprenoids, bind to fiber.

You get them in cereal products like oats, rice, and barley, as well as palm and olive oil. And you get similar substances in fruits and vegetables.

Tocotrienols are structurally very close to vitamin E. "They're closer in structure than a golden retriever is to a Labrador retriever," says Charles Elson, Ph.D., a researcher at the University of Wisconsin at Madison. "They differ in just one small chain of molecules."

Dr. Elson notes that plants produce some of these substances when a fungus or an insect attacks. In the laboratory, combinations of isoprenoids offer more protection against disease than individual isoprenoids. "This suggests that you're better off eating a variety of the foods rich in isoprenoids, especially tocotrienols," Dr. Elson says. "It's not a very exciting concept—doing what your grandmother told you to do—but we think it works."

fat in the diet is probably the major factor in cholesterol control. In addition, soluble fiber may trap bile, which must be replaced. The replacement material is cholesterol, which is drawn out of the blood and tissues," says Dr. Newman. That cholesterol-laden bile heads on down the intestinal highway and out of the body.

But the benefits don't stop there. Elsewhere on the digestive route, bacteria break down soluble fiber to create short-chain fatty acids. When these are absorbed back into the body, they restrict the body's ability to synthesize cholesterol, reducing your blood's cholesterol levels still more.

Researchers note that some people can lower cholesterol much more cheaply and just as effectively with fiber than with cholesterol-lowering medication.

At the University of Minnesota, researchers looked at 10 studies of oat bran and found that eating just 3 grams of soluble fiber a day (what you would get in 1 cup of ready-to-eat oat bran cereal) can drop cholesterol levels by 2 to 3 percent. In people whose levels were over 230 mg/dl, cholesterol declined more steeply, an average of 6 to 7 percent. And it seems that the more oat bran people eat, the more cholesterol goes down. In one study, 6 to 9 grams of soluble fiber brought cholesterol levels of over 260 down by 23 percent.

James W. Anderson, M.D., world-renowned professor of medicine and clinical nutrition at the Veterans Affairs Medical Center, recalls that he began eating oat bran in 1977. A pioneer in oat bran research, he couldn't even get the stuff from food suppliers. Oat bran's main use in those years? Face powder.

But he found that just a bowl of cereal and three to four oat bran muffins a day lowered his cholesterol from 285 to 175 in five weeks. He also lost 8 pounds in that same time. He has been researching (and eating) oat bran ever since.

Cleans out your arteries. Researchers theorize that soluble fiber may also be an arterial housecleaner, helping to reduce the risk of the plaque buildup in your arteries that can lead to heart attacks and strokes. Soluble fiber helps lower the levels of cholesterol that circulates in your body—and that automatically drops your risk of an artery-clogging buildup.

Controls blood sugar. Soluble fiber improves the body's ability to maintain normal blood sugar, by slowing absorption of starchy foods. This helps forestall plaque buildup in the arteries, which can lead to a heart attack or stroke.

Fights high blood pressure. Researchers studied 850 Yi people, members of an ethnic minority in southwest China. They found that the Yi diet, high in oats and buckwheat, resulted in lower blood pressures and lower levels of the harmful low-density lipoprotein cholesterol.

(continued on page 58)

Play the Numbers for Protection

You don't have to play a food lottery, guessing which foods give you the most heart-protecting soluble fiber. Here's a list of the top foods for soluble fiber and the amount they contain.

Food	Portion	Soluble Fiber (g.)
Vegetables		
Artichoke, cooked	1 medium	2.2
Celery root, fresh, chopped	½ cup	1.9
Sweet potato, cooked	½ cup	1.8
Parsnip, cooked	½ cup	1.8
Turnip, cooked	½ cup	1.7
Acorn squash, baked	½ cup	1.6
Potato with skin, baked	1 medium	1.6
Brussels sprouts, cooked	½ cup	1.4
Cabbage, fresh	1 cup	1.3
Green peas, cooked	½ cup	1.3
Broccoli, cooked, chopped	½ cup	1.2
Carrots, cooked, chopped	½ cup	1.1
Carrot, raw	7½" long	1.1
Cabbage, cooked	½ cup	1.1
French-style green beans, cooked	½ cup	1.1
Cauliflower florets, cooked	¾ cup	1.0
Asparagus, cooked	¾ cup	1.0
Fruits		
Mango, sliced	1 cup	2.9
Strawberries, whole, capped	1 cup	2.0
Figs	2	1.7
Kiwifruits	2	1.4
Orange	1	1.4
Plums	2	1.4
Pear	1 small	1.1
Grapefruit	½ medium	1.1
Blackberries	¾ cup	1.1
Apricot halves, dried	7	1.1
Apple with skin	1 small	1.0
Prunes	3	1.0
Peach	1 medium	1.0

Food	Portion	Soluble Fiber (g.)
Cereals		
Quaker Oat Bran	1 cup cooked ($\frac{1}{2}$ cup dry)	3.0
Quaker Oat Bran Cereal, ready-to-eat	1$\frac{1}{4}$ cups	3.0
SmartBeat High Fiber Oatmea,	1 packet, instant	3.0
H-O Super Bran High Fiber Cereal	$\frac{3}{4}$ cup	3.0
Kellogg's Bran Buds	$\frac{1}{3}$ cup	3.0
Quaker Oatmeal, cooked	1 cup	2.0
Health Valley Healthy Crunch	$\frac{1}{2}$ cup	1.4
Raisin bran	1 cup	1.2
Quaker Instant Oatmeal	1 packet	1.0
Nabisco 100% Bran	$\frac{1}{3}$ cup	1.0
Kellogg's All-Bran	$\frac{1}{2}$ cup	1.0
Post Oat Flakes	$\frac{2}{3}$ cup	1.0
Kellogg's Common Sense Oat Bran	$\frac{3}{4}$ cup	1.0
Cheerios	1$\frac{1}{4}$ cups	1.0
Nabisco Shredded Wheat 'N Bran	$\frac{2}{3}$ cup	1.0
Post Bran Flakes	$\frac{1}{2}$ cup	1.0
Grains		
Pearl barley	$\frac{3}{4}$ cup cooked	1.8
Oat flour	$\frac{1}{4}$ cup	1.6
Rye flour	$\frac{1}{4}$ cup	1.3
Wheat germ	4$\frac{1}{2}$ tablespoons	1.0
Legumes		
Large lima beans, canned	$\frac{1}{2}$ cup	5.7
Kidney beans, cooked	$\frac{1}{2}$ cup	2.8
Cranberry beans, cooked	$\frac{1}{2}$ cup	2.7
Butter beans, cooked	$\frac{1}{2}$ cup	2.7
Baked beans, canned, cooked	$\frac{1}{2}$ cup	2.6
Black beans, cooked	$\frac{1}{2}$ cup	2.4
Navy beans, cooked	$\frac{1}{2}$ cup	2.2
Lentils, cooked	$\frac{1}{2}$ cup	2.0
Pinto beans, cooked	$\frac{1}{2}$ cup	1.9
Great Northern beans, cooked	$\frac{1}{2}$ cup	1.4
Chick-peas, cooked	$\frac{1}{2}$ cup	1.3
Split peas, cooked	$\frac{1}{2}$ cup	1.1

Soluble Fiber: A Plan for 10 Grams

Here's how to get 10 grams of soluble fiber a day, the amount researchers recommend for lowering your cholesterol, says Belinda Smith, R.D., research dietitian at the Veterans Affairs Medical Center in Lexington, Kentucky. (We're counting grams of soluble fiber only here—remember that you still need a total of 25 to 35 grams of fiber a day.)

For breakfast, eat a bowl of high-soluble-fiber cereal (for instance, ⅔ cup cooked oatmeal) and fruit (say, an orange) for approximately 3.4 grams.

With lunch or dinner, have a serving of cooked legumes for another 2.5 grams. You will get what you need from any of the following choices.

- ¾ cup bean soup made with navy beans
- ¾ cup vegetarian chili made with pinto beans
- 1 cup of three-bean salad made with kidney beans, chick-peas and green beans
- 1¼ cups lentil soup
- 1½ cups split pea soup
- ¾ cup minestrone soup made with kidney beans

During the course of the day, eat two more fruits or vegetables that are high in soluble fiber for an additional 2 grams of soluble fiber. (See "Play the Numbers for Protection" on page 56 for a list of the best choices.)

Chances are, you get 3 grams of soluble fiber from the rest of the foods you eat.

So without breaking a sweat, you have made it to 10.

Slashes cancer risk. In one laboratory study, researchers used a modified form of pectin, a soluble fiber. They found that this special kind of pectin helped prevent cancer from spreading. It kept cancer cells from sticking to the walls of the lungs, keeping lung tumors from getting a start.

Cut Cholesterol with This Three-Stage Plan

Soluble fiber is a mighty cholesterol-buster. James W. Anderson, M.D., professor of medicine and clinical nutrition at the Veterans Affairs Medical Center in Lexington, Kentucky, recommends this three-stage program for use of soluble fiber to cut your blood cholesterol. Stay at each level for four to six weeks.

- Level I: Adjust your diet so that you take in 10 grams of soluble fiber a day. You will probably get a 5 to 10 percent drop in cholesterol levels. Generally, the higher the levels, the bigger the drop.
- Level II: Consume 15 grams of soluble fiber per day for a 10 to 15 percent cholesterol reduction.
- Level III: Combine 15 grams of soluble fiber with a psyllium supplement (under your doctor's supervision). This will give you a 15 to 20 percent cholesterol reduction.

In Search of the Soluble

Most foods contain much more insoluble fiber than soluble. But you can increase your intake of soluble fiber by making small changes in how you approach foods that you're probably already eating.

Leave the liquid. The liquid that comes with canned beans contains a lot of dissolved soluble fiber (the reason why it is soupy instead of watery). Unless you have salt-sensitive high blood pressure or congestive heart failure, the salt in the liquid should not bother you. Save the liquid and combine it with soups. Or, for a low-salt or no-salt substitute, cook your own beans and save the leftover liquid, says Dr. Anderson.

Put away the peeler. The peels of many fruits and vegetables are rich in soluble fiber. Don't peel apples, pears, peaches, or potatoes. Eat the white inner rind of oranges, which is high in pectin. For grapefruit sections, spoon out the membrane with the pulp for extra soluble fiber, says Dr. Anderson.

Eat it whole. While you get concentrated nutrients from fruit juice, you lose out in the fiber department. An 8-ounce glass of extracted carrot juice contains just 2 grams of fiber, compared with the 14 grams you would get from the six carrots (1 pound) that went into the juicer, says Dr. Adelman.

Get supplemental protection. "A lot of people find that it's easier to take a soluble fiber supplement than to adjust their diets," says Dr. Adelman. The main ingredient in fiber supplements like Metamucil is psyllium, which comes from the ground-up seed husks of a plant grown in India. It has been used as a laxative for more than 60 years. You get the most benefit if you take psyllium with a meal.

While taking a supplement is the easy way out, it may not be the best way to reward your taste buds. "My patients who use a supplement tell me that it tastes like powder mixed with water. They make it palatable by mixing it with orange juice or apple juice," says Dr. Adelman.

Psyllium is also available in cereals. In one study people with mildly high cholesterol levels ate Bran Buds, a cereal high in psyllium, for two weeks. Their cholesterol levels dropped by 8 percent.

Don't supplement without your doctor's okay, since psyllium can interfere with other medicines that you may be taking.

Make substitutions. Look for products containing substances such as TrimChoice, formerly known as Oatrim, a fat substitute that is made from oat flour, which is rich in soluble fiber. Produced by Mountain Lake Manufacturing, it appears as hydrolyzed oat flour in cheese, baked goods, confections, and meat, as well as a variety of other low-fat products.

While it is touted for its low-fat benefits, Oatrim also cuts cholesterol. In a U.S. Department of Agriculture study, 24 people with high levels of cholesterol who ate products containing Oatrim experienced a 16 percent drop in total cholesterol in five weeks. Their levels of protective high-density lipoprotein cholesterol were unchanged. To add to the benefits, blood pressures went down and their blood sugar levels became more stable.

Prescription for Prevention

Eating more fiber can substantially lower your cholesterol levels, greatly reducing your risk of heart disease and stroke. High-fiber diets also slash your risk of some forms of cancer, including breast, colon, pancreatic, and prostate cancer.

Do:

- *Eat wheat products and vegetables for insoluble fiber.*
- *Get soluble fiber from fruits, oats, and beans.*
- *Increase your fiber intake by adding beans to soups, lasagna, casseroles, and salads.*
- *Eat brown rice instead of white rice and replace refined flour with whole-wheat flour.*
- *Choose whole-grain bread products.*
- *Drink 8 to 12 (8-ounce) glasses of water or juice each day. Fiber draws liquids out of your system.*

Don't:

- *Peel apples, pears, peaches, or potatoes.*
- *Add a high-fiber psyllium supplement if you're on other medications without first checking with your doctor.*

Chapter 3

The Power of Plants

Scientists Cheer for Fruits, Vegetables, and Grains

Imagine an array of well-armed forces battling heart disease, cancer, and stroke, catching cancerous invaders and throwing them out of your system before they destroy healthy cells. Shrinking any tumors that get started. Sending blood pressure tumbling down. Cleaning out the fat in your arteries. Keeping your arteries clear of the blood clots that lead to strokes. Protecting cells against DNA damage. Even slowing down the aging process.

Sounds like the antics of superheroes in your grandchildren's video games?

It's also what goes on in your body when you eat fruits, vegetables, and grains. Scientists have discovered that when you eat food made from plants, you get the benefits of all those powerful defenses. They come from *phytochemicals,* a term that simply means chemicals in plants. Scientists once thought that these largely nonnutritional, noncaloric substances were just plain useless. It looked as though they were just along for the ride.

But the picture is changing as experts sift through the thousands of phytochemicals in plants. Think of phytochemicals as a bureaucracy that works—most phytochemicals work in groups, but no one knows exactly what each one does. Most have unpronounceable names and produce a cascade of chemical reactions that resemble a Rube Goldberg drawing. But the phytochemicals that you consume can help ward off cancer, heart disease, and stroke. In fact, more than 200 studies have shown that diets high in fruits and vegetables cut cancer risk. That becomes even more important as you get older and your risk of heart disease, cancer, and stroke increases.

Sometimes protective phytochemicals make their presence known: You can see their calling cards in the bright orange color of carrots or sweet potatoes. Or you get a whiff of phytochemicals in action when you come nose-to-clove with garlic. You taste them in the sharp bite of freshly cut watercress. But many are undetectable.

"These chemicals are there to protect the plants, not you," says James Duke, Ph.D., an ethnobotanist, formerly with the U.S. Department of Agriculture Research Service in Beltsville, Maryland. Researchers theorize that some antioxidant phytochemicals evolved to protect plants from oxygen (since plants feed on carbon dioxide, with oxygen as waste), as well as wind, weather, and insects. "These substances keep plants from oxidizing under the hot sun's ultraviolet radiation. They protect bulb plants that grow underground from an onslaught of microbial and insect hazards," says Suzanne Paxton Pierson, a pharmacy doctor and president of Preventive Nutrition Consults in Woodinville, Washington.

"But you can borrow the protective benefits," notes Dr. Duke.

Slash Your Cancer Risk

Up to 33 percent of potential cancers might be prevented just by eating a diet rich in fruits and vegetables, according to scientists at the National Cancer Institute.

"We can save more than 150,000 lives a year, right now, with no treatments, no medical costs, no long-term recovery—if people just eat the foods that protect them," says Edward Miller, Ph.D., professor of biomedical sciences in the Department of Biomedical Sciences at Baylor College of Dentistry in Houston, who researches oral cancer.

"Studies worldwide show that phytochemicals protect against cancer," says Paul Lachance, Ph.D., chairman of the food science department at Rutgers University in New Brunswick, New Jersey, and an internationally known researcher in the field. But, he cautions, "there is no panacea phytochemical, no one thing you can take or eat for protection."

If you eat lots of plant foods (and thus plenty of phytochemicals), you

(continued on page 66)

How I Did It: Now She Knows Beans—And Carrots

Diagnosed with breast cancer at age 49, Grace Maloney recalls, "I knew I would beat it. I just put one foot in front of the other mentally. But, back then, I didn't really make any big changes in my life, with one exception—I stopped smoking."

But when the Jackson Heights, New York, resident reached menopause, she did change her diet. "I always loved meat and fruit but hated cooked vegetables. With menopause, I noticed that I put on another 10 pounds. That wasn't healthy, so I knew that I had to change."

Now she is in her sixties and volunteers three days a week at SHARE in New York City, an organization of breast and ovarian cancer survivors. Maloney says that her downfall wasn't a sweet tooth. It was cheese and other high-fat foods. "It was a real sacrifice to give those foods up," she sighs, recalling a special treat—cheese and pâté.

"I can't say that it made my life better right away, but switching to more fruits and vegetables made my life a lot easier. I've always hated cooked vegetables. In fact, I cook them for my husband, but I can't stand to eat them. So I tried them raw. I discovered that I liked raw carrots and fresh string beans."

Each week, Maloney bought several bunches of carrots and a pound or so of beans. She peeled and sliced the carrots, pulled the strings and the ends off the beans, and stored them in separate, sealed containers in the refrigerator to keep them fresh. "I realized that the string beans, in particular, are delicious, with a crunchy, fresh taste. I would bring things like that to work with me and just eat on the run. Why sit down and have lunch when you can run errands and never waste a minute?"

She added tomatoes to her assortment and stocked up on fruit. "I've always loved fruit, and it was wonderful to have an excuse to buy more," Maloney says. She started buying watermelons, cutting them up and storing them in the refrigerator, along with her vegetable assortment. "I'd just nosh on that when I wanted a snack. Pretty soon, eating fruits and vegetables got to be a routine.

"But I haven't given everything up. I have my wine with dinner every night," she adds. "My husband, Robert, and I eat out twice a week. We try to order sensibly, but I figure that because I eat carefully almost all the time, I'm entitled to an occasional treat. The other day at a French restaurant, I even had pâté."

Around the time she turned 60, Maloney started to worry about other ailments. "I was scared of debilitating things like strokes," she says. "Several friends died. I realized that I could affect the quality of my life." Still, she didn't act until her gynecologist remarked about her borderline high blood pressure.

"Hypertension runs in my family. I worried about that, and I was angry that my internist never talked with me about high blood pressure. My gynecologist suggested that I stop in a couple of times. She said that she had to take several readings to check for accuracy. I did have high blood pressure. I thought that I was worth more than the information I was getting, so I changed internists. I went to see several before deciding on one. When you've had cancer, you don't worry about tact with a doctor. You just say, 'I want this and this and this.'

"My new internist told me to limit my salt intake, which worked a little. She also put me on a very low dose of medication."

That's when Maloney made even more lifestyle changes to keep her heart healthy. "I'm doing a lot of bicycle riding, just for flexibility. Although I ignore it, I have arthritis of the spine. I've found that movement helps my arthritis. Plus, I do weight-bearing exercises. And I started playing tennis an hour a day on the handball wall. The wall never yells at me, and I never have to wait for it to show up."

The effort has paid off. Now when she travels, she has more stamina. "I didn't behave myself when I was young, and it's nice not to have to pay too much for your past sins when you get older," Maloney says. "It has been a sacrifice, but I'm glad for the result—I don't think that I look my age, and I feel great. It keeps me going."

have a lower risk for cancers that attack the lungs, bladder, cervix, mouth, larynx, throat, esophagus, stomach, pancreas, colon, and rectum. Scientists that also believe plant foods may help protect you from breast and prostate cancer.

In the laboratory, phytochemicals keep cancer-forming substances and defective cells—which are turning into cancers—from getting a foothold or spreading. Some contain hormones that disrupt the growth of breast cancer and prostate cancer cells.

Cure Cardiovascular Problems

Phytochemicals keep your heart healthy, too. "The 60-to-80 age group has a much greater risk of heart disease than younger people do. If your diet is rich in fruits and vegetables, you can reduce risk," notes Dexter Morris, M.D., vice chairman of the Department of Emergency Medicine and a heart researcher at the University of North Carolina at Chapel Hill School of Medicine.

Some plant chemicals help your cardiovascular system by neutralizing harmful low-density lipoprotein (LDL) cholesterol that, if left unchecked, can lead to hardening of the arteries. Others act on the walls of your blood vessels and in the process lower your blood pressure or make blood platelets less sticky and less likely to clot so that you're not as vulnerable to strokes.

In a study begun in 1973, researchers kept track of 1,883 men ages 35 to 59 who had high cholesterol levels. Over the next 20 years, the men who had the highest levels of carotenoids (a phytochemical) in their blood had 60 percent fewer heart attacks and deaths.

Fight Free Radicals

Many phytochemicals also do double-duty as antioxidants, neutralizing free radicals, which are unstable molecules that damage or destroy the body's healthy cells. "Antioxidants are particularly important for people ages 60 to 80 because they reduce the effects of aging—system-wide," says Joanne Slavin, Ph.D., professor in the Department of Food Science and

Nutrition at the University of Minnesota in St. Paul.

Your body produces harmful free radicals routinely. You also get them from a variety of exterior sources, including cigarette smoke, pollutants, medications, pesticides, and household cleaners.

Free radicals have been linked to more than 60 diseases and medical problems. Beyond heart disease, cancer, and stroke, these include premature aging, stiff joints, wrinkled skin, arthritis, diabetes, and liver cirrhosis.

Here is a breakdown of the major groups of phytochemicals that seem to provide the most protection and how scientists think they work. In this relatively new field, research is still underway.

Organosulfur Compounds: Scents That Protect

The aromatic clout and pungent flavor that you get from plants belonging to the allium family—garlic, onions, leeks, chives, and shallots—are actually signs that protective phytochemicals are at work. You also get these compounds in cruciferous vegetables such as broccoli and cauliflower.

Cancer. Foods rich in organosulfur compounds could be called dietary anticarcinogens, according to John Potter, M.D., Ph.D., head of the Cancer Prevention Research Program at the Fred Hutchinson Cancer Research Center in Seattle.

Studies have shown that some of the powerful organosulfur compounds in these plants, such as diallyl disulfide, block or suppress carcinogens. Plus, they help the body intercept and eject cancer-causing agents before they can do any damage.

Another important organosulfur compound, alliin, works as a powerful antioxidant, disposing of the free radicals that damage healthy cells and play a part in both cancer and atherosclerosis. In animals, alliin interferes with tumor growth and prevents the molecular changes that lead to cancer.

Some of these chemicals also help the immune system stay strong, increasing the number of your body's infection-fighting T cells. Researchers at the University of Minnesota School of Public Health looked at the eating habits of more than 41,830 Iowa women ages 55 to 69. Those who ate garlic, a particularly rich source of organosulfur compounds, had a one-third reduction in risk of colon cancer.

In other studies researchers note that the bacteria-fighting organosulfur compounds may also fight off cancer. They disarm *Helicobacter pylori*, a bacteria found in the stomach that can lead to stomach cancer.

Danish scientists have discovered that chemicals in garlic not only block the growth of cancer cells but also delay the normal aging process of healthy cells.

Heart disease and stroke. Organosulfur compounds found in onions, garlic, and other members of the allium family also defend your heart. "When you eat a hearty meal, you get an influx of fats into the bloodstream. This makes your blood more likely to clot. The alliums, particularly onions, will help your body manufacture substances to get rid of the fat quickly," says Isabella Lipinska, Ph.D., a nutritional counselor for the Cardiac Rehabilitation Program at St. Elizabeth's Medical Center in Boston. This means that you're less at risk for heart disease and stroke.

Organosulfur compounds contribute to lower blood pressure without the common side effects, such as headaches and impotence, that some people get from prescription medication.

Experts theorize that these compounds dilate the muscle cells in the arteries, opening up blood vessels and lowering blood pressure. They may also help the blood circulate to the smaller vessels more efficiently, lowering blood pressure even more.

They also decrease levels of harmful LDL cholesterol that can narrow artery walls. And they increase levels of the beneficial high-density lipoprotein (HDL) cholesterol that keeps your arteries free of plaque and protects against heart disease and stroke.

Scientists in Australia examined the results of eight trials with a total of 415 people. Those who consumed a commercial dried garlic powder for one to three months lowered their blood pressure. Project researchers speculate that if long-term studies of garlic eaters sustain this same rate of lowered blood pressure, the studies might show 30 to 40 percent fewer strokes and 20 to 25 percent less coronary heart disease.

Another study measured cholesterol levels, revealing an 11 percent drop in harmful LDL cholesterol and a 6 percent drop in total cholesterol in people who took 900 milligrams a day of garlic powder tablets (the equivalent of about three cloves) over a 12-week period. That's important because researchers estimate that every 1 percent drop in total cholesterol could translate into a decrease in heart attack risk of 2 percent.

You get protection against stroke from these phytochemicals, too. At Brown University, men ages 30 to 70 who had cholesterol levels of 230 to 290 consumed 700 milligrams of garlic a day. Total cholesterol and LDL cholesterol levels declined by 8 percent. The levels of beneficial HDL cholesterol did not change.

Here are some ways to get the most benefit from organosulfur compounds. You should check with your doctor before you increase intake if you are on anticlotting medicines or aspirin, according to Dr. Lachance.

Get souped up. As you get older, your body doesn't absorb food as easily, a problem compounded if you have dentures and don't chew your food properly. Dr. Lipinska advises using a blender to liquefy vegetables, then making cream of vegetable soups, complete with onion and garlic.

Put away two to three a day. "For health benefits, based on retrospective epidemiologic studies, eat two to three cloves of garlic a day," advises Dr. Paxton Pierson.

Yu-Yan Yeh, Ph.D., professor of nutrition science at Pennsylvania State University in University Park, conducted a study of men ages 35 to 55 with high LDL ("bad" cholesterol) levels. They received supplements equal to two to three cloves, and their LDL cholesterol levels dropped. Still, Dr. Yeh says, "it's better to incorporate fresh garlic into daily cooking and to eat healthy foods instead of taking a supplement. You get extra benefits from vegetables you eat with garlic."

Pass up the riches. Adding garlic or other foods rich in phytochemicals may tempt you toward the wrong kinds of food. A garlicky sauce, for instance, is hardly a wise choice if it's also rich in butter or other animal fats, advises Dr. Yeh. "The benefits won't offset the health hazards of rich food."

Sauté for health. "You'll get the most benefit out of alliums (garlic and its relatives) by chopping them up and then sautéing them in a little oil," says Dr. Yeh. He adds that chopping activates some phytochemicals while heat gets others going. "Use olive oil or canola oil, because they're high in

monounsaturated fat and don't seem to contribute to higher LDL cholesterol levels the way other oils do."

Say good-bye to heartburn. Garlic and other alliums don't agree with
everyone's digestive tract. If you get heartburn, try deodorized garlic such
as aged garlic extract, says Dr. Yeh. People who participated in one study
consumed the deodorized supplemental equivalent of three cloves a day.
They got the benefits, and no one felt the burn.

Keep it cooked. Avoid raw garlic because, like other bulb vegetables, it
grows underground in close contact with bacteria that may be harmful to
you. (So don't mix raw garlic in oil, for instance, and store it in the refrigerator.) Raw garlic also gives some people intestinal irritation, says Dr. Yeh.

Use condiments for flavor only. Condiments such as onion or garlic
powder may add flavor to your food, but processing techniques have probably cost them just about all of their protective benefits. So just be aware
that the payoff doesn't go any farther than your taste buds.

Use it or lose it. The enzymes that activate protective phytochemicals
get busy when you chop or press the garlic, but they dissipate within 12
to 24 hours. So you'll get the most benefit when it's freshly chopped, according to Dr. Lachance. If you cut up a garlic clove and save it for another day, all you'll get is the taste.

Isothiocyanates: Leaves That Stem Cancer

You get plant chemicals called isothiocyanates in leafy green vegetables such as watercress, arugula, cabbage, Chinese cabbage, and brussels
sprouts, as well as broccoli and cauliflower.

These compounds help the body get rid of cancer-causing substances.
"They take the trash out, to put it in the simplest terms. Fewer carcinogens
reach their cellular targets," says Stephen Hecht, Ph.D., professor of cancer
prevention at the University of Minnesota Cancer Center in Minneapolis.
These chemicals also make it difficult for cancer-causing substances to zero
in on the DNA (genetic material) of healthy cells. In the laboratory, they
have kept tumors from forming and have detoxified carcinogens.

In a laboratory experiment, watercress-eating rats that ate a diet containing an isothiocyanate from watercress and a carcinogen from tobacco

were 50 percent less likely to develop lung tumors than those exposed only to the carcinogen.

Here is how to get the most benefit from the isothiocyanates in your food.

Eat it raw. "Isothiocyanates are released when you chew the raw vegetable or chop it up," says Dr. Hecht. "You know it's happening because of the sharp taste. Cooking reduces some of the compounds, but the vegetables still contain a lot of beneficial chemicals."

Keep it fresh. While the phytochemicals in these vegetables are fairly stable, you'll get more if you eat fresh vegetables, adds Dr. Hecht.

If, for example, you chop up watercress or broccoli and use it the next day, the taste will be subdued—and the benefits will be slightly less, according to Dr. Duke.

Put it high on the list. "The National Cancer Institute recommends at least five helpings a day of fruits and vegetables. While you won't be immune to cancer if you eat a lot of cruciferous vegetables, they do contain a large number of compounds that we strongly suspect to be anticarcinogens," says Dr. Potter.

Eat the leaves. "Phytochemicals are most concentrated in the broad leaves of many vegetables in order to protect the plant, although we also see some concentration in seeds," says Dr. Duke.

Indoles: Part of the One-Two Punch

Like Laurel and Hardy, indoles and isothiocyanates go together. Eat the leafy greens of cruciferous vegetables like broccoli, cauliflower, and cabbage, and you get the benefits of both, says Dr. Duke.

Cancer. Indoles protect against breast cancer because they alter the body's estrogen metabolism. But it's not for women only—it has the potential for use as a treatment for prostate cancer.

"In humans, they stop the growth of small virus-caused tumors. In animals, these vegetables prevent breast cancer," says Leon Bradlow, Ph.D., director of the Murray Rayburn Laboratory of Biochemical Endocrinology at Strang Cancer Research Laboratory in New York City. "This makes us optimistic that we'll see similar results in humans. We al-

Fight Disease While You Eat

Ever think that you could protect yourself from disease every time you put food to your lips? You can, if you eat foods rich in the phytochemicals. Here is how to get more of the foods that protect you from cancer, heart disease, and stroke.

Keep it varied. No one knows why, but vegetables grown in different plots of ground can have very different concentrations of beneficial chemicals—even when they are raised right next to each other under closely monitored research conditions.

How do you compensate for those differences? "Vary what you eat," says Leon Bradlow, Ph.D., director of the Murray Rayburn Laboratory of Biochemical Endocrinology at Strang Cancer Research Laboratory in New York City. By choosing lots of different fruits and vegetables, you ensure yourself maximum phytochemical coverage.

Minimize meats. Gradually decrease the amount of meat and other high-fat items on your plate and increase the amounts of vegetables. Suppose a slice of meat usually occupies half your dinner plate. Slowly cut back until your meat serving is the size of a deck of cards or smaller, and the rest of the space is filled with vegetables, pasta, or rice, says John Potter, M.D., Ph.D., head of the Cancer Prevention Research Program at the Fred Hutchinson Cancer Research Center in Seattle. Try meatless meals using recipes from cuisine of the Mediterranean, India, Japan, China, Indonesia, Southeast Asia, and North Africa.

If you make your changes gradually, you won't be as aware of the changing proportions. The shift will be easier to tolerate.

"Work on your own or enroll in cooking classes," suggests Dr. Potter. "You get to meet new people and eat more healthy foods."

Count on mistakes. Tell your family and friends that you're trying

ready know that people in China and Korea, who eat cabbage all their lives, have much lower breast cancer rates than people in the West."

You get added benefits from broccoli, a rich source of indoles. It also

new foods for health and enlist their psychological support. "Learning new styles of cooking takes time, and you will screw up," says Dr. Potter. "It's easier if your friends and family are tolerant of your failures. I sometimes think that cooking is a skill that has gone the way of the horse and buggy. I would like to see people get it back."

Make it a party. Get together with friends for "moving dinners," perhaps held once a week at a different person's home. That way, you can all learn together, Dr. Potter says.

Crack open a cookbook. Get ideas for new foods by checking out cookbooks from the library or buying a few. Look for books that promote fruits and vegetables and other plant foods, suggests Dr. Potter.

Eat in company. Whether you pop a clove or a pill, you'll get maximum benefit if you consume phytochemicals with a meal of plant foods, because the intake of protein, fat, and carbohydrate helps your body absorb and use the phytochemicals more effectively, says Paul Lachance, Ph.D., chairman of the food science department at Rutgers University in New Brunswick, New Jersey, and an internationally known researcher in the field.

Eat what you like. "If you don't like something, you probably won't eat it," says Dexter Morris, M.D., vice chairman of the Department of Emergency Medicine and a heart researcher at the University of North Carolina at Chapel Hill School of Medicine. If you only like tomatoes and hate other vegetables, just eat more tomatoes. "There are probably enough different kinds of phytochemicals in every vegetable to do you some good," he says. "It's not like there is only one kind in a tomato and another kind in a carrot. There are mixtures in all. It's more important to eat vegetables than to worry about which ones."

contains sulforaphane, a phytochemical that prevents mammary tumors in rats.

Heart disease and stroke. Because indoles are phytoestrogens, estrogen-like substances from plants, they may help lower the risk of heart disease and stroke. Estrogen has been linked to lower levels of harmful LDL cholesterol and may even help control high blood pressure and reduce the blood's tendency to clot.

Here's how to benefit the most from indoles.

Get a quarter a day. For maximum protection Dr. Bradlow suggests that you eat the equivalent of a quarter head of cabbage a day or an equal amount of broccoli (about half a bunch), brussels sprouts, or cauliflower. "We have found the highest levels of indoles in savoy cabbage, the crinkly looking type, and in purple broccoli," he says.

Isoflavones: Tofu to the Rescue

Isoflavones are a group of plant estrogens found in soy products. "In countries where people consume a lot of soy, the rate of breast and prostate cancer is very low," says Clare Hasler, Ph.D., director of the Functional Foods for Health Program at University of Illinois at Urbana-Champaign.

Cancer. The powerhouse isoflavones in soy are genistein, daidzein and equol. In laboratory tests they keep cancerous cells from growing. Some studies on animals show genistein also keeps tumors from growing and getting the blood supplies they need. And, in fact, when leukemia cells divide, genistein also helps them to return to their original healthy state.

In laboratory studies the phytoestrogens in soy reduce the number of mammary tumors in rats and prevent the growth of human breast cancer cells. Researchers also think that phytochemicals such as isoflavonoids may slow the growth of prostate cancer.

In a Japanese study, the diets of 142,875 women were followed for 17 years. Breast cancer risk was lowest in women whose diets included miso soup, made from soybean paste. Researchers theorize that the isoflavones do the job.

Studies also show that soy consumption is tied to a lower rate of colon and rectal cancers.

Soy also is a good source of saponins, another group of phytochemicals that, in the laboratory, fight cervical, pancreatic, gastric, colon, breast, and prostate cancers.

Heart disease and stroke. "Studies have shown that soy can bring cholesterol from the high-risk to moderate- or low-risk range," says Dr. Hasler.

"Soy contains a variety of chemicals that probably interact. Even independently, some of them do lower levels of harmful cholesterol," says Susan Potter, R.D., Ph.D., associate professor of nutrition at the University of Illinois at Urbana-Champaign.

Scientists believe that plant estrogens in the diet lead to the low levels of heart disease in Asian countries. Scientists speculate that phytoestrogens also slow down atherosclerosis, protecting the arteries.

Soy may taste bland, but it is unique among plants. The important protectors, genistein and daidzein, are only found to any significant extent in soybeans and the foods that come from them. They may keep LDL cholesterol from oxidizing so that it can't easily attach to artery walls. Genistein may also keep artery walls from thickening and keep platelets from clumping together, reducing the risk of heart disease and stroke.

A study conducted by the University of Kentucky reviewed 38 previous studies to show that soy protein lowers LDL cholesterol and triglyceride levels but does not affect levels of the beneficial HDL cholesterol. In some experiments soy-rich diets have reduced total cholesterol by 10 percent and LDLs by 13 percent. Cardiologists estimate that a cholesterol reduction of 10 percent lowers risk of death by 30 percent.

Dr. Susan Potter conducted a study to examine the blood cholesterol and bone density of women ages 50 to 70. Findings showed that women who consumed 40 grams a day of soy protein isolate, the powerful stuff in soy foods, ended up with a drop in LDL and an increase in HDL cholesterol levels.

"We also found that bone density improved in those women taking a soy protein isolate with slightly higher levels of isoflavones," adds Dr. Susan Potter. "Soy consumption may possibly be an alternative to estrogen therapy."

How I Did It: Supermarket Savvy

Manhattanites Claire and Stanley M. were struck by the double whammy of cancer and heart disease several years ago. Claire, then age 68, was diagnosed with breast cancer, while an electrocardiogram revealed that her husband had previously suffered a silent heart attack.

"I realized that we could do more to control our health, especially by adding fiber and decreasing fat to help reduce the risk of heart problems and cancer," says Claire. "So I started to read labels carefully. I stayed away from processed foods, especially ones that contain a lot of chemicals. I spend much more time in the supermarket now because I read the labels. I look for high fiber, low fat, and serving size. For instance, one brand will call three crackers a serving and another will call six a serving. It often makes a big difference when you add up the total in fiber, fat, and calories."

Before label reading became part of her shopping routine, Claire says, "I used to buy foods that contained chemicals and preservatives. Now I'm more careful. We really emphasize fresh fruits and vegetables. We make it a point to get broccoli, apples, and oranges for fiber and other nutrients."

Stanley wasn't as careful about his diet before his heart attack. "We've both come to enjoy the high-fiber, low-fat diet," Claire says. "I never had any problems with constipation, but Stanley really knows the difference when he doesn't take in enough fiber."

Unfortunately, the typical American diet is virtually soyless. Use these methods to increase your soy consumption.

Go ahead, try tofu. Tofu isn't the most appealing food to look at, but it absorbs the taste of spices and other foods with which it is cooked. This means that you can easily transform the bland into the sublime.

Look for Asian main-course and soup recipes. For grilling and sautéing, use extra-firm tofu—it won't crumble. Add small cubes of tofu

The healthy diet has become a habit. "These days, we maybe eat meat twice a month. When we first tried to change our diet, we used to say to each other, "What is there to eat?" It was just hard to figure out what we could eat. We bought low-fat cookbooks and concocted recipes of our own using a lot of pasta, vegetables, and beans. Now, if we go off our diet, both of us feel guilty."

Claire had just retired from her job as a controller at a New York advertising agency when her cancer was diagnosed. "One of my best survival tactics centered on making attitude changes. After my illness, I was very tense and anxious. I learned to meditate, using breathing exercises to relax."

Exercise helps, too. "I always walk a lot, mostly because my husband and I like to go to museums, movies, theaters, and concerts. I started doing floor exercises for my back. I must be in better shape now, because when I started, I'd get so exhausted that I'd almost be nauseated. Now I can do them with ease."

Claire does volunteer work with SHARE, a New York organization that helps women fight breast and ovarian cancers. She found an important sense of community in helping others. "I led discussion groups and worked on the hotline. It's been very meaningful.

"Facing mortality has made us stronger—more appreciative of the time we have. It has underscored how precious life is and that you can make changes in your life if you go step by step and do what you can."

to salads (under a light dressing or with a topping of nuts or seeds, you won't even know it's there), says Dr. Hasler.

Keep it firm. Fermented soy products such as tempeh are available in dense, firm blocks. Researchers theorize that fermented soy products are easier for your body to use. Tempeh, firmer than tofu, is perfect for grilling or stir-frying.

Stick to low-fat. Look for low-fat (1 percent) tofu, tempeh, and soy

Visit an Exotic Aisle

As you work on adjusting your diet for disease prevention, it is likely that you will want to change your shopping habits as well. So grab a grocery cart and be prepared to take a few turns off the beaten path.

Fill 'er up with produce. When you shop in a supermarket, head straight for the fruits and vegetables section and fill up your cart there. That way, you'll be less likely to head for the more familiar aisles of the store filled with less nutritional foods, suggests Isabella Lipinska, Ph.D., a nutritional counselor for the Cardiac Rehabilitation Program at St. Elizabeth's Medical Center in Boston.

Find strength in numbers. Lots of cities have co-op food stores, where members buy food in bulk and split up the distribution chores. Usually, you get top-quality fruits and vegetables at a lower price. If you and your friends organize a combined "buying and cooking" club, you'll reap benefits in taste, health, and finances, notes John Potter, M.D., Ph.D., head of the Cancer Prevention Research Program at the Fred Hutchinson Cancer Research Center in Seattle.

Buy it off the truck. Make your shopping more fun by frequenting farmers markets, where local produce often has more taste than the prepackaged stuff in the big stores, suggests Dexter Morris, M.D., vice chairman of the Department of Emergency Medicine and a heart researcher at the University of North Carolina at Chapel Hill School of Medicine. With some extra charm in your shopping expedition and a tastier time in the dining room, you'll be more likely to stick to the fruits-and-vegetables habit.

milk products. Avoid high-fat varieties, advises Dr. Hasler.

Drink bean milk. "I drink soy milk," says Dr. Hasler. "The beany flavor is great on whole-grain cereals or granola." Soy milk also comes in vanilla and carob flavors. You can find it in some grocery stores. Soy protein can also be found as a supplement in health food stores.

Eat a burger. Some vegetarian hamburger substitutes are made with soy products. Check the label, says Barbara P. Klein, Ph.D., professor of foods and nutrition at the University of Illinois at Urbana-Champaign. Look at the fat content as well: Some contain more than their fair share. If you just can't do without your meat, try one of the vegetarian sloppy joe mixes available at grocery stores and use half meat and half soy substitute.

Lay off the sauce. You won't get much help from soy sauce—it contains very little soy, says Dr. Lachance. Most products are also loaded with salt, which can raise your blood pressure. Other condiments, such as Bac-Os, contain soy, but in such small amounts that they won't do you any good.

Make a substitution. When you bake, trade 25 percent of your regular flour for soy flour. You'll get those soy benefits, and most recipes will come out the same, says Mark Messina, Ph.D., a nutritionist and soy expert in Port Townsend, Washington, and author of *The Simple Soybean and Your Health.*

Lignans: A Little Flax'll Do Ya

Lignans are powerful plant estrogens that are most plentiful in flaxseed, something that you probably don't normally include in your diet. You do get small amounts in cereals and vegetables.

"Some baking companies add small amounts of flax, or linseed, to give breads and other baked goods a nutty flavor. You can get products made with flax in health food stores, too," notes Dr. Hasler.

"This is a new area for research, and we don't know that much about it yet," cautions Dr. Hasler. She suggests that if you want to add flax to your diet, do so very slowly, perhaps sprinkling a little fortified flax (no more than a teaspoon) on your breakfast cereal. It's available at health food stores.

Cancer. Lignans, especially in flaxseed, also seems to prevent breast cancer, at least in the laboratory. In addition to working as phytoestrogens, which means they provide the body with estrogen, lignans are antioxidants, helping to prevent cell damage and stop cancers before they start.

Heart disease and stroke. As antioxidants, lignans may help prevent the dangerous LDL cholesterol damage that can lay the groundwork for heart disease.

In a study at the University of Western Ontario, rats ate flax and flaxseed oil—and their blood pressures held stable, while blood pressures rose in the rats that got no flax in their diets. In another study, people ate three slices of bread containing flaxseed and 15 grams of ground flaxseed a day and saw drops in LDL cholesterol levels and in the clotting action of their blood.

Carotenoids Show Their Colors

You see evidence of carotenoids in the bright red, orange, and yellow pigments of some plants. They're also in leafy green vegetables. You'll find them in carrots, tomatoes, sweet potatoes, cantaloupe, winter squash, parsley, pink grapefruit, Swiss chard, spinach, beet greens, pumpkin, watermelon, broccoli, mangoes, oranges, papaya, and tangerines. They're also in fish liver oil.

Cancer. "Study after study shows that diets rich in carotenoids fight disease," says Dr. Lachance. In one study a high-carotenoid diet reduced the risk of lung cancer in nonsmokers. Researchers studied the diets of 1,197 people in Hawaii. Those who ate a variety of fruits and vegetables and consumed high amounts of three carotenoids had less lung cancer. The European Institute of Oncology in Milan looked at rates of oral cancer in Beijing, China, and found that carotenoid consumption reduced risk.

In a survey of 3,000 northern Italians, people who ate seven or more servings of raw tomatoes a week ended up with a 50 to 60 percent lower risk for cancers of the mouth, esophagus, stomach, colon, and rectum. Researchers also think that carotenoids reduce the risk of cancers of the cervix and pancreas.

A particularly powerful carotenoid, lycopene, comes in tomatoes and everything made from them, including pizza sauce and ketchup. Plus, watermelon, guava, and pink grapefruit have lycopene.

In the laboratory, tomato juice extract, for example, has prevented the formation of cancer-causing compounds. An Israeli study showed that lycopene knocks out human endometrial, breast, and lung cancer cells in the laboratory. It also affects the systems that allow the cells to grow into tumors.

Researchers at Harvard Medical School found that people who ate tomatoes, tomato sauce, tomato juice, and pizza—all foods rich in lycopene—had lower rates of prostate cancer.

But lycopene isn't the only carotenoid that protects. Beta-carotene is another potent disease preventer. You get it in sweet potatoes, carrots, apricots, spinach, collard greens, cooking pumpkins, and cantaloupe.

Your body converts beta-carotene into some vitamin A and retinoic acid, which thwarts precancerous and cancerous cells while it enhances T cells, a key part of your body's immune system. As antioxidants, beta-carotene and lycopene root out the dangerous free radicals that can turn cells cancerous.

Researchers note that beta-carotene seems to help reduce the risk of cancers of organ linings, including colon cancer. Researchers think that precancerous colon polyp tissue that contains beta-carotene is less likely to turn malignant. In a combined Swiss and Italian study, beta-carotene in the diet protected against endometrial cancer.

The carotenoids work together, too. In a study conducted by the University of Hawaii, diets rich in beta-carotene, alpha-carotene, and lutein resulted in lower risks of lung cancer in a study of more than 1,200 people. You get lutein in broccoli, green peas, celery, spinach, kale, collard greens, Swiss chard, mustard greens, red peppers, okra, and romaine lettuce.

Heart disease and stroke. Researchers agree that the more carotenoids you eat, the lower your risk will be for chronic heart disease. "They work as antioxidants and prevent the formation of LDL cholesterol," says Dr. Morris.

Use these methods to get the biggest boost from carotenoids.

Use a little fat. "Since most of the carotenoids are fat soluble, eat them with other foods that contain a hint of fat," says Dr. Morris.

Cook 'em up. Most carotenoids aren't damaged by cooking, says Dr. John Potter.

Go for color. Reds, oranges, and deep greens tell you that carotenoids are present, even in fruits and vegetables where you might not expect them. For instance, red-leaf lettuce has more carotenoids than iceberg lettuce, and you get more carotenoid benefit from pink grapefruit than from white grapefruit. If you're a meat-and-potatoes sort of person, put some yams or sweet potatoes on your plate for an extra carotenoid boost. (Not that there is anything wrong with white potatoes—they are a good source of potassium, an important mineral, says Dr. Lipinska.) If your lunch features a piece of broiled chicken and potatoes, add a slice of red pepper or tomato, she adds.

Snack on vegetables and crackers. Raw vegetables plus a high-fiber, low-fat cracker or two give you the most phytochemical benefit, says Dr. Lipinska. The small amount of fat in the cracker enables your body to take in fat-soluble phytochemicals as well as the water-soluble kind. Make your snack even more beneficial by choosing a bright orange or green vegetable, high in carotenoids.

Try concentration. You'll get more carotenoids from some concentrated products, says Dr. Morris. Tomato paste, ounce for ounce, contains twice as many carotenoids as do fresh tomatoes, for instance. Tomato puree contains 20 percent more.

Don't turn orange. Carotenoids are fat soluble, which means that your body stores them until they are used. If you take in too much, the side effects will be obvious to everyone you see.

"You can turn orange. This doesn't happen if you get carotenoids in food, because you'd have to eat an awful lot. But it's easy to take too many supplements," says Dr. Morris. Beyond keeping your normal skin tone, Dr. Morris says, you're better off getting your carotenoids from food—not from a bottle—for other reasons: It's hard to know the quality of supplements and how well your body can use the substances they contain. And researchers haven't yet figured out whether the carotenoids themselves help your body or whether other substances linked with them in fruits and vegetables are providing the real benefit.

Flavonoids: Can't-Miss Protection

You're in luck—flavonoids occur in just about every plant, from apples to onions to soy.

Cancer. Even black tea (the kind that you get at the grocery store) and Japanese green tea contain flavonoids that help ward off cancer.

"Flavonoids dissipate the substances that cause cancer. They prevent— they don't cure," says Dr. Lachance. Studies at Rutgers University have shown that, at least in laboratory mice, green tea blocks the development of cancer tumors by 90 percent. Black tea, says Dr. Lachance, performs only a little less impressively.

Many flavonoids are also powerful antioxidants. Researchers have found that the process used to make the green tea leaves activates a key antioxidant, epigallocatechin gallate. In the lab, it prevents tumors of a broad range of cancers.

Researchers have found that some flavonoids, such as quercetin in onions and kaempferol in leeks and garlics, fight off the earliest stages of cancer.

In a Dutch study involving 58,279 men and 62,573 women ages 55 to 69, scientists found that onion eaters decreased their risk of stomach cancer.

Heart disease and stroke. In a Canadian laboratory study, a flavonoid called purpurogallin protected the heart against the injuries that occur during a heart attack.

Another Dutch study followed 805 men ages 65 to 84 over a 25-year period. Researchers found that those who ate a flavonoid-focused diet (mostly from black tea, but also from onions and apples) had a 58 percent drop in risk of dying of a heart attack. Average daily tea consumption? About 3.4 cups.

That study was part of a larger, seven-country study which revealed that, all in all, a high-flavonoid diet was the reason for a 25 percent variance in coronary heart disease among the countries studied. Researchers in Israel discovered that red wine, which is high in flavonoids, lowers LDL cholesterol levels, which when raised leads to hardening of the arteries. Laboratory research shows that flavonoids can reduce the tendency of blood platelets to stick together and cause clots.

To get the most of flavonoids, try these tips.

Look to the vine. Researchers are actively scrutinizing "the French paradox," the fact that people who drink wine regularly seem to have lower rates of heart disease even when they dine on a rich cuisine like France's. "We think that the chemicals in wine are potent antioxidants, and they may keep blood from clotting," says Andrew Waterhouse, Ph.D., a researcher in the Department of Viticulture and Enology at the University of California, Davis. The people who benefit, studies show, drink just a little wine on a daily basis.

Turn to tea. Dr. Lachance says that tea will give you an effective dose of flavonoids—but you have to drink it regularly. "I drink a cup of coffee in the morning and then drink black tea the rest of the day," he says. "I drink around a half-dozen cups. It's safer than coffee, too, because it's not as stimulating."

Triterpenes, Monoterpenes: Put the Squeeze on Cancer

Triterpenes are a group of compounds that include limonoids, found in the seeds, fruit, and juice of citrus plants. Monoterpenes also are found in citrus but in the skin or peel. Monoterpenes are also present in caraway seeds in the form of D-carvone.

Cancer. "We're excited about these substances as possible anti-cancer agents because people consume them at high levels anyway," says Dr. Miller. "We used to think that vitamin C was the protective component in citrus, but studies suggest other agents. For this reason it's better to drink the glass of orange juice than to take a vitamin tablet." Epidemiological studies show that citrus consumption is linked to protection against a whole slew of cancers—oral, esophageal, and pancreatic, among others.

In laboratory rats, some of the phytochemicals in citrus reduce the number of tumors by up to 60 percent. This is only at very high dosages and with side effects. They also help your body increase the production of enzymes that dispose of cancer-causing substances.

Dr. Miller is studying limonoids, a group of cancer-fighting phytochemicals that fend off oral cancer in animals. Two substances, limonin and limonin 17-beta-D-glucopyranoside, actually block and suppress tumors.

Heart disease and stroke. A University of Wisconsin at Madison study shows that monoterpenes can decrease the harmful LDL cholesterol that contributes to heart disease and stroke.

Here's how to get the most benefit out of monoterpenes. It's definitely worth making the effort because you get a lot of other good things from citrus, too (such as vitamin C and fiber).

Make salad surprising. Combine fruits to make a fruit salad (avoid canned fruits—they lose vitamin C during storage). Buy a variety of fruits and, every day, serve them in different combinations—a slice of plum, apricot, peach, and apple, for example.

Use the peel. Use orange or lemon peel as a flavor enhancer in fruit drinks and carbonated beverages. It's rich in protective d-limonene. For limonoids, keep away from the watered-down citrus drinks or the carbonated citrus drinks. Eat the actual fruit or drink the real juice, recommends Dr. Miller. In one study, researchers applied orange-peel oil to skin tumors and found that the tumors grew much more slowly.

Tannins: Stains That Sustain

You might think of tannins as colorful concoctions used in dying, making inks, and even in the tanning process. One tannin, ellagic acid, is in the kinds of foods that stain your clothing—strawberries, raspberries, blackberries, and loganberries. And it may make a lasting impression on your body, too, by protecting you from cancer.

Cancer. Research on tannins (and ellagic acid, in particular) is getting underway in laboratory studies. Researchers believe ellagic acid may keep cancerous substances from altering the DNA of healthy cells. In the laboratory, it neutralizes cancer-causing substances and helps prevent cancers in tissues of the lung, liver, skin, and esophagus.

Heart disease and stroke. In the laboratory, ellagic acid works as an antioxidant, preventing oxidation of the fats that turn into LDL cholesterol.

Here's how to get more tannins into your system, says Dr. John Potter.

Go straight to the source. Grape juice may be a sweet refreshment, but you're better off eating the grape itself to get the benefit of the phytochemicals clustered in the grape peel.

Get jamming. You're better off eating the whole fruit and nothing but the fruit. But if your tastes run to jellies, take a close look at the contents listed on the label. Pick products listing a higher content of real fruit.

Top it off. Find inventive ways to work berries into your daily eating pattern. Use berries to top off desserts like sherbet, for instance, or sprinkle them over a slice of melon.

Prescription for Prevention

When you eat a diet rich in fruits, vegetables, and grains, you stoke up your defenses against heart disease, cancer, and stroke. You may cut your disease risk in half.

Do:

- *Eat at least five helpings a day of fruits and vegetables.*

- *Choose bright orange or dark green vegetables.*

- *Add vegetables rich in organosulfur compounds to soups. Choose garlic, onions, leeks, chives, shallots, broccoli, and cauliflower, for example.*

- *Enjoy raw vegetables with a cracker to get the benefits of both water-soluble and fat-soluble phytochemicals.*

- *Eat the leaves, seeds, and peel, where many phytochemicals are concentrated.*

- *Drink milk made from soybeans and try soy-based vegetarian hamburger substitutes.*

- *Drink tea, which is rich in phytochemicals, instead of coffee.*

Don't:

- *Add more than just a teaspoon of flax to your cereal.*

- *Rely on canned fruits, because they lose valuable nutrients during storage.*

Chapter 4

The Top 100 Foods for Your Health

From Almonds to Yogurt, Your Edible Allies

Good news: You can easily get cheap, good-tasting medicine that helps ward off cancer, heart disease, and stroke—without even going to the pharmacy. These disease-preventing substances are in the everyday, garden-variety foods available in any grocery store.

The secret lies in eating a wide variety of foods that contain an assortment of disease-fighting substances. That way, you create a protective mosaic of vitamins, minerals, enzymes, and other substances that help you stay disease free. So be sure you get the five-plus servings of fruits and vegetables recommended by the National Cancer Institute and leading nutritionists.

The following 100 foods stand out as top-notch disease fighters, easily found in the supermarket.

A note about serving sizes: The standard serving size for cooked vegetables or chopped raw vegetables is ½ cup and, for raw leafy vegetables, the serving size is 1 cup. For fruit a serving is one medium apple, banana, or orange or ½ cup of chopped, cooked, or canned fruit. A serving of cooked cereal, rice, pasta, or cooked dried beans is ½ cup.

A note about the Daily Value: The Daily Value is the amount of a nutrient that scientists figure you need each day if you eat a 2,000-calorie diet. If you eat more or fewer calories, your Daily Value will be higher or lower accordingly.

A note about vitamin A: Actual vitamin A is found in animals, not plants. A source of vitamin A in our bodies, however, is beta-carotene, which is found in plants. Throughout this chapter you will note that certain vegetables or fruits are a good source of vitamin A because, through a simple process, the body converts beta-carotene into a usable form of vitamin A.

Almonds

Not what you would expect to head up a list of healthy foods—almonds weigh in like sumo wrestlers in calories and fat. Fortunately, most of the fat is monounsaturated, the kind that may actually reduce high blood pressure and cholesterol.

Cancer. A serving of almonds (the amount that fits in your hand, about an ounce, or 24 whole kernels) gives you 13.5 percent of the Daily Value for copper.

Almonds deliver copper to power up your immune system, which needs more of a boost as you get older. Plus, they provide some fiber (1.9 milligrams) and calcium to help lower your risk of colon cancer.

Heart disease and stroke. In one study, people eating 3½ ounces of almonds a day reduced cholesterol levels by 20 points. Almonds are a good source of riboflavin, which has been associated with lower heart disease rates. In addition, a handful of almonds is high in magnesium—it provides 21 percent of the Daily Value, which may help prevent blood clots and lower blood pressure.

Apples

Whole, sliced, juiced, cooked, or sauced, apples deliver protection from disease.

Cancer. Take a bite and take in some glutathione (well, it does sound as if you're talking with your mouth full when you try to say it). This tongue twister protects your mouth because it cuts the risk of oral and throat cancer by up to 50 percent in comparison to the risk in people who don't eat apples. It also makes your immune system work as though it belongs to someone much younger. The problem is that most people over 60 have blood levels of glutathione 17 percent lower than people under 40.

This antioxidant is available only from raw vegetables and fruits, so eat your apples raw. You'll have to think of another excuse to eat apple pie. Apples are a great source of another mouth-saver—vitamin C, which helps guard your mouth against cancer.

Apples also provide you with flavonoids, antioxidants that help stop cancer's start-up process. A medium-size apple, with peel, gives you a little more than 2.5 grams of total fiber, protection against both cancer and heart disease.

Heart disease and stroke. When researchers in the Netherlands studied 805 men ages 65 to 84, they found that the apple eaters had a 32 percent lower risk of dying from heart disease, in part because of flavonoids concentrated in the apple peel.

Researchers think that the vitamin C in apples also performs such feats as lowering your blood pressure, which could help protect your arteries and heart. Vitamin C also helps prevent oxidation of blood cholesterol and, therefore, slows clogging of the arteries. Apples are high in flavonoids, which have antioxidant properties. One small apple with skin gives you 1 gram of soluble fiber, which can aid heart health.

Apricots

The taste is tart, but the benefits are sweet. This tiny low-fat, low-cal, zero-cholesterol fruit packs a lot of protection in the form of beta-carotene, dietary fiber, and vitamin C. And remember that apricots in the dried form contain even greater concentrations of their beneficial nutrients.

Cancer. A serving of three fresh apricots boosts your body's defenses as a source of more than half of the Daily Value of vitamin A. People who eat a lot of vitamin A/beta-carotene have lower rates of breast, cervical, and uterine cancer. They may also get protection against cancer of the esophagus, stomach, colon, and mouth. Vitamin A also helps keep invaders out by strengthening the mucous membranes that line the digestive, respiratory, reproductive, and urinary tracts.

The vitamin C helps lower your risk of cancer of many vital organs. More than 1 gram of insoluble fiber is in a ½-cup serving of canned apricots, and there are 5 grams of total fiber in ¼ cup of dried apricots, which helps fend off colon and breast cancer.

Heart disease and stroke. Proof that good things come in small packages, seven dried apricot halves give you 1.1 grams of soluble fiber to help bring down high cholesterol and high blood pressure.

Apricots provide potassium, which helps lower your high blood pressure. One serving of three fresh apricots is the source for more than half the Daily Value of vitamin A, which may protect you from the harmful low-density lipoprotein (LDL) cholesterol buildup that can lead to hardening of the arteries. Stroke victims in Belgium fared better when their diets included lots of sources of vitamin A.

Artichokes

Perhaps the ancient Romans were thinking about taste, not disease protection. Regardless, they paid more for artichokes than any other garden vegetable.

Cancer. A ½-cup serving of artichoke hearts gives you 4.5 grams of total dietary fiber for protection against colon cancer. Plus, you get 10 percent of your Daily Value of copper to boost your immune system. And 14 percent of the Daily Value of vitamin C helps protect you against a variety of cancers.

Heart disease and stroke. One medium cooked artichoke gives you 2.2 grams of soluble fiber for heart health. Vitamin C also fights the hazardous LDL cholesterol and other fats in the blood by keeping them from latching onto artery walls where they can do their dirty work.

A serving provides almost 11 percent of the Daily Value for folate (the natural form of the supplement folic acid), which helps prevent rises in homocysteine levels. Elevated homocysteine may increase the risk of heart disease. Researchers estimate that if people took in more of the B vitamin folate, between 13,500 and 50,000 deaths from coronary artery disease could be prevented every year. A ½-cup serving of artichoke hearts provides you with more than 12 percent of your Daily Value of magnesium, which may prevent the blood clotting that increases your risk of a heart attack or stroke. It also helps lower blood pressure.

Asparagus

It's a stand-up kind of vegetable. Next time you see a bunch of asparagus upright in a pan of water in the grocery store, think about how these low-cal, cholesterol-free little green spears stand up to disease.

Cancer. According to research, asparagus could actually help block tumor development. Obviously, you wouldn't want to go on an all-asparagus diet, but these laboratory findings make it clear that your body will benefit from a regular helping of these great defenders. In the laboratory, compounds in asparagus keep cells from mutating and keep tumors from forming.

Weighing in with 1.4 grams of insoluble fiber, a single serving of cooked fresh asparagus (about six spears) beefs up your defenses against colon cancer. Asparagus also provides vitamin C to protect you from a variety of cancers and copper to help strengthen your immune system.

Asparagus is a very good source of an antioxidant called glutathione, which has been found in animal studies to inhibit tumor growth. Asparagus gives you almost 33 percent of a day's requirement for folate, which keeps your cells healthy. Studies show that people who eat a diet rich in folate have lower levels of cancer of the cervix, colon, and rectum, and folate may help prevent cancer of the esophagus.

Heart disease and stroke. The ingredient list for asparagus reads like a who's who of heart protection: It's a source for nearly 10 percent of your Daily Value of vitamin A, which helps prevent buildup of the harmful LDL cholesterol in your arteries. At the same time, people with high amounts of beta-carotene have higher levels of the protective high-density lipoprotein (HDL) cholesterol than people with low amounts of beta-carotene.

As you age, it becomes harder for your body to absorb the B vitamins, so you have to take in more than you used to. B vitamins are plentiful in asparagus: Folate and vitamin B_6 protect your heart, partly by lowering levels of the harmful amino acid homocysteine. Homocysteine is associated with high risk of heart attack and stroke. Riboflavin boosts the other B vitamins.

The soluble fiber in asparagus lowers the levels of LDL cholesterol and fats in your blood.

Go Light on Meat

Meat tends to be high in calories, fat, and iron—but some cuts fit easily into a healthy diet. Here are top choices for meat dishes. All give you over half your Daily Value of protein.

Eye round roast. A lean 3-ounce serving (the size of a deck of cards) has 143 calories, 59 milligrams of cholesterol, and just over 4 grams of fat. Protective nutrients include vitamin B_{12}, zinc, niacin, vitamin B_6, potassium, riboflavin, and magnesium.

Top loin steak. One lean 3-ounce serving with fat trimmed, contains 168 calories, 65 milligrams of cholesterol, and 7 grams of fat. Protective nutrients include vitamin B_{12}, zinc, niacin, vitamin B_6, potassium, riboflavin, and magnesium.

Lamb foreshank. One lean 3-ounce serving gives you 159 calories, 88 milligrams of cholesterol, and 5 grams of fat. Protective nutrients include vitamin B_{12}, zinc, niacin, riboflavin, magnesium, and potassium.

Pork tenderloin. One lean 3-ounce serving gives you 139 calories, 67 milligrams of cholesterol, and 4 grams of fat. Protective nutrients include vitamin B_{12}, riboflavin, vitamin B_6, zinc, and magnesium.

Avocados

Avocados contain a lot of protective nutrients, but they're also high in fat. One avocado leaves you with almost 31 grams of fat. And that's a bigger problem now that you're older and trying to slow the buildup of the body fat that leaves you more at risk for heart disease, some cancers, and excessive weight. But there's a silver lining: About two-thirds of the fat is monounsaturated, which may actually lower cholesterol levels. Plus, you can use mashed avocados or guacamole as a healthy mayonnaise substitute.

Cancer. Heading up the protective roster are 5.3 grams of insoluble fiber—a lot of protection from colon cancer. You get as much insoluble fiber from one avocado as you do from 5 tablespoons of toasted wheat germ.

A standard serving, half of an avocado, gives you 14 percent of the Daily Value of vitamin B_6. If you're low on vitamin B_6, your immune system gets sluggish—something you can't afford to have happen as you get older. But studies show that increasing your intake of vitamin B_6 will reverse that slump. You also get 14 percent of the Daily Value of copper, important to help shift your immune system into high gear. Beta-carotene in avocados helps disable cancer-causing agents before they strike. Avocados also provide vitamin C to guard against a variety of cancers and glutathione to help strengthen your immune system.

A serving of avocado provides more than 15 percent of the Daily Value of folate. Researchers think that this nutrient protects healthy cells from cancerous invasion. High levels of folate are also linked to low rates of cancer of the cervix, colon, rectum, lung, and possibly of the esophagus. In the laboratory, substances in avocados even keep tumors from getting started.

Heart disease and stroke. In one study people who ate ½ to 1½ avocados each day reduced cholesterol levels from an average of 236 milligrams per deciliter (mg/dl) of blood to 217. Even better, the levels of the beneficial HDL cholesterol, which lowers your risk of heart attack, didn't go down.

Researchers note that certain B vitamins can reduce heart disease risks by 10 to 25 percent. And avocados are loaded with B vitamins, including folate and vitamin B_6. Studies show that folate and vitamin B_6 may help keep the levels of homocysteine low, which means lower risk of heart disease. Homocysteine tends to accumulate in the blood of people who eat meat, and it may harm artery walls. Half an avocado gives you more than 9 percent of the Daily Value for magnesium, which also bolsters heart health.

Avocados are rich in soluble fiber, which helps control cholesterol. Plus, avocados contain potassium, which helps to lower blood pressure and reduces your risk of stroke.

Bananas

Voted America's favorite fruit, bananas are almost fat-free.

Cancer. The B vitamins—one banana has 33 percent of the Daily Value of vitamin B_6—help strengthen your immune system to fight off cancer-causing interlopers.

Scientists think that a healthy helping of other substances in bananas—vitamin C and the powerful antioxidant glutathione—can help cut your risk of cancer of the mouth and strengthen your immune system. When glutathione was added to the white blood cells of both older and younger people, it increased their infection-fighting ability. The benefit was especially strong in the white blood cells from the older people. The 1.4 grams of insoluble fiber, found in one banana, helps reduce your risk of colon cancer. In the laboratory, substances in bananas keep tumors from developing.

Heart disease and stroke. In a study of 859 men and women, those who ate just one potassium-rich fruit, such as bananas, per day had a 40 percent lower risk of stroke.

Folate, a B vitamin that protects against cancer, also safeguards your heart by lowering levels of the harmful amino acid homocysteine, a risk factor in heart disease and heart attack. Vitamin C increases beneficial HDL cholesterol while it reduces harmful LDL cholesterol and triglycerides. You get 17 percent of the Daily Value of vitamin C from one banana.

Barley

Barley has been a staple of good health from time immemorial, even getting a "thumbs-up" in the Bible, which describes the good land as one of "wheat and barley." With that kind of endorsement, what are you waiting for?

Cancer. One serving of barley (½ cup cooked) gives you almost 2 grams of insoluble fiber to fight cancer.

Heart disease and stroke. A ½-cup serving of cooked barley gives you 1.2 grams of soluble fiber, which is great news for your heart.

Beans

The butt of many jokes, beans are superheroes of disease protection. Take your pick: black, garbanzo, cranberry, navy, pink, pinto, kidney, white, or yellow. You can't beat them.

Cancer. Research shows that women who eat a diet rich in beans have lower rates of breast cancer, thanks to substances in beans that block estrogen. Natural chemicals in green and wax beans, and even in the juice from beans, keep cells from mutating. They also destroy enzymes that give cancer its start.

Beans boost your immune system. One-half cup of canned garbanzo beans (chick-peas), for instance, gives you 10 percent of your Daily Value of copper and 8.4 percent of your Daily Value of zinc. You get protection from colon cancer with almost 4 grams of insoluble fiber in ½ cup of cooked beans.

Heart disease and stroke. A high-bean diet cuts the risk of heart disease because it lowers cholesterol levels. Even bean sprouts help your heart. In one study people with very high cholesterol levels ate 1½ cups of cooked beans daily for three weeks and made no other dietary changes. Their cholesterol levels fell by an average of 60 points.

One-half cup of cooked garbanzo beans gives you 1.3 grams of soluble fiber, the heart-protecting stuff. And 35 percent of the Daily Value of folate further cuts your risk of heart disease and stroke. Plus, you get magnesium and potassium. These nutrients help prevent blood clots and reduce high blood pressure.

Beets

On the surface, beets don't look all that remarkable. But research reveals that beets are rich in the protective plant compounds known as phytochemicals.

Cancer. Sure, beets have an impressive lineup of vitamins, minerals, and fiber. Just ½ cup canned beets gives you a very beneficial 1.5 grams of insoluble fiber and 6.4 percent of the Daily Value for folate to protect your cells and DNA coding.

But that isn't what has been impressing lab researchers. What's in the beet? At least 11 (and probably more) phytochemicals that fight cancer, including genistein, a substance that keeps estrogen from linking up with cancer cells to start tumor construction. It also keeps blood vessels from getting supplies to tumors. But beets have even more cancer-fighting properties that researchers have yet to explain.

Heart disease and stroke. One serving (½ cup) gives you more than 0.5 gram of the soluble fiber that helps lower your cholesterol levels and keeps plaque in the arteries from getting out of hand. Plus, you get 6.4 percent of your daily needs for the ever-important folate, lowering your risk of heart disease.

Don't forget the green stalk and leaves that top the beet itself. One-half cup of the cooked greens (especially when they're young) will give you 2.2 milligrams of beta-carotene, 2 grams of dietary fiber, plus some calcium, to lower mild blood pressure and cholesterol, magnesium to ease heart arrhythmia, and vitamin C to lower blood pressure and prevent oxidation of blood cholesterol. What's more, that same serving of beet greens provides 9 percent of the Daily Value of copper—a boon to your immune system.

Blackberries and Blueberries

Black or blue, you can't go wrong. Ever notice that when blueberries are exposed to acid (in lemon juice or yogurt, for example), they turn red? Exposed to baking soda, they turn a little green. But fear not—the change in color won't affect the change in protection.

Cancer. Blackberries pack more fiber than any other summer fruit (3.6 grams in ½ cup). Blueberries and blackberries contain important cancer fighters, including the phytochemicals catechins, flavonoids, and phenolic acids. Blackberries also contain ellagic acid, which neutralizes three different cancer-causing agents. Blackberries are high in vitamin C, which helps reduce your risk of cancers of the breast, cervix, esophagus, lung, mouth, pancreas, rectum, and stomach.

Heart disease and stroke. One-half cup of blackberries gives you more than 25 percent of the Daily Value of vitamin C. (Blueberries contain a little less vitamin C.) The vitamin C in these berries helps keep your HDL cholesterol levels high, which lowers the risk of your arteries becoming plagued by plaque.

Breads and Cereals

The name of the game is whole grain. Get out your reading glasses and check the fine print on packages. Look for the words "whole wheat" as the first ingredient on your bread wrapper—that means the bread contains whole-wheat flour.

Other good ingredients to look for are things like oat bran, soy flour, seeds, nuts, or whole grain. About 22 nutrients are diminished due to processing. And manufacturers only put a few nutrients back in. For example, enriched flour has had niacin, riboflavin, thiamin, and iron added to it.

Cancer. Two studies have found that something in oats keeps cells from mutating, but they haven't yet identified the compounds that provide the protection.

The consumption of breads and cereals made from whole grains may help lower the risk of colon cancer. Insoluble fiber speeds up the time it takes food to travel through the intestinal tract. So potential cancer-causing substances may be moved out of the body more quickly. Or, it could be that insoluble fiber lowers colon cancer risk because the fermentation of the fibers in the colon lowers the pH levels. Lower pH in the colon has been associated with lower colon cancer risk.

Heart disease and stroke. One slice of whole-wheat bread contains about 2 grams of dietary fiber. Fiber lowers cholesterol levels partly because it slows the absorption of cholesterol. Oats, rye, and barley are good sources of soluble fiber.

While there's little calcium in breads, yeast makes it easy for your body to take full advantage of what's there, according to a study at Creighton University in Omaha, Nebraska. Some bread and cereal products are fortified with vitamins and minerals for added protection against disease. Look for cereals fortified with folic acid, the supplemental form of folate, as well.

Broccoli

This is the workhorse of the food world. A serving (½ cup) of chopped raw broccoli contains only 12 calories and just a tiny bit of fat.

Cooking destroys a few nutrients, but broccoli is worth its weight in gold in just about any form.

Cancer. One serving (½ cup) of cooked broccoli gives you 97 percent of the Daily Value of vitamin C, an effective fighter against cancer of the breast, cervix, esophagus, lung, mouth, pancreas, rectum, and stomach.

You also get a sizable portion of folate to help keep your cells healthy and able to fight off cancerous agents. Researchers have found that folate plays an important role in cell division. It also helps keep the genetic coding in DNA intact. People whose diets are rich in folate have lower rates of cervical, colon, rectal, lung, and possibly esophageal cancer.

Cancer-fighting substances in broccoli also include such tongue twisters as flavonoids, isothiocyanates, sulphoraphane, indoles, carotenoids, dithiolthiones, glutathione (in uncooked broccoli), monoterpenes, plant sterols, phenolic acids, glucobrassicin. Whew! In fact, researchers have cataloged—and they're not done yet—more than 30 substances in broccoli that seem to have cancer-fighting abilities.

Heart disease and stroke. A lot of the cancer-fighting substances also help your heart. Vitamin C can prevent the LDL particles in blood from becoming oxidized, which helps lessen the risks were for of heart disease. A 13-year study of men with high cholesterol levels revealed that the higher their carotenoid levels were, the lower their risk were for heart disease and strokes. Flavonoids lower your risk of heart disease and heart attack. Carotenoids shoot down harmful LDL cholesterol.

Cooked broccoli gives you 1.2 grams of heart-saving soluble fiber, which lowers LDL cholesterol levels and helps control blood sugar.

Broccoli is a source for a high amount of vitamin A, which may help decrease your risk of heart disease. Unlike some foods, broccoli contributes calcium that your body can use easily, which is important because calcium helps reduce mild high blood pressure and reduce harmful LDL cholesterol. The higher your LDL levels, the bigger your risk of heart disease.

Brussels Sprouts

A close relative of broccoli, brussels sprouts deliver many of the same low-fat, low-cal benefits.

Cancer. A serving (about four sprouts) gives you 3 grams of insoluble fiber for protection from colon cancer.

You also end up with an array of protectors with long, complicated names. Indoles destroy the estrogen that helps breast cancer get started. They also helps activate your body's protective forces. Isothiocyanates help eliminate or neutralize cancer-causing agents. Flavonoids inhibit hormones that help cancer grow. Sulforaphane bolsters the body's natural defenses. Carotenoids work as antioxidants to stop damage to healthy cells.

Eat a serving of fresh cooked brussels sprouts and get 80 percent of the Daily Value of vitamin C. More than 30 studies have shown that if you eat foods rich in vitamin C, you cut your risk of cancer. They're also a good source of cancer-fighting vitamin A and folate. Its vitamin B_6 helps maintain your immune system.

Heart disease. Heading the list of protective compounds are the 1.4 grams of soluble fiber that you get in ½ cup, helping to reduce cholesterol in your blood.

You also get a good amount of folate, which lowers your blood levels of homocysteine, an amino acid in the blood that seems to add to the buildup of harmful cholesterol in your arteries.

Vitamin C also reduces the artery-clogging LDL cholesterol while keeping levels of the protective HDL cholesterol high. Vitamin A weighs in to protect your heart. Some studies show that even some people with heart disease may be able to cut their risks when they add foods that are sources of vitamin A to their diets.

Cabbage

In Lewis Carroll's *Through the Looking Glass,* a talking walrus speculates about cabbages and kings. It might have sounded like nonsense to put the two together, but the walrus had a point. Cabbage is a king of disease protection.

Any way you slice it, coleslaw it, steam it, boil it, or soup it, cabbage is a powerful disease-fighting food. And savoy cabbage, the crinkly stuff, is the leader of the protective pack.

Cancer. Researchers at the Strang-Cornell Cancer Research Lab in

New York City found that women who eat lots of cabbage and other cruciferous vegetables have lower levels of a kind of estrogen that stimulates breast cancer. The estrogen declined just five days after the women started eating more cruciferous vegetables. And the levels stayed down for the three months of the study. Those who ate the equivalent of one-third of a head of cabbage daily got the most benefit. Researchers attribute the drop to one substance, indole-3-carbinol.

The list of heavy-duty cancer fighters in cabbage also includes flavonoids, indoles, monoterpenes, phenolic acids, plant sterols, and sulforaphane. This long list of the hard-to-pronounce natural chemicals stops cancer at every stage of its development. Some substances keep cancerous agents from getting the slightest toehold in cells. Others keep healthy cells from mutating, block tumor development, or cut off the blood supply to tumors.

Cruciferous vegetables such as cabbage also contain glutathione, which helps counter cellular destruction by free radicals.

Heart disease and stroke. One cup of shredded raw cabbage gives you 37.6 percent of the vitamin C that you need each day, increasing your protective HDL cholesterol and lowering hazardous LDL cholesterol levels.

That cup of shredded raw cabbage provides some folate, which helps decrease the risk of heart disease.

Cantaloupe

One of the food world's Southern belles, cantaloupe looks sweet but gets tough in your system. You get a mouthful of protection in every bite.

Cancer. You get a healthy 1.5 milligrams of beta-carotene from ½ cup of cubed cantaloupe or about 2.5 milligrams from a quarter of a melon.

Plus, that ½ cup of cubed cantaloupe gives you a little over 50 percent of the Daily Value of two heavy hitters against cancer: vitamin A and vitamin C. And folate weighs in for the fight against cancer. (Folate may help ward off cancer of the cervix, colon, rectum, lung, and possibly the esophagus.) It also helps keep cells healthy and DNA—the substance that makes each person different—from getting damaged and passing on mutations to new cells. Glutathione may cut your risk of oral cancer and helps your immune system work as well as it did when you were a whole lot younger.

Heart disease and stroke. Beta-carotene may help clear your arteries of the harmful LDL cholesterol that can clog up the works and run up your risk of heart disease and stroke. In one major study, people whose diets included high levels of beta-carotene had half the number of fatal heart attacks and strokes as those whose levels were low.

Its potassium helps lower your blood pressure. Cantaloupe provides more than 56 percent of the Daily Value of vitamin C, which increases the good cholesterol, drops the bad, and helps lower your risk of developing arterial plaque.

Carrots

In the 1800s, an art critic predicted a revolution in painting, all because of the way Paul Cézanne painted some simple little carrots. The result? Modern art. Now carrots are at the center of another revolution—the discovery of important disease fighters.

Cancer. The orange color highlights carrots' protective compounds. Bright oranges, yellows, reds, and greens signal the presence of carotenoids, a powerful class of cancer-fighting substances. A single raw carrot gives you more than 12 milligrams of the carotenoid called beta-carotene, which in turn provides 405 percent of the Daily Value of vitamin A. Scientists note that beta-carotene may actually reverse cancers of the cervix and uterus that have started. And it protects against cancer of the lung, breast, cervix, uterus, esophagus, stomach, colon, and mouth. Vitamin A is an essential component of the mucous membranes that line the digestive, respiratory, urinary, and reproductive tracts, your body's first lines of defense against many invaders.

Researchers at Johns Hopkins University in Baltimore discovered that people who have little beta-carotene in their blood have four times the risk of developing lung cancer. The Harvard Nurses' Study found that women who eat less than one serving a day of foods rich in beta-carotene have a 20 percent higher risk of breast cancer.

Carrots contain other protective substances, including limonene, to protect against cancer of the mouth. In studies this substance has actually reduced the size of tumors. So far, more than 50 cancer-fighting compounds have been isolated in Bugs Bunny's favorite food.

Heart disease and stroke. Beta-carotene and its chemical cousin vitamin A do wonders for your heart. Studies show that people who get a lot of this nutrient suffer fewer heart attacks. One theory is that the beta-carotene may keep dangerous LDL cholesterol from attaching to artery walls. In the Physicians Health Study, men who took in high levels of beta-carotene had half as many strokes and fatal heart attacks as those who didn't. One-half cup of cooked carrots also gives you 1.1 grams of soluble fiber, which lowers blood cholesterol levels.

Carrots carry vitamin B_6 for possible heart protection and some copper to help maintain heart structure. One raw carrot gives you 11 percent of the Daily Value for vitamin C.

Cauliflower

The plain Jane of the vegetable world, cauliflower looks and tastes, well, pretty colorless. But the lackluster exterior is just a front—the substances in cauliflower go a long way toward protecting you from disease.

Cancer. Researchers have identified a bunch of substances that are powerful cancer fighters (and bestowed upon them names that would bring any Pictionary game to a halt). Some of these substances help the body counteract substances that cause mutations in DNA. Others make it hard for cancer-causing agents to zero in on healthy cells. And they cut off supplies to tumors. Talk about leading the resistance. Cauliflower is a good source of glutathione, an antioxidant, which in the lab has increased the ability of white blood cells to divide.

You also get the usual suspects for cancer prevention: insoluble fiber, folate, and vitamin C. A cup serving of raw cauliflower has 2 grams of insoluble fiber, and ½ cup of cooked cauliflower has almost 1 gram. There's also some vitamin B_6 in a serving of raw cauliflower, which keeps your immune system strong.

Heart disease and stroke. Here's a good lineup for protection: vitamin B$_6$, which helps lower your risk of heart attack and stroke, plus folate, an important B vitamin that helps reduce your levels of homocysteine, an amino acid linked to plaque buildup in the arteries, heart attack, and stroke.

One-half cup of cooked cauliflower has nearly 0.5 gram of soluble fiber, which lowers LDL cholesterol levels and heart attack risk. It also provides about 40 percent of the Daily Value of vitamin C, which helps increase levels of the good HDL cholesterol while it shoots down the bad LDL stuff.

Celery

A dieter's delight, a serving of celery (three stalks or 1 cup diced) gives you only 19 calories, less than 0.1 gram of fat, and no cholesterol.

Cancer. Studies have shown that compounds in celery actually neutralize toxic substances and prevent tumors from developing. There's a group of chemicals called the phthalides that may protect you from stomach cancer. When researchers in Minneapolis looked closely at one form of the chemical, 3-n-butyl phthalide, they found that it (along with another substance in celery, sedanolide) interferes with the development of tumors and helps activate an enzyme that detoxifies harmful substances in the body's tissues.

You also get protection from cancer thanks to insoluble fiber, folate, vitamin C, and vitamin B$_6$.

Heart disease and stroke. Butyl phthalide may also lower blood pressure by helping to relax the muscles that line the blood vessels. In the laboratory the chemical seems to reduce stress hormones that cause blood vessels to constrict and blood pressure to rise.

The vitamin C in celery also helps raise your beneficial HDL cholesterol levels, lowering your risk of heart disease and stroke.

Cherries

"Life is just a bowl of cherries," goes the song first belted out by Ethel Merman in 1931. Eat them and you sing a song of disease protection.

Cancer. A cup serving of sour cherries gives you almost 1 milligram of protective beta-carotene and is a source of 26 percent of the Daily Value for vitamin A, which may combat cancer-causing substances and disable them before they can invade your body's cells. Scientists discovered that a diet high in beta-carotene–rich foods helps reduce the risk of lung cancer in smokers and nonsmokers.

One-half cup of canned red sour cherries gives you almost 1 gram of protective insoluble fiber. There is some vitamin C in canned sweet cherries. And vitamin C protects you from cancer of the breast, cervix, esophagus, lung, mouth, pancreas, rectum, and stomach. There is also some cancer-fighting beta-carotene. Sour cherries contain more beta-carotene than sweet cherries, and they're lower in calories, too.

Heart disease and stroke. Vitamin C in cherries also helps raise your beneficial HDL cholesterol levels and lower your risk of heart disease and stroke. At the same time, it cuts the amount of the harmful LDL cholesterol and triglycerides that leave you vulnerable to a plaque buildup in your arteries. Its potassium helps keep your blood pressure under control.

Chestnuts

You probably remember a song about chestnuts, open fires, and holidays. Mel Torme penned the lyrics in 1946. As a disease fighter, chestnuts will help you enjoy many holidays to come.

Cancer. Just eight chestnuts give you 9 grams of dietary fiber for protection against colon cancer and only 1.5 grams of fat. Additionally, chestnuts contain copper to protect your immune system and vitamin C to help lower your risk of cancer of the breast, cervix, esophagus, lung, mouth, pancreas, rectum, and stomach.

Heart disease and stroke. Heart helpers in chestnuts include potassium; magnesium; vitamin C; and the beneficial B vitamins folate, riboflavin, and vitamin B_6. Altogether, you end up with lower blood pressure, less risk of a clot that could lead to a heart attack or stroke, lower levels of the harmful LDL cholesterol, and higher levels of the protective HDL cholesterol.

Chicken Breast

It's a deal you shouldn't pass up: This part of the chicken (without the skin) gives you half the fat that you would get from a trimmed, choice-grade T-bone steak.

Cancer. Your immune system gets a boost, thanks to zinc and vitamin B_6. Chicken breasts are rich in niacin, which some scientists think may help prevent cancer.

Heart disease and stroke. Half a breast gives you a lot of vitamin B_6, which, when combined with folate, can drop your risk of heart disease by 10 to 25 percent, doctors say.

You also get smaller amounts of other B vitamins such as riboflavin. Chicken provides potassium, which helps lower high blood pressure; and magnesium, which may also protect your heart by helping lower blood pressure.

Chicory Greens

Time to do a little exploring of the unfamiliar. On your next visit to the vegetable aisle of your supermarket, keep an eye peeled for chicory greens, also known as curly endive or, simply, endive. If your cashier picks it up and asks, "What's that?" you can reply, "It's protection against disease."

Cancer. You get 72 percent of the Daily Value of vitamin C in 1 cup of raw endive, decreasing your risk of a variety of cancers. Almost half of the Daily Value of folate is found in endive, which helps protect you against cancer of the cervix, colon, rectum, lung, and possibly the esophagus. Folate also helps keep cells healthy, making it harder for cancerous invaders to attack. Plus, the calcium in endive seems to give you protection from colon cancer.

Heart disease and stroke. Why leave the tried and true to experiment with this strange food? Because it's a hotbed of heart protection. A rich supply of vitamin C means that your levels of good HDL cholesterol get a boost while you beat down levels of the harmful LDLs and blood fats. Chicory greens also give you 18 percent of the Daily Value of calcium, which may help lower high blood pressure and LDL cholesterol levels, and potassium, which helps lower high blood pressure.

Chinese Cabbage and Bok Choy

They come from different groups within the oriental cabbage family, but both protect you from diseases that kill.

Cancer. Researchers note that people in Asia have lower rates of some forms of cancer. They theorize that compounds such as indole-3-carbinol in cabbages change the body's estrogen metabolism and stop the growth of small virus-caused tumors.

These cabbages give you some fiber: A 1-cup serving of shredded raw bok choy gives you 0.7 gram. And it gives you the important B vitamin folate, which may protect against cancer of the cervix, colorectum, lung, and possibly the esophagus. You also need folate to keep your cells healthy.

One-half cup of boiled boy choy is a source for more than 42 percent of the Daily Value of vitamin A, which strengthens your body's defenses against cancer. Almost 8 percent of the Daily Value of calcium in that ½ cup of bok choy helps lower your risk of colon cancer. Your body absorbs calcium from bok choy slightly more easily than it does calcium from milk.

Heart disease and stroke. You get potassium to help lower your blood pressure. Vitamin A lowers your risk of stroke—one theory is that it keeps LDL cholesterol from getting a grip on artery walls. Plus, with ½ cup of boiled bok choy, you get 37 percent of the Daily Value of vitamin C to further lower LDL and harmful fat levels in the blood and increase the beneficial HDL cholesterol.

Clams

Remember when people used to call money "clams"? Well, for their disease-preventing benefits, clams are worth a lot—especially since, when canned, they're less expensive than a lot of other seafoods. But don't go overboard: One 3-ounce serving of canned clams gives you 23 milligrams of iron or 264 percent of your requirements for iron. Men and post-menopausal women should aim for 9 milligrams or less of iron a day. Your body stores more iron as you age, so you don't want to risk too big a buildup, which potentially can be serious.

Cancer. One serving gives you 29 percent of your Daily Value of copper and almost 16 percent of your Daily Value of zinc to help strengthen your immune system. You'll also get more than 31 percent of your Daily Value of vitamin C, which helps reduce your risk of cancer of the breast, cervix, esophagus, lung, mouth, pancreas, rectum, and stomach. And the calcium in clams helps cut down your risk of colon cancer.

Heart disease. You get big-time heart protection from the B vitamins. One serving of clams gives you more than 1,400 percent of your Daily Value of vitamin B_{12}, plus some folate. Researchers theorize that these B vitamins can lower your risk of heart disease by 10 to 25 percent. They help reduce levels of homocysteine, an amino acid linked to high risk of heart disease.

Researchers say that clams and some other foods from the sea are high in omega-3 fatty acids, which may protect the heart. Omega-3's seem to lower the body's production of triglycerides, fats in the blood that are harmful in excess amounts. Plus, omega-3's help get the triglycerides out of the bloodstream. Scientists have linked low levels of triglycerides to high levels of the HDL cholesterol that may help protect you from heart disease.

Collards

A member of the cabbage family closely related to kale, collards give you disease-fighting benefits along with a mild taste.

Cancer. Indoles, isothiocyanates, sulforaphane, and quercetin—that's not the name of some blue-chip law firm. It's a lineup of cancer-preventing substances that get into your system when you take a bite of collards.

You also build up your body's first line of defense with vitamin A, which helps strengthen the membranes that line your body's vital organs and helps keep cancerous invaders at bay. A serving of collards provides a decent amount of the antioxidant vitamin E, which protects red blood cells and cells of the lungs. A deficiency of vitamin E may cause the initiation of some cancers.

107

Some studies show that the consumption of high levels of vitamin E decreases the levels of prostaglandin E$_2$, a substance that limits the efficiency of the immune system. Although these studies used supplements, food sources of vitamin E like collards help.

Heart disease. Collar heart disease with collards. One serving (½ cup, frozen, chopped, and cooked) provides more than 3 grams of beta-carotene, plus it's a source for 101 percent of the Daily Value of vitamin A. These important nutrients may help keep your arteries from getting clogged up with dangerous cholesterol. It also contains more than 37 percent of the Daily Value of vitamin C, which helps increase the protective HDL cholesterol while it lowers the harmful LDLs that can clog your arteries. Collards are also a source of vitamin E. A lack of vitamin E has been associated with the early stages of heart disease.

Corn

In Mitchell, South Dakota, people know how to show some appreciation for corn. Each year, the outside of the Corn Palace in Mitchell is covered in patterns, colors, and designs, all made from ears of corn. It's a big building. More than 3,000 bushels go into the project. And why not? In terms of disease protection, corn deserves a palace.

Cancer. Scientists have identified substances in corn that fight off cell mutations, the first step in cancer production. You get a number of other cancer protectors, too. One ear gives you almost 9 percent of the folate that helps your cells stay healthy. High folate levels are also linked to lower rates of cancer of the cervix, colon, rectum, lung, and possibly the esophagus. Vitamin C cuts your risk of cancer of the breast, cervix, esophagus, lung, mouth, pancreas, rectum, and stomach. Almost 2 grams of insoluble fiber protect against colon cancer.

Heart disease and stroke. Potassium in corn helps lower high blood pressure. You get a helping of the heart-protecting B vitamins and more than 14 percent of the Daily Value of vitamin C to help keep HDL cholesterol levels high and the harmful LDL stuff on the low side, in addition to helping to prevent the buildup of plaque in your arteries.

Cranberries

In pies, sauces, or juices, cranberries do more than give a tang to your taste buds. Most people probably think of cranberries only at Thanksgiving and Christmas, but they provide year-round disease protection.

Cancer. It's time for a reprise on the song of disease prevention called ellagic acid, a polyphenol. In the lab this substance fights cancer of the lung, skin, esophagus, and liver. It decreases the number of tumors and even keeps cancers from forming. Among fruits and nuts tested for ellagic acid content, cranberries have high amounts. Polyphenols also work as antioxidants to fight cancer-causing agents and may even counteract some of the effects of aging.

Cranberries also belt out 1.2 grams of insoluble fiber per ½ cup of chopped raw berries to protect against colon and breast cancer.

Heart disease and stroke. A serving contains more than 0.5 gram of soluble fiber, which helps keep high blood pressure down. Plus, it has 12 percent of your Daily Value of vitamin C, which keeps your arteries clear of the nasty fats and cholesterol that clog things up and lead to heart attacks and strokes. Also, the same polyphenols that protect you from cancer may help stave off heart disease.

Cucumbers

Cool as a cucumber, so the saying goes. But cucumbers are definitely hot stuff when it comes to disease prevention.

Cancer. Chlorogenic acid—this tongue twister may be the substance in cucumbers that makes them a powerful weapon against cell mutation. Cucumbers contain other important chemicals that protect you from cancer—coumarins, phenolic acids, monoterpenes, and triterpenes.

About a third of a cucumber (an average serving) gives you close to 9 percent of the Daily Value of vitamin C to help protect against cancer of the breast, cervix, esophagus, lung, mouth, pancreas, rectum, and stomach.

Heart disease and stroke. The boost from vitamin C also helps keep your levels of protective HDL cholesterol high.

Currants

Run against the current of disease with currants. (We're talking about the berries, not dried currants, a type of raisin that is made from the Black Corinth grape.)

Cancer. One-half cup of raw red currants gives you more vitamin C than ½ cup of blackberries, or about as much as in a tangerine, to help lower your risk of cancer of the breast, cervix, esophagus, lung, mouth, pancreas, rectum, and stomach. Add to that more than 1.5 grams of insoluble fiber to guard against colon and breast cancer. Studies in Germany found that currants can prevent genetic damage to cells. There is evidence that vitamin E in currants gives a boost to the immune system.

Heart disease and stroke. You get heart protection, thanks to almost 0.5 gram of soluble fiber per serving, helping to lower your cholesterol. One cup of fresh black currants provides you with 11 percent of the Daily Value for vitamin E. There is evidence that this nutrient fights heart disease.

Figs

The fig leaf provided Adam and Eve with coverage of one kind. And figs still keep you covered against disease. Two fresh medium-size figs contain only 74 calories and less than 0.5 gram of fat.

Cancer. Two fresh medium figs give you almost 1.5 grams of insoluble fiber to protect you from colon and breast cancer. (A serving of five dried figs gives you almost 4 grams of insoluble fiber.) Those five dried figs supply you with 15 percent of the Daily Value for copper to help your immune system stay strong and fend off invaders. The calcium in figs helps protect against colon cancer.

Heart disease and stroke. You get a lot of cholesterol-lowering soluble fiber from two fresh figs (1.7 grams). Plus, the potassium in figs helps lower your blood pressure.

A serving of five dried figs gives you even more: more than 3.5 grams of soluble fiber, more than 13 percent of the Daily Value for calcium, and 11 percent of the Daily Value of the heart-saving vitamin B_6.

Flounder and Family

From a health standpoint, you just can't go wrong with flounder or its popular relatives sole, turbot, and fluke. Beyond providing nutrients that protect you from disease, they're also low in fat. One average serving of 3 ounces weighs in with 1.3 grams of fat and 100 calories.

Cancer. These flat-bodied bottom-feeding fish are full of disease prevention. One 3-ounce serving (the size of a deck of cards) gives you vitamin B_6 to keep your immune system working effectively.

Heart disease and stroke. Flounder have a good amount of omega-3 fatty acids, which may help lower your risk of heart attack by lowering triglyceride levels. You get the heart-protecting B vitamins, namely vitamin B_6 and B_{12}. These nutrients reduce your risk of heart disease by up to 25 percent. Add to that magnesium to help prevent clots that can cause heart attacks or strokes. Magnesium also helps bring down high blood pressure.

Garlic

In World War II, Russian soldiers used garlic as an antiseptic. Not the sort of information that you'd care to share over dinner, but it should give you an inkling that garlic powers up more than your breath.

Cancer. In lab animals garlic reduces tumor growth by 60 percent. Researchers note that it even keeps cells from mutating. Antioxidants in garlic help keep harmful substances in the body from damaging healthy cells. The anti-tumor–promoting activity in garlic may be due to ajoene, quercetin, or other phytochemicals in the bulb. In the lab, researchers at Penn State University showed that a compound in garlic, DATS, slowed the growth of lung cancer cells. Aged garlic extract inhibited the growth of human breast cancer cells in the test tube.

Heart disease and stroke. Study after study has shown that people who eat one-half to one clove of garlic a day see their cholesterol levels drop by an average of 9 percent.

When scientists studied the results of eight previous garlic powder tests, they found that in half the tests, the people who ate garlic powder had a significant reduction in blood pressure readings.

How to Be a Crack Snacker

Remember: The terms *snack* and *junk food* are not at all the same. Here's how to satisfy your munchies and get disease prevention at the same time.

Plant the seeds for disease prevention. Seeds don't seem like healthy foods. They're pretty high in fat. But, in moderation, they offer you a lot of protection from cancer, heart disease, and stroke.

Sunflower seeds. They're a good source of fiber and vitamin E, an important nutrient that in supplement form protects against heart attacks, cancer, and stroke. Although it's hard to get vitamin E in most of the foods you eat, eating foods that contain vitamin E can only help in the fight against heart disease. A ¼-cup serving provides almost 3 grams of fiber. But here's the problem: You also get almost 16 grams of fat from that ¼ cup.

Sesame seeds. There's that trade-off again: High calories, high fat (1 ounce gives you 13 grams). You also get iron that you probably don't need, since your body stores more iron as you get older. On the positive side, in a 1-ounce serving, you get almost 4 percent of the Daily Value of calcium, 20 percent of the Daily Value of copper, almost 5 grams of fiber, almost 25 percent of the magnesium that your heart needs daily, and 115 milligrams of your potassium needs, helping to control your blood pressure. Plus you get an assortment of

A study at Tulane University Medical Center in New Orleans found that people who took a special garlic tablet experienced a 6 percent drop in their total cholesterol levels compared to those who did not take the tablet.

Grapefruit

It wasn't given the scientific name *Citrus paradisi* for nothing. Grapefruit is the fruit of paradise in terms of disease protection.

riboflavin, niacin, and folate (the natural form of the supplement folic acid).

Ice the fruit. Make fruit ices. Put a serving of your favorite fruit in a blender and mix it until smooth. Pour it into a bowl or shallow pan and put it in the freezer. Stir every 15 minutes or so to break up ice crystals and keep it from freezing solid too fast. It will take 1 to 1½ hours (and six to eight vigorous stirrings).

Pop the corn. Three cups of air-popped, unbuttered popcorn—enough to get you through even the longest movie—gives you 92 calories, 1 gram of fat, and more than 3 grams of fiber.

Soiree with sorbet. If you're on the prowl for a healthful after-dinner treat, try fruit sorbet with some fresh fruit thrown in. Not only will you stoke up on the goodness of the fruit, you also will take in less fat and cholesterol than you would with ice cream.

Pear it down. Grate a crispy Bosc pear and put it on hot breakfast cereal for a taste treat. Slice the Comice pear and use it in cereals or even for dessert.

Eat potato chips. Do what? Surprise—fat-free potato chips are readily available these days, so you can have the snack that you crave without the high fat, sodium, and calories. Look for brands with zero fat and low sodium and calories.

Cancer. Lycopene, carotenoids, limonene, flavonoids, glutathione, terpenes. Sounds like the mutterings of a mad scientist. But these natural chemicals all show cancer-preventing promise, and you get a healthy dose of them in ruby red grapefruit. This is especially good since lycopene levels decrease as you age.

All grapefruit contain terpenes, substances that encourage enzymes in your system to block carcinogens. Grapefruit of all colors are also rich in vitamin C to protect you from cancer of the breast, cervix, esophagus, lung, mouth, pancreas, rectum, and stomach. Half of a white grapefruit gives you nearly 69 percent of the Daily Value of this important nutrient (you get about 13 percent more from red). You'll get extra fiber if you eat your grapefruit like an orange. Eat the membrane that encases each segment as well as the pulp. You get 1.3 grams of insoluble fiber from half a pink grapefruit with the membrane, to fight off colon and breast cancer. If you spoon the grapefruit out, without eating the membrane, you'll still get 0.5 gram of insoluble fiber.

Heart disease and stroke. The amount of the flavonoid naringin found in half a grapefruit may help prevent excessive clumping of red blood cells in your arteries. That same serving size of any grapefruit equips you with just over a gram of the soluble fiber to help lower your cholesterol. It also contains some potassium, which downs another hazard to your heart by reducing high blood pressure. The vitamin C helps lower the harmful LDL cholesterol levels to keep arteries clear of the plaque that paves the way for heart attacks and strokes. It also helps keep protective HDL cholesterol levels high.

Grapes

Dionysus, the Greek god of wine, supposedly sailed in a ship outfitted with grape vines flowing from the mast. Gods didn't need disease protection, but you do. And the grape provides it.

Cancer. Grapes are a good source of flavonoids, substances that scientists theorize may fight cancer.

Plus, there's vitamin C to further cut your risk. Vitamin C seems to lessen the risk of certain cancers, including those of the cervix, breast, lung, mouth, pancreas, rectum, and stomach.

Heart disease and stroke. Flavonoids in grapes protect you from heart disease. In a study of 805 men ages 65 to 84, researchers found that those whose diets were highest in flavonoids had a 32 percent lower risk of dying of heart disease than those who ate the least. Researchers believe that flavonoids keep blood platelets from clumping together and forming a clot.

One-half cup of grapes (that's about 16 grapes) gives you a good amount of vitamin C, which helps raise the good cholesterol, lower the bad, and keep arteries clear. You get more than 0.5 gram of heart-protecting soluble fiber, which helps lower cholesterol.

Green Beans

They're just immature beans, still in the pod (or just out of it). Left in the garden, they would eventually grow up to be Great Northern, kidney, or pinto beans, depending on the variety. But immaturity is a plus (with beans, anyway). They're richer in beta-carotene and vitamin C than dried mature beans.

Cancer. Researchers have found that juice from the beans keeps cells from mutating.

Beta-carotene, which becomes vitamin A in our bodies, works as an antioxidant, fighting cancer-causing substances that your body produces and that come from things like car exhaust and tobacco smoke. In one study of lung cancer in nonsmokers, high intakes of the carotenes in green vegetables and fruits, which include beta-carotene, seemed to help protect against lung cancer. Vitamin A helps disable hazardous substances that can cause cancer—before they go to work in your body. A ½-cup serving of beans also gives you 1 gram of insoluble fiber to help prevent colon cancer.

Heart disease and stroke. Green beans are a source for some vitamin A, which does double duty. Not only does it help protect you against cancer, but it also helps lower your risk of heart attack and stroke. Beta-carotene, which gets converted into vitamin A, works as an antioxidant that may help keep the harmful LDL cholesterol from forming. This is the stuff that forms plaque buildup on artery walls and can pave the way for heart attacks and strokes.

Guavas

These tropical fruits are available in varying quantities, almost all year-round, especially during the late fall and early winter.

Cancer. Guavas look like limes with smooth skin, but they contain six times more vitamin C. In one fruit you get more than 275 percent of the Daily Value of this important nutrient to help sideline your cancer risk.

115

One guava also gives you more than 4 grams of insoluble fiber to help reduce your risk of colon and breast cancer.

Heart disease and stroke. In one doctor-supervised study, 120 people on medication to lower their blood pressures cut out the medicine and scarfed down several guavas a day. Their blood pressures went down and their levels of cholesterol and triglycerides dropped even further on guavas than on medication.

A guava gives you nearly 1 gram of soluble fiber and is a source of 14 percent of the Daily Value of vitamin A and vitamin B_6 to cut cholesterol, drop blood pressure, and help keep your heart healthy.

Halibut

Get in the halibut habit, and you'll be swimming in heart protection. One 3-ounce serving gives you less than 3 grams of fat and only 35 milligrams of cholesterol.

Cancer. A study found that lab animals had smaller breast tumors when fed omega-3 fatty acids from fish than those fed a fatty acid from corn oil.

Heart disease and stroke. Several studies show that eating one to two servings of fish a week (one serving is the size of a deck of cards) may cut your risk of stroke in half.

A lot of the benefit comes from a particular kind of fat in oily fish. Researchers have found that people who eat one to two servings of fish a week have less heart disease than people who eat less, and they think that it may be partly due to the omega-3 fatty acids that fish are rich in. An Australian study showed that a fish-rich diet may actually get rid of the dangerous triglycerides that pave the way for coronary heart disease.

Halibut also protects your heart with potassium, helping to lower high blood pressure.

B movies may be second rate, but the B vitamins are the Academy Award winners for heart protection. One serving of halibut writes a new script for your heart with almost 20 percent of the Daily Values for vitamins B_6 and B_{12}. As you get older, you need more of these important B vitamins. One serving contains 22 percent of the Daily Value for magnesium, which may help prevent blood clots and helps lower blood pressure. Calcium plays a bit part in this food, and it may help lower blood pressure in some people.

Honeydews

Whether at a summer roadside stand or in the grocery store, people looking for honeydew melons do a strange dance as they pick up melon after melon to shake them and poke them. And it's worth going to all the trouble because honeydews protect you.

Cancer. One-half cup of cubed honeydew provides you with 35 percent of the Daily Value of vitamin C, an antioxidant that helps protect your body from various cancers.

Heart disease and stroke. Just a sliver of this melon packs a punch: Its vitamin C helps keep the heart-protecting HDL cholesterol levels high while sending the harmful LDL levels into the cellar. Studies show that high levels of vitamin C keep your arteries from getting clogged and make you less vulnerable to strokes and heart attacks. Honeydew also provides potassium, which helps lower your blood pressure.

Kale

You know the plot line—Joe Average gets a chance and becomes a hero. Sort of like kale. This disease fighter doesn't often get the opportunity to show its stuff. You will often find it relegated to ornamentation at restaurant salad bars.

Cancer. Kale is one of the best sources of lutein, an antioxidant associated with lower rates of lung cancer. Isothiocyanates activate protective enzymes that carry carcinogens out of the system before they can do damage to cells. In the lab they have kept tumors from forming and neutralized cancerous agents.

Other disease fighters, among them indole-3-carbinol and sulforaphane, may protect against breast cancer. You also shore up your vitamin and mineral defenses with beta-carotene, vitamin A, dietary fiber, and vitamin C. Kale gives you calcium in a form that your body can use to protect against colon cancer. Kale is a good source of vitamin E. Some studies show that the consumption of high levels of vitamin E decreases the levels of prostaglandin E_2, a substance that limits the efficiency of the immune system. Although these studies used supplements, dark green leafy vegetables like kale are known sources of vitamin E.

Heart disease and stroke. Kale is rich in flavonoids, linked to lower rates of fatal heart attacks. One-half cup of frozen kale, cooked, provides 27 percent of the Daily Value for vitamin C and 2.5 milligrams of beta-carotene.

With ½ cup of cooked kale, you get almost 9 percent of the Daily Value of calcium, which helps lower blood pressure. Studies show that people with high levels of vitamin E are less likely to suffer heart attacks.

Kiwifruit

What taste would you get if you crossed a banana with a strawberry and added a touch of tartness? The kiwifruit—a brown, fuzzy-skinned fruit with emerald green pulp that hails from California and New Zealand.

Cancer. Kiwifruit are packed with vitamin C—in an ounce-for-ounce contest, the kiwi even beats out oranges. One large fruit gives you almost 150 percent of the Daily Value of that cancer-fighting nutrient. You also get a gram of insoluble fiber to guard against colon and breast cancer. Research has found that substances in the kiwifruit also keep cells from mutating. Studies show that high intakes of vitamin C lower the risk of breast cancer.

Heart disease and stroke. Vitamin C may be the food world's workaholic. Not content with protecting against cancer, it also helps your heart by lowering the levels of harmful fats and triglycerides in your blood. This means less buildup of debris to narrow arteries and increase your risk of a heart attack or stroke. Kiwifruit are loaded with vitamin C.

Plus, you get more than 0.5 gram of soluble fiber and some other nutrients that keep your heart healthier: 6.8 percent of the Daily Value of magnesium, plus some potassium to help lower blood pressure.

Kohlrabi

Kol-rab-ee. If you think that pronouncing kohlrabi is a brainteaser, just wait until you get a load of the science-speak that sums up how substances in the wonder food can protect you.

Cancer. On the cancer front, let's sample this strange use of the English language: Antimutagenic, desmutagenic, and inducers of glutathione-S-transferease. Translation: All are methods by which your body fights off tumor initiation.

You also get the usual lineup of protection that comes with any cruciferous vegetable. One-half cup cooked kohlrabi contains 74 percent of the Daily Value of vitamin C to help protect you from cancer of the breast, cervix, esophagus, lung, mouth, pancreas, rectum, and stomach. You also pump up your immune system with copper and vitamin B_6. If you like to nibble your kohlrabi raw, a 1-cup serving provides some folate, which may protect against cancer of the cervix, rectum, colon, lung, and possibly the esophagus.

Heart disease and stroke. Beyond weighing in with the vitamin C that helps block the formation of the LDL cholesterol that can build up in your arteries, kohlrabi helps lower your blood pressure with potassium.

Leeks

Okay, these relatives of onions and garlic are a nuisance. You have to clean them really well, or you end up eating dirt, literally. But it's worth it—their taste is sweeter and milder than onions, but their protective qualities are just about as strong.

Cancer. A close relative of garlic, leeks give off a mildly pungent scent. You'll get a lot of protection against cancer. Two studies identified compounds in leeks that may help to stop or reduce tumor growth. Among them are the important sulfur compounds that stop carcinogens before they can start to do damage. When researchers in Belgium looked at the eating habits of 3,669 people, they found that those who ate leeks were 66 percent less likely to develop colon cancer than those who did not eat leeks.

Other substances take the fight out of dangerous free radicals, substances that damage healthy cells. Plus, you get more than 0.5 gram of insoluble fiber to help protect against colon and breast cancer.

Heart disease and stroke. The same sulfur compounds that cancel car-

119

cinogens also help cut down blood pressure. Substances in leeks called flavonoids neutralize LDL cholesterol to help keep your arteries from clogging up. They also seem to help keep levels of the beneficial HDL cholesterol high. You get heart protection from 1.3 grams of soluble fiber per serving.

Lemons

"I would like a medium vodka dry martini—with a slice of lemon peel. Shaken and not stirred, please." Leave it to James Bond, master of high-tech weaponry, to figure out the protective qualities of even the lowly lemon and its peel.

Cancer. That spray from the lemon twist releases limonoids, powerful substances that, in animal studies, prevent oral cancer. But the twist isn't the only way to get protection. You can grate the zest (the colored part of the peel) and use it as a flavor enhancer.

Lemons put the squeeze on cancer: Flavonoids inhibit the hormones that promote cancer. Monoterpenes work as antioxidants to neutralize harmful substances. Phenolic acids keep dangerous nitrosamines from forming. Terpenes help enzymes block carcinogens.

Vitamin C gets into the act, too—eat a wedge, one-quarter of a lemon, and you get close to 13 percent of the Daily Value, lowering your risk of oral cancer. And you pick up just under 0.5 gram of dietary fiber to guard against colon cancer.

Heart disease and stroke. Lemons fight heart disease with a payload of vitamin C, which helps prevent cholesterol from building up to block your arteries.

Lentils

Whether you chose red, brown, or green lentils, this bean is such a star that it deserves to shine on its own, rather than get lumped with the rest of the beans. Lentils are often sold as "dahl," but this isn't the best buy for protection, since the fiber-rich outer skins have been removed.

Cancer. One-half cup serves up more than 4.6 grams of insoluble fiber to help protect against colon cancer. You also get almost 45 percent of the Daily Value of folate, which may protect you against cancer of the cervix, colon, rectum, lung, and possibly the esophagus. Folate also helps your cells stay healthy, making it harder for cancers to attack, and keeps the important DNA intact. Plus, you get 12.5 percent of the Daily Value of copper and 8.4 percent of the Daily Value of zinc to help strengthen your immune system.

Heart disease and stroke. This little bean is a beacon of heart protection. In one study people with high cholesterol who added 1½ cups of lentils or other legumes to their diets each day for three weeks experienced an average 60-point drop in cholesterol. Add to that some soluble fiber to help lower your LDL cholesterol and 9 percent of the Daily Value of vitamin B$_6$, which may help keep homocysteine levels low. The magnesium and potassium in lentils work together to lower high blood pressure and keep blood from clotting, which could lead to a heart attack or stroke.

Lettuce

Lettuce is a mixed bag in terms of benefits. You don't get many nutrients from the pale green stuff that most of us put on our sandwiches, although even that contains protective substances. The more exotic lettuces with big, dark leaves give you a lot of protection. Rule of the green thumb: The darker green the leaf, the more protection you'll get from it.

Cancer. Scientists have found that even the juice of lettuces contain substances that fight cell mutation and interfere with the development of tumors.

Romaine lettuce, with broad, dark leaves, is a noble cancer fighter. One-half cup, shredded, gives you more than 9 percent of the Daily Value of folate. This valuable B vitamin may protect you against cancer of the cervix, colon, rectum, lung, and possibly the esophagus. It also helps cells stay healthy and able to fight off cancerous agents.

Romaine also gives you 11 percent of the Daily Value of vitamin C, reducing your risk of cancer of the breast, cervix, esophagus, lung, mouth, pancreas, rectum, and stomach. More good news: Endive does just as well.

Heart disease and stroke. One cup of romaine weighs in with potassium. Arugula is a heavyweight in beta-carotene, a substance that may block the harmful LDL cholesterol and reduces your risk of stroke, packing 2 milligrams into a 1-cup serving.

Limes

In the 1700s, British ships packed limes to protect the troops from scurvy. Thus, British sailors earned the nickname "limeys." Scurvy's not a disease that we worry about anymore, but limes protect against diseases that we do fret over.

Cancer. Limes are rich in a lot of substances that keep cancer from getting a foothold: flavonoids that inhibit hormones that help cancers get started, limonoids that trigger enzymes to protect you, monoterpenes that work as antioxidants, phenolic acids that keep dangerous nitrosamines from forming, and terpenes that block carcinogens. Limes also give you vitamin C, which helps decrease the risk of breast cancer.

Heart disease and stroke. Like other citrus fruits, limes are particularly rich in vitamin C, which lowers the risk of stroke, especially in people age 65 and over.

Lobster

Who says that healthy eating can't be fun? Steamed or boiled, lobster contains 0.5 gram of fat and just 83 calories per serving.

Cancer. Eat lobster and you do a favor for your immune system as well as your taste buds. Three ounces of lobster (about the size of a deck of playing cards) gives you 83 percent of your Daily Value for copper and more than 16 percent of your Daily Value for zinc, both of which keep your immune system at its best. Calcium in lobster helps in the fight against colon cancer.

Heart disease and stroke. It's the catch of the day in terms of heart protection. A rich helping of omega-3 fatty acids may help lower your risk of heart attack by lowering triglyceride levels. Plus, you get a lot of nutrients that may help lower high blood pressure: 5 percent of the Daily Value of calcium, more than 7 percent of the Daily Value of magnesium, and some potassium.

High levels of homocysteine in the blood are linked to high risk of heart attack. Some B vitamins such as B_{12}, plentiful in lobsters, counteract them. You get 44 percent of the Daily Value of vitamin B_{12} in a serving.

Mackerel

You know the routine: On one hand, the benefits; on the other, the problems. Mackerel is that kind of fish, swimming in both directions. On the plus side, mackerel is rich in disease preventers. It is also rich in calories, fat, and cholesterol. One 3-ounce serving loads you up with 15 grams of fat. Fortunately, more than a third of that is monounsaturated fat, the kind that helps, not hurts. You also pull in 64 milligrams of cholesterol and 223 calories. But from a disease-prevention standpoint, mackerel has a lot going for it.

Cancer. Zinc builds up your body's defenses by strengthening the immune system and disabling substances that could cause cancer.

Heart disease and stroke. Several studies have revealed that people who eat one serving of fish a week may cut their risk of stroke in half.

Part of the reason may be that high levels of protective omega-3 fatty acids are tied to lower rates of heart disease. Researchers note that the higher the fat content of a fish, the more omega-3 fatty acids it provides. You also get close to 21 percent of the Daily Value of magnesium and some potassium to help keep your blood pressure low.

Plus, one serving of mackerel gives you 269 percent of the Daily Value of vitamin B_{12}. That's important because, as you age, you don't absorb this important nutrient as efficiently as you used to. You also get vitamins B_6 and B_{12} to help keep your heart healthy.

Mangoes

A taste sensation, mangoes remind some people of a fruit assortment of apricots and melons. Others characterize it as a cross between peaches and pineapple. But however you slice it, you get the taste of a fruit cocktail in just one fruit.

Cancer. Vitamins A and E turn out to be heavyweights in cancer protection, protecting your body from cancer-causing substances such as nitrosamines. Vitamin E lodges in cell membranes, where it fights off cancerous agents. And just half a mango is an excellent source of vitamin A, providing you with almost 78 percent of its Daily Value and almost 6 percent of the Daily Value for vitamin E.

A serving of half a mango gives you more than 2.3 milligrams of beta-carotene. Researchers have also discovered that a diet high in beta-carotene–rich foods protects both smokers and nonsmokers from lung cancer. You'll find about 5 percent of the Daily Value for copper in half a mango, boosting your immune system.

Heart disease and stroke. Half a mango gives you 1.5 grams of the soluble fiber that keeps high blood pressure down. The same nutrients that lower your cancer risk also help your heart: Vitamin E helps disarm fats before they can latch onto artery walls and clog up the works. Vitamin A and beta-carotene also work to protect your arteries from the plaque buildup that leaves you at risk for heart attacks and strokes. In addition, you get 46 percent of the Daily Value for vitamin C, which helps decrease the risk of stroke among elderly people.

Milk

It has a well-deserved rep for building bone, but that's not all it does. Skim milk deserves a place high on your list of protectors against cancer, heart disease, and stroke.

Okay—you've tried it, and it tastes watery and looks worse. You can fix that. Try decaf café latte. It's pretty much hot milk with a little espresso mixed in. Less than 80 calories and 0.5 gram of fat are in it, plus you bone up and protect your heart with 264 milligrams of calcium.

Or give the milk a richer taste and creamier look by stirring 2 to 4 tablespoons of instant nonfat milk powder into each cup of skim. You also get extra calcium that way.

Cancer. The skim in skim milk isn't something to take lightly. One study links high rates of breast cancer in mice to a high-fat and low-calcium diet.

Beyond cutting out the fat for cancer protection, skim milk provides calcium, which may reduce your risk of colon cancer; and zinc, which helps your immune system stay strong. Skim milk is a source of vitamin A and beta-carotene, which may help disarm the cancerous agents that invade your cells. One study suggests that beta-carotene, derived from foods, reduces the risk of lung cancer in nonsmokers.

Heart disease and stroke. One cup of skim milk fortified with vitamin A gives you almost 10 percent of the Daily Value for vitamin A and a little beta-carotene, which may help keep cholesterol from attaching to your artery walls and increasing your risk. (Buy milk in cardboard cartons that block the light—fluorescent lights in supermarket display cases can cost you up to 90 percent of vitamin A after 24 hours.)

Skim milk makes a three-pronged attack on high blood pressure: You get more than 30 percent of the Daily Value of calcium (which many researchers believe to be a countermeasure to mild high blood pressure), close to 7 percent of the Daily Value of magnesium, and more than 405 milligrams of potassium. Calcium may also help lower levels of the harmful LDL cholesterol.

You also get a sampling of the B vitamins riboflavin, B_{12}, and B_6, which are important for reducing your risk of heart disease, heart attack, and stroke.

Mushrooms

The mushroom may be a lowly fungus, but it has been a favorite of royalty since ancient Egypt. And it defends your body nobly with antibacterial and medicinal substances.

Cancer. Mushrooms contain antibacterial substances that help keep tumors from growing.

Shiitakes are also rich in other nutrients. Four cooked mushrooms (72 grams) give you almost 33 percent of the Daily Value of copper to make your immune system's defenses, well, mushroom. You also get almost 2 grams of dietary fiber to help protect you from colon cancer and heart disease, and you receive more than 6 percent of the Daily Value of zinc to help protect your immune system.

Button mushrooms also give you immunity-building protection: ½ cup gives you 8.5 percent of the Daily Value of copper.

Heart disease and stroke. Just four cooked shiitake mushrooms equip your system with more than 84 milligrams of potassium, lowering your blood pressure. Its vitamin C does double duty against both cancer and heart disease as it raises your blood levels of beneficial HDL cholesterol and drops the levels of the harmful LDL cholesterol and triglycerides, or fats, in the blood. You end up with a lower risk of the plaque buildup in the arteries that can lead to a heart attack or stroke. You also get small amounts of the heart-helping folate and vitamin B_6, which have been shown to lower the production of homocysteine—a substance that activates a clotting system, making blood more prone to adhere to arterial walls.

Regular mushrooms, served raw, aren't nearly as powerful as cooked shiitakes, but with a quarter cup of them you still end up with a very respectable 42 milligrams of potassium to fight heart disease.

Mussels

Mussels muscle up your body's protective systems.

Cancer. One serving of 3½ ounces of cooked mussels provides vitamin A, which may help strengthen your body's defenses and protect against lung cancer. Its vitamin C helps ward off cancer of the breast, cervix, esophagus, lung, mouth, pancreas, rectum, and stomach. Almost 18 percent of the Daily Value of zinc and a helping of copper assist your immune system. You get almost 19 percent of your Daily Value of folate, which may lower your risk of cancer of the cervix, colon, rectum, lung, and possibly the esophagus. Folate also helps cells stay healthy.

Heart disease and stroke. Mussels are rich in the omega-3 fatty acids, which may help keep your cholesterol levels low and fight heart disease. Some studies have found that vitamin A and beta-carotene block the harmful LDL cholesterol and lower your risk of stroke. Vitamin C keeps the beneficial HDL cholesterol levels high and also helps knock down the nasty LDLs and triglycerides, fats in the blood. Potassium weighs in with almost 266 milligrams, keeping your blood pressure low.

The innards of these deep blue shells are rich in the B vitamins. High levels of B_{12}, B_6, and folate in the blood have been shown to lower the production of homocysteine—a substance that activates a clotting system, making blood more prone to adhere to arterial walls. So getting the proper daily dose of these vitamins helps lower your heart disease risk. Mussels contain almost 19 percent of the Daily Value of folate, 397 percent of the Daily Value of the important vitamin B_{12}, and 5 percent of vitamin B_6. These tasty mollusks also contain more than 24 percent of the Daily Value of riboflavin, which has been shown to control cholesterol levels.

Mustard Greens

Hey, the seeds that make mustard have to come from somewhere. As you might expect from the mother of mustard, this leafy green vegetable has a tangy taste.

Cancer. Researchers working with the National Cancer Institute have been busy isolating substances in mustard greens that, at least in the lab, put a lid on cancer. Here's what some of these substances do: They interfere with cancer's start-up process, propelling your protective enzymes into action. They even get in the way of estrogen, which helps reduce the likelihood of breast cancer.

A good source of fiber when eaten raw, mustard greens lower the risk of colon cancer. A ½-cup serving, cooked and chopped, is a source of almost 42 percent of the Daily Value of vitamin A and a respectable amount of beta-carotene, which may strengthen the mucous membranes that keep cancer-forming agents from damaging healthy cells. Also, there is nearly 30 percent of the Daily Value for vitamin C, lowering your risk of cancer of the breast, cervix, esophagus, lung, mouth, pancreas, rectum, and stomach.

You get almost 13 percent of the Daily Value of folate, which may protect you from cancer of the cervix, colon, rectum, lung, and possibly the esophagus. This vitamin also protects DNA's genetic codes. At the most basic level, your cells rely on folate to help them divide and

From Condiments, A Dash of Protection

How nice—what's good for your taste buds is also great for your body. The spices that transform bland foods into sublime culinary treats also protect you from cancer, heart disease, and stroke.

Chilies. Hot peppers, the source of dried chilies and cayenne, contain capsaicin, a chemical that not only gives your taste buds a buzz but also fights bacteria and mutes your system's pain receptors. Chilies are rich in vitamin C—½ ounce of the red variety gives you more than 57 percent of the Daily Value. It never hurts to keep your taste buds happy by using chilies or cayenne when you eat low-salt and low-fat foods.

Curry. Tumeric, derived from a plant root, gives the characteristic flavor to Indian curry dishes. It contains curcumin, which in the lab prevents cancerous lesions of the skin, breast, and colon. It also helps keep blood platelets from sticking together and causing clots and helps stop fats in the blood from oxidizing and turning into harmful low-density lipoprotein cholesterol.

Horseradish. This condiment will not only wake up your taste buds, but may also provide disease prevention. A cruciferous vegetable (meaning it's a cousin to broccoli and cauliflower), fresh horseradish contains beta-carotene and vitamin C, along with the phytochemical isothiocyanate that gets the body's protective enzymes working to root out cancerous agents. Remember, fresh is best—prepared horseradish that you buy in the store is not very nutritious.

Parsley. Two sprigs offer more than 4 percent of the Daily Value of vitamin C, 2 percent of the Daily Value of vitamin A, and a little fiber. They're also a good source of the protective flavonoids and beta-carotene. You benefit most from dried parsley, with its concentrated nutrients like copper and magnesium. Don't go wild: 1 tablespoon gives you 7 percent of the Daily Value for iron; you probably don't need extra.

replicate properly. Doctors note that damaged cells are easy prey for carcinogens.

Heart disease and stroke. Mustard greens are a source of vitamin E, an important antioxidant that some studies say helps reduce your risk of heart attack and stroke. Researchers at Harvard Medical School looked at 1,795 women who'd had a heart attack or angina. Over a 10-year period, they found that the women who ate the most foods containing vitamin E, beta-carotene, vitamin C, and riboflavin had a 71 percent lower risk of a stroke and a 33 percent lower risk of a second heart attack. You get all these nutrients in mustard greens.

The benefits continue with more than 141 milligrams of potassium to lower your blood pressure, a healthy dose of magnesium to help keep blood pressure down and prevent the blood clots that could lead to a heart attack or stroke. Calcium may help by lowering mild high blood pressure and the harmful LDL cholesterol levels. Mustard greens contain B_6 and folate, which help lower your risk of heart disease by lowering high blood pressure and dropping levels of homocysteine.

Nectarines

The name probably comes from the Greek word for "drink of the gods." The nectarine should be celebrated for its disease-fighting capabilities as well as its taste.

Cancer. Researchers working with the National Cancer Institute found substances in nectarines that help prevent cancers from getting started and growing.

Your immune system will like the taste of nectarines—one fruit is a source of copper, vitamin B_6, and vitamin A to help keep cancerous agents away. More than 12 percent of the Daily Value of vitamin C is in a nectarine, which helps protect you against cancer of the breast, cervix, esophagus, lung, mouth, pancreas, rectum, and stomach. And it has close to 2 grams of insoluble fiber to help you cut your risk of colon and breast cancer.

Heart disease and stroke. Eat a nectarine and give high blood pressure a downward thrust, thanks to more than 288 milligrams of potassium. Nearly a gram of soluble fiber helps you send your cholesterol down, too. Vitamin C helps lower the levels of LDL cholesterol that tend to build up plaque in your arteries.

Olive Oil and Canola Oil

Wait a minute—how can oils be on a healthy foods list? Easy.

Cancer. Next time you measure out a tablespoon of olive oil, look at it this way: You're getting almost 8.5 percent of the Daily Value of vitamin E, which helps your infection-fighting T cells do their job. You're also keeping the rest of your immune system up to par. Plus, vitamin E seems to reduce the risk of oral cancer.

Heart disease and stroke. When researchers at the University of Milan examined the relationship between the Mediterranean diet and low rates of heart disease, they decided to investigate oleuropein, a component of olive oil. They found that it blocks the start-up of chronic heart disease.

Canola oil is rich in omega-3 fatty acids (the same stuff that makes fish the dish of protective choice) that may combat cholesterol and protect you from heart disease.

Both olive and canola oil are good sources of vitamin E. Several large studies have shown that vitamin E reduces the risk of heart disease by preventing the oxidation of cholesterol and the formation of blood clots. Although these studies used vitamin E supplements, foods that contain vitamin E can always help.

Not surprisingly, both of these oils are high in monounsaturated fat, the kind that doesn't clog up your arteries. In fact, it's been linked to lower levels of both cholesterol and blood pressure.

Onions

Shakespeare had nothing nice to say about onions. In "A Midsummer Night's Dream," a character advises, "Eat no onions nor garlic, for we are to utter sweet breath." Maybe that's good advice for a romantic evening, but not for a disease-free life.

Cancer. Onions come in all shapes, sizes, and colors. You'll get more cancer protection from red onions because they contain the most flavonoids, substances that studies show help fight cancer.

But any onion contains a wealth of cancer protection. Compounds in onions block or suppress carcinogens, help keep cells from mutating, and interfere with tumor growth. They have even been reported to protect against radiation damage.

Heart disease and stroke. Substances in onions called flavonoids may lower blood pressure. They also help neutralize the LDL cholesterol that leads to clogged arteries (and increases your risk of a heart attack or stroke).

Oranges

Christopher Columbus carried orange seedlings with him across the Atlantic. What would Florida and California look like if he had forgotten that part of his cargo?

Cancer. Orange juice is loaded with limonoid glucosides, natural chemicals that reduce the growth of cancer in animals. You also get glutathione, which may lower your risk of oral and throat cancer and help your immune system work more efficiently. Eat an orange and get almost 2 grams of insoluble fiber to help prevent colon and breast cancer. You take in more than 116 percent of the Daily Value of vitamin C to protect against cancer of the breast, cervix, esophagus, lung, mouth, pancreas, rectum, and stomach. Look for calcium-fortified orange juice, which may combat colon cancer.

Heart disease and stroke. Calcium-fortified orange juice gives you about 33 percent of the Daily Value of calcium. In some studies, calcium has been shown to also help lower your blood pressure. Plus, that healthy dose of vitamin C lowers the bad LDL cholesterol levels and raises the good HDL levels. Another good reason to reach for orange juice is for the fiber it contains. A ¾-cup serving gives you almost 0.5 gram of the soluble fiber that protects your heart.

Oranges give you 237 milligrams of potassium to help keep your blood pressure in check. Eat the white part just under the outer peel and the center core of the orange for an extra dose of heart-protecting flavonoids, a group of phytochemicals.

Oysters

"Why, then the world's mine oyster, / Which I with sword will open," wrote Shakespeare. Crack open that stubborn little shell, and you will discover an abundance of disease protection, too.

Cancer. Oysters help make your immune system a hard shell for cancer to crack. Six medium steamed oysters provide you with 159 percent of the Daily Value of copper and 509 percent of the Daily Value of zinc. Talk about defenses. Plus there's vitamin C to contribute to the cause of protection. They are also a source of vitamin A, which may cut your risk of cancer.

Heart disease and stroke. Oysters defend your heart, too. Just six oysters give you a lot of the important B vitamins that reduce risk of heart disease: 245 percent of the Daily Value of vitamin B_{12}, plus some riboflavin. Vitamin B_{12} is harder for your body to absorb as you age, making it especially important that your diet give you enough.

Magnesium in oysters helps prevent the blood clots that can lead to a stroke. Oysters also provide potassium, which can help lower high blood pressure.

Papayas

Sweet and refreshing, these large fruits contain little black, peppery-tasting seeds (and, yes, they're fine to eat—some people actually use them as a substitute for capers).

Cancer. One serving, about 1 cup of cubed papaya, gives you 144 percent of your Daily Value of vitamin C, important to help cut your risk of cancer of the breast, cervix, esophagus, lung, mouth, pancreas, rectum, and stomach. It's also a source of beta-carotene and vitamin A, which may help strengthen your body's defenses. You get more than 13 percent of the Daily Value of folate to help ward off cancer of the cervix, colon, rectum, lung, and possibly the esophagus. Folate helps keep cells healthy so that they're less easily invaded by carcinogens.

Heart disease and stroke. Vitamin C raises the levels of HDL cholesterol, protecting you from heart disease and heart attacks. It also lowers the harmful blood fats that attach to artery walls and increase your risk of a heart attack or stroke.

Vitamin A gets into the act and has been found in some studies to block LDL cholesterol before it can become a permanent (and unwelcome) fixture in your arteries. Vitamin B$_6$ helps lower levels of the harmful LDL cholesterol, decreasing your risk of heart problems.

You also get a little magnesium to reduce the blood's tendency to clot where it shouldn't. Calcium in papayas may help lower mild high blood pressure and LDL cholesterol levels. And a serving of papaya gives you 359 milligrams of potassium, which helps keep high blood pressure down, too.

Parsnips

How food fashions change. Most people today probably couldn't tell you what a parsnip looks like. In the 1700s they were one of the most commonly consumed vegetables in America. These now-exotic vegetables look like pale and oversized carrots with a celery-like scent and a vaguely nutty taste.

Cancer. Eat parsnips and you get an array of protective phytochemicals such as coumarins, phenolic acids, monoterpenes, and phthalides. What's more, ½ cup of boiled parsnips contains 1 gram of insoluble fiber to guard against colon and breast cancer. Plus, it provides copper, which helps strengthen your immune system.

Heart disease and stroke. Parsnips aren't parsimonious when it comes to heart protection: The same phytochemicals that help prevent cancer also lower your risk of heart disease. They prevent harmful LDL cholesterol from sticking to artery walls.

You get a healthy, heart-saving helping of the B vitamins, including folate, riboflavin, and vitamin B$_6$. You also get almost 2 grams of soluble fiber to lower LDL cholesterol levels, 286 grams of potassium to help lower blood pressure, and more than 16 percent of the Daily Value for vitamin C to raise levels of HDL cholesterol and lower LDL levels. That's hearty protection.

Peaches

When settlers from Spain came to the New World, they brought peaches with them. "Just peachy," you might say, especially when you consider what peaches do to protect you.

Cancer. In the lab, substances in peaches make it hard for cancerous tumors to get started. Peaches contain glutathione, which may reduce the risk of oral and throat cancer.

One fruit gives you nearly a gram of insoluble fiber, lowering your risk of colon and breast cancer. Its vitamin C protects important organs from cancer. Vitamin A in peaches may help keep cancerous agents from getting into your system.

Heart disease and stroke. One peach gives your heart all-purpose protection. It's a source of more than 9 percent of your Daily Value of vitamin A, which may help keep the harmful LDL cholesterol from getting a lock on artery walls.

Peaches provide you with more than just one LDL-fighting weapon—think of it as gang warfare on your behalf. Along with vitamin A, vitamin C clobbers the LDL cholesterol that leads to clots. It also increases the levels of the HDL cholesterol that keeps the bad stuff from getting a grip. Potassium in peaches protects against high blood pressure.

Pears

If you're shaped like a pear, you're in luck: Your risk for disease is lower than your apple-shaped friends. For those of you who don't sport the pear shape, and for those "pears" who want to remain healthy, eating pears—the fruit—has some considerable disease-fighting effects.

Cancer. In the laboratory, substances in pears prevent cell mutations and may trip up cancer's first steps in your body. In one medium pear, you get more than 3 grams of insoluble fiber to protect against colon cancer and a helping of copper to help keep your immune system up to par.

Heart disease and stroke. A pear gives you almost 2 grams of soluble fiber to protect your heart. Add to that more than 350 milligrams of potassium to help drop your blood pressure.

And about 11 percent of the Daily Value of vitamin C is found in a pear, which cuts harmful LDL cholesterol and raises the beneficial HDL cholesterol levels. (You'll get less benefit from canned pears because they have been peeled. The canning process also saps away some of the vitamin C.)

Peas

Remember the story that you read to your children about the princess and the pea? If her highness had been thinking about disease prevention, she would have banished the servant who put the pea under the mattress instead of on the dinner table.

Cancer. While the princess of the story did discover the pea, today's researchers remain puzzled. Peas do seem to prevent cells from mutating, although no one yet has a clue why that happens.

But we do know that peas are a good source of vitamins A and C. One-half cup of snow peas gives you about 64 percent of the Daily Value of vitamin C, protecting you from cancer of the breast, cervix, esophagus, lung, mouth, pancreas, rectum, and stomach.

Heart disease and stroke. Peas give you princely protection—one serving, about ½ cup of green peas, provides almost 17 percent of the Daily Value of vitamin C to help slash the LDL cholesterol that leads to clots. This nutrient also helps raise levels of the HDL cholesterol that keeps the LDLs from getting a grip. They are also a good source of vitamin A, which may help keep LDL cholesterol from attaching to arterial walls. There's some vitamin B_6 and folate, which help lower the blood levels of homocysteine, a substance that activates the blood's clotting system. The magnesium in peas helps lower mild high blood pressure, and the soluble fiber keeps cholesterol down.

Pecans

Okay—they're really high in calories. Of the nuts that you are likely to see in the grocery store, only macadamia nuts pack in more. They're high in fat, too, although 55 percent is monounsaturated, the kind of fat that doesn't contribute to clogs in the arteries. But pecans also wield some mighty weapons against cancer, heart disease, and stroke.

Cancer. The answer? Ellagic acid. In a study using laboratory mice, it has been shown to be a powerful adversary that fights cancer of the lung, skin, esophagus, and liver. It detoxifies carcinogens and scavenges substances that carcinogens need to do their nasty work. It might even keep cancerous substances from damaging DNA.

One ounce of pecans—that's about a handful—also gives you almost 18 percent of the Daily Value of copper, an essential nutrient for your immune system. It provides almost 11 percent of the Daily Value for zinc, another key mineral for immunity.

Heart disease and stroke. That single ounce does a lot for your heart. You get 105 milligrams of potassium and more than 9 percent of the Daily Value of magnesium to lower high blood pressure. Magnesium also helps keep your blood from clotting. The monounsaturated fat in pecans helps lower cholesterol and high blood pressure.

Peppers

You know John Wayne didn't talk much in films—just mowed down villains and saved the town (or country). Bell peppers are a lot like that. They don't get the attention, but boy do they come to the rescue.

Cancer. Red peppers are really just green ones that got to spend more time on the vine—and in the process stocked up on extra nutrients that protect you.

You get more vitamin C in one red pepper than you do in two oranges. Low vitamin C levels have been linked to a higher risk of developing breast, cervical, esophageal, lung, oral, pancreatic, rectal, and stomach cancer. Plus, you get 2.5 milligrams of beta-carotene (more than in a cup of apricots and nine times more than in a green bell pepper). Researchers have found that beta-carotene may help cut your risk of oral cancer. You also get carotenoids and flavonoids for added anti-cancer protection.

Heart disease and stroke. The flavonoids that protect against cancer also help you steer clear of heart disease and stroke. In a five-year Dutch study, older men with diets high in flavonoids had a lower risk of heart attack and stroke.

Peppers are loaded with other nutrients for your heart: ½ cup sweet green peppers gives you 74 percent of your Daily Value of vitamin C to help keep your arteries clear of debris.

Eating peppers gives you some vitamin B_6 and folate, which a study involving older adults found may reduce the risk of heart disease.

Persimmons

Persimmons are the Jekyll and Hyde of the food world: Bite into an unripe persimmon, and you'll get a taste more bitter than three-day-old coffee. When ripe, persimmons turn sweet and spicy.

Cancer. One medium-size Japanese persimmon weighs in with a lot of disease protection. You get more than 2 milligrams of beta-carotene, and they are a source of almost 73 percent of the Daily Value of vitamin A. Several studies have shown that these nutrients may protect against cancer. You get 9.5 percent of the Daily Value of copper to help your immune system. And more than 6 grams dietary fiber to lower your risk of colon cancer.

Heart disease and stroke. The vitamin C in persimmons helps keep the levels of the HDL cholesterol high while it decommissions the harmful LDL cholesterol. Your arteries get the benefit: There is less plaque buildup, which can lead to a stroke or heart attack. Persimmons also have some potassium, helping to lower high blood pressure.

Pineapple

Pop quiz: Where do pineapples come from, really? South America. By the time Columbus arrived, they had spread to the Caribbean. Other explorers soon carried them to China and the Philippines. Finally, they landed happily in Hawaii.

Cancer. This globe-trotting fruit packs a lot of disease-preventing power. Researchers working with the National Cancer Institute have discovered that substances in pineapples fight cell mutations as shown in laboratory studies.

One-half cup of diced raw pineapples gives you almost a gram of dietary fiber to help protect against colon and breast cancer. There's also a little folate to help keep your cells healthy and less vulnerable to a cancerous attack. Folate may also help reduce your risk of cancer of the cervix, colorectum, lung, and possibly the esophagus. You get some copper to help strengthen your immune system.

Heart disease and stroke. One helping gives you almost 20 percent of

137

the Daily Value of vitamin C. It helps raise levels of the beneficial HDL cholesterol, the stuff that keeps the harmful LDL cholesterol from doing damage. Having a low HDL level may be the most accurate indicator that you're at risk for a heart attack or stroke.

Plums

When you think "plum," you think "purple," right? Not so—colors range from almost green to red to so-purple-they-look-black. And they have great names, such as President, Empress, Tragedy, Freedom, and Elephant Heart, which is mainly used for cooking. Take your pick—they're all plum protection.

Cancer. One medium plum gives you close to 1 gram of insoluble fiber to help fight colon and breast cancer. Vitamin C in plums protects against cancer of the breast, cervix, esophagus, lung, mouth, pancreas, rectum, and stomach. A little vitamin B_6 helps round out the anti-cancer forces by boosting your immune system.

Heart disease and stroke. Plums give you some of the cholesterol-lowering soluble fiber that protects your heart. They're also a source of riboflavin, vitamin B_6, and vitamin C for a cornucopia of heart protection. The result? Higher amounts of protective HDL cholesterol, lower levels of the harmful LDL cholesterol that clogs your arteries, and less risk of blood clots that trigger heart attacks and strokes.

Pollock

Sometimes the imitation is just as good as the original, and even better if it saves you money. Pollock often masquerades as a low-cost imitation crabmeat (often labeled "surimi"). One 3-ounce serving gives you just over 1 gram of fat and 77 milligrams of cholesterol.

Cancer. Pollock provides a healthy helping of vitamin B_6, weighing in at 14 percent of your Daily Value, which helps strengthen the defenses of your immune system. Folate, another B vitamin in pollock, may help lower your risk of cancer of the cervix, colon, rectum, lung, and possibly the esophagus. You need folate to protect DNA's genetic codes and to help cells divide and multiply properly. Damaged cells are attractive targets for cancerous invaders.

Heart disease and stroke. People who eat one serving of fish a week can lower their risk of stroke by about half. A 3½-ounce serving of Atlantic pollock, for example, gives you 421 milligrams of omega-3 fatty acids, along with just a bit over 1 gram of fat. In some studies, omega-3 has been shown to fight heart disease. A healthy 77 milligrams of calcium in a serving of pollock contributes close to 7 percent of your Daily Value and may help to lower your levels of hazardous LDL cholesterol while at the same time help drop your blood pressure.

One 3-ounce serving deals out disease protection in the form of 19 percent of the Daily Value of magnesium to help get your blood pressure down. It also helps keep blood from clumping and forming clots that increase your risk of a heart attack or stroke.

Potatoes

Pop quiz: What food makes up the leading source of vitamin C in the American diet?

Yup—potatoes.

Cancer. Eat one medium baked potato with its skin and you will take in more than 43 percent of the Daily Value of vitamin C to help stave off cancer of the breast, cervix, esophagus, lung, mouth, pancreas, rectum, and stomach. There are also substances in potatoes that fight off cell mutation.

Heart disease and stroke. That baked potato also gives you 844 milligrams of potassium to help bring down high blood pressure. (To get the full benefit, eat the skins.) And its vitamin B_6 helps lower your risk of heart disease.

Prunes

Why all the fuss? Prunes are just dried-up plums, right? When water gets removed during processing, nutrients become more concentrated. If foods got Academy Awards for disease protection, prunes would be working on an acceptance speech.

Cancer. One-half cup of these dried delectables contains more than 2 grams of insoluble fiber to help prune your risk of colon and breast cancer. They are a source of vitamin A and beta-carotene, which may help keep cancers from invading healthy cells. Some studies also suggest that these nutrients help protect against lung cancer. You get 10 percent of the Daily Value of copper to strengthen your immune system.

Heart disease and stroke. In an ounce-per-ounce comparison, prunes contain more fiber than most dried beans, fruits, and vegetables. A lot is soluble, protecting your heart. You get 354 milligrams of potassium, plus an assortment of powerful protectors against heart disease: calcium, folate, magnesium, riboflavin, vitamin A, vitamin B$_6$, and vitamin C.

Pumpkins

The kind of pumpkin that you and your grandchildren carve out at Halloween isn't the kind that usually goes into a pie, bread, or soup. Smaller, sweeter (and less stringy) sugar pumpkins get used instead.

Cancer. A variety of nutrients protect: A mug full of pumpkin soup can give you about 1.4 grams of fiber. One-half cup of mashed pumpkin is a source of more than 26 percent of the Daily Value of vitamin A and some beta-carotene, which may reduce your risk of cancer of the esophagus, stomach, colon, breast, cervix, uterus, and lung. You get cancer-fighting, immune-strengthening copper, too. Researchers working with the National Cancer Institute also note that substances in pumpkins keep cells from mutating.

Heart disease and stroke. A 10-year study of 1,795 women heart-attack or angina survivors found that those who ate the highest amounts of beta-carotene, vitamin C, vitamin E, and riboflavin had 71 percent less risk of stroke and a 33 percent reduced risk of a second heart attack. Fortunately, pumpkins contain all these nutrients.

They're one of the few foods that give you even a moderate amount of vitamin E. Several large studies show that vitamin E may reduce the risk of heart disease. It helps prevent the oxidation of cholesterol and helps prevent clumping of platelets in blood vessels. These studies used vitamin E supplements, but foods that contain vitamin E will help, too. One-half cup of canned pumpkin gives you more than 251 milligrams of potassium, along with magnesium, to help keep your blood pressure from going through the roof.

Radishes

What movie features the star brandishing a radish? Here's a clue: "As God is my witness, I'll never be hungry again." Sure, you remember: Vivian Leigh, Scarlett O'Hara, *Gone with the Wind.* And the vegetable that many of us use to garnish salads.

Cancer. Radishes kept Scarlett going, and the substances in them will help your body fight off cancer. Researchers working with the National Cancer Institute have found that eating just a little more than one radish a day may keep tumors from developing and cells from mutating. They're a rich source of vitamin C for protection against cancer.

Heart disease and stroke. Just ½ cup of sliced radishes gives you 22 percent of your Daily Value of vitamin C to raise the levels of the important HDL cholesterol that helps keep your arteries clean. HDL levels are often used as an indicator of whether you're likely to suffer a heart attack—the lower the levels, the greater your risk. Vitamin C also helps lower the dangerous LDL cholesterol that grabs onto artery walls and, over time, leaves them narrow and easily clogged.

Raisins

People have been drying grapes in the sun to make raisins for more than 3,000 years. Talk about wisdom of the ages!

Cancer. A ½-cup serving gives you almost a gram of insoluble fiber to help prevent colon cancer. You get 11 percent of the Daily Value of copper and more than 9 percent of vitamin B_6 to help your immune system.

Heart disease and stroke. Imagine a David and Goliath setup: Little raisins battle big diseases. The winner? The little guys, of course. A ½-cup serving of raisins gives you more than 544 milligrams of potassium to help keep your blood pressure low. You get a bit of heart protection from magnesium. Riboflavin and vitamin B_6, among others, gang up on LDL cholesterol and substances in your body that can damage your heart.

141

Raspberries

These delicate berries won't keep for long in the refrigerator, so what are you waiting for? Pop them in your mouth for disease protection.

Cancer. Like other berries, raspberries give you a healthy dose of ellagic acid. In the lab it fights cancer of the lung, skin, esophagus, and liver. It may even keep cancerous substances from damaging DNA, the first step in cancer's growth.

One-half cup also gives you a lot of additional cancer protection. You get more than 1 gram of insoluble fiber to help protect against colon and breast cancer. More than a quarter of your Daily Value of vitamin C goes a long way to protect you against cancer of the breast, cervix, esophagus, lung, mouth, pancreas, rectum, and stomach.

Heart disease and stroke. A healthy dose of vitamin C helps protect your heart by raising your HDL cholesterol levels, preventing buildup of plaque in your arteries. It also helps reduce levels of LDL cholesterol and other blood fats that lodge in your arteries. You will also get almost 0.5 gram of soluble fiber to help fight bad cholesterol.

Rhubarb

Talk about a confused plant. Those stalks that look like pink celery protect you from disease—but its leaves are poisonous. Most people don't eat the roots, but they were prized for medicinal use in ancient China.

Cancer. Ummm, smell that rhubarb pie. And think about how healthy it is. One-half cup of raw rhubarb gives you more than 1 gram of dietary fiber to help protect you from colon cancer.

You get some vitamin C that helps lower your risk of cancer of the breast, cervix, esophagus, lung, mouth, pancreas, rectum, and stomach.

Heart disease and stroke. One-half cup of cooked rhubarb gives you more than 17 percent of your Daily Value of calcium, which may help lower mild blood pressure and reduce harmful LDL cholesterol, which can stick to your artery walls.

Vitamin C takes care of more than one matter of the heart, as it raises your HDL cholesterol and lowers LDL cholesterol and other blood fat.

Rice

The big question: Is there really a difference between white rice and brown rice? The big answer: Yes.

Cancer. Let's do a little math. Copper protects you from cancer because it helps build up your immune system. Eat ½ cup of cooked long-grain brown rice, and you get 5 percent of the Daily Value. If, instead, you go for white rice, you get 3.5 percent. Brown rice gives you almost 2 grams of total dietary fiber, which protects you from colon cancer. The long-grain white stuff gives you 0.4 gram.

Researchers working with the National Cancer Institute have also found that brown rice neutralizes dangerous substances that play havoc with your system and allow cancer to make inroads.

Heart disease and stroke. Eat ½ cup of cooked brown rice and get double protection—vitamin B_6 and magnesium. Both help lower risk of a blood clot, while magnesium also helps lower high blood pressure.

Rutabagas

If the name sounds a little foreign to your ear, there's a reason: It comes from a Swedish word that means "round root."

Cancer. These round roots harbor a lot of protective substances: indoles, isothiocyanates, sulforaphane, and some genistein—cancer fighters all. Compounds in rutabaga keep cells from mutating and block the formation of tumors. More than 26 percent of the Daily Value of vitamin C, found in ½ cup of cooked rutabaga, protects you from oral cancer. As a source of vitamin A, rutabaga may help prevent cancerous agents from getting into your system.

Heart disease and stroke. Eat a ½-cup serving of cooked rutabaga and take in more than 26 percent of the Daily Value of vitamin C, which helps lower levels of LDL cholesterol while raising the HDL. More than 277 milligrams of potassium helps keep your blood pressure low. As a source of almost 10 percent of the Daily Value of vitamin A, rutabaga may help keep LDL cholesterol from getting a grip on artery walls.

Salmon

As one of the much-touted sources of omega-3 fatty acids, salmon swims against the current of disease.

Cancer. Half of a filet of fresh cooked coho salmon has high levels of vitamin B_6 along with some copper and zinc, which have been shown to heighten cancer-resisting immunity. More than 7 percent of the Daily Value for calcium is available, which may help fight colon cancer.

Heart disease and stroke. Eating fish once a week will cut your risk of stroke in half, researchers say. Make it salmon, and you get plenty of omega-3 fatty acids, which some studies have associated with reduced risk of heart attacks and strokes.

One 3-ounce serving of fresh cooked coho salmon dishes up almost 387 milligrams of potassium, helping to lower your blood pressure. You get almost 63 percent of the Daily Value of vitamin B_{12}, one of the important B vitamins that can help to reduce your risk of heart disease by lowering the amount of homocysteine, a substance that activates the clotting system in the blood. Other B vitamins include riboflavin (more than 8 percent of the Daily Value) and vitamin B_6 (almost 24 percent of the Daily Value). Your body doesn't absorb vitamin B_{12} very well now that you're older, so it's important to make sure that you get a good supply through your diet.

Salmon also gives you magnesium (almost 8 percent of the Daily Value) and a little folate, which, combined with B_{12} and B_6, may lower the homocysteine levels in your blood, to help prevent clogged arteries. Eat salmon and you're going to get calcium, which in some studies has been shown to lower mild high blood pressure. Get extra calcium by eating canned sockeye salmon, which contains edible chunks of bone.

Sardines

When you peel back the lid on a can of sardines, you let out a crowd of disease fighters.

Cancer. That canned cluster of tightly packed fish gives you a healthy dose of zinc and copper to help your immune system function at its peak and to neutralize dangerous invaders. The contents in one can gives you

144

more than 5 percent of your Daily Value of calcium, which may help lower your risk of colon cancer.

Heart disease and stroke. The calcium in sardines also may help keep your blood pressure and levels of harmful LDL cholesterol down. One can, or about 3 ounces, gives you a heart-helping assortment of the B vitamins that cut down your risk of a heart attack or stroke: 137 percent of the Daily Value of vitamin B_{12} and almost 8 percent of the Daily Value of vitamin B_6, to help control blood clots in the blood vessels.

Sea Bass

Sea bass, or grouper, swim in just about any ocean and include a lot of species, most of which have firm, white, lean meat. One 3-ounce serving contains just over 2 grams of fat.

Cancer. A little zinc helps protect you against cancer by keeping your immune system strong.

Heart disease and stroke. One 3-ounce serving of sea bass gives you 650 milligrams of omega-3, which some studies have found to fight cholesterol. You get almost 279 milligrams of potassium to help lower blood pressure. A generous helping of magnesium helps keep clots from forming and lowers high blood pressure. As a source of vitamin A, sea bass may help raise the levels of the beneficial HDL cholesterol. You get an assortment of the valuable B vitamins, which help reduce your overall risk of heart disease, heart attack, and stroke.

Shallots

Shallots look like a cross between a garlic and an onion. So you won't be surprised to find out that they offer just about as much protection as their close relatives.

Cancer. In the lab, substances in shallots block and suppress cancer-causing carcinogens. Shallots also contain beta-carotene and are a source of vitamin A, which may keep cancerous agents from invading healthy cells, stopping cancers before they get started. In one study, beta-carotene is linked to lower rates of lung cancer in nonsmokers. Some scientists believe that they also protect other important organs from cancer invasion.

Heart disease and stroke. The same vitamin A and beta-carotene that may help protect you from cancer might also help your heart. One study found that beta-carotene keeps the harmful LDL cholesterol from oxidizing, the first step in latching onto the walls of your arteries where it can turn into dangerous plaque that increases your risk of heart attack and stroke.

Soybeans

Yes, we're talking about tofu and sprouts. But before you roll your eyes toward the ceiling, consider all of the good things that these products do.

Cancer. Soy products contain genistein, a chemical that attacks cancer the way that Arnold Schwarzenegger goes after bad guys. It blocks the formation of blood vessels around new tumors, stops cancer cells from multiplying, and prevents the absorption of tumor-promoting estrogen. In the lab it keeps breast cancer cells and precancerous prostate cells from growing.

You get protection from other foreign-sounding substances: isoflavones, phytosterols, protease inhibitors, saponins, and phytic acid. The bottom line? They keep cancer-causing substances from getting a grip in your body, stop cancerous cells from reproducing, and slow down tumor growth. One-half cup of boiled soybeans gets you a healthy helping of calcium, 13 percent of the Daily Value, which may help protect you from colon cancer.

Heart disease and stroke. Soybean products give you just about as much protection from heart disease as they do from cancer. Calcium may help lower your blood pressure and reduce the nasty LDL cholesterol that leads to clogged arteries, heart attacks, and strokes. In ½ cup of boiled soybeans, you get almost 14 percent of your Daily Value of magnesium to help keep blood from clotting and gumming up your arteries. Magnesium also helps lower high blood pressure. The beans weigh in with 485 milligrams of potassium to quiet down your blood pressure, too.

Vitamin C in soybeans (more than 25 percent of your Daily Value) helps raise your HDL cholesterol, which keeps fatty deposits from blocking your arteries.

Spinach

Popeye was no fool. Spinach is high on disease prevention and low in calories. Plus, fresh spinach can keep in the refrigerator for 10 to 14 days.

Cancer. Researchers working with the National Cancer Institute note that some of the stuff in spinach keeps cells from mutating. Antioxidants also neutralize the substances that help cancer get started.

One cup of raw spinach (green and tender, not brown and wilted) gives you more than 27 percent of the Daily Value of folate, which protects you against cancer of the cervix, colorectum, lung, and possibly the esophagus. Folate also helps keep cells strong and healthy, so they are better able to fend off a cancerous attack. Some studies show that the consumption of high levels of vitamin E decrease the levels of prostaglandin E_2, a substance that limits the efficiency of the immune system. Although these studies used supplements, dark green leafy vegetables are a known source of vitamin E.

Heart disease and stroke. When Popeye fought Bluto, he may have looked as though his blood pressure was about to go through the roof, but the potassium in spinach probably helped keep it down. Other heart-helping nutrients include vitamin C, magnesium, folate, and vitamin E. Several large studies note that vitamin E can actually slow the development of heart disease by preventing the oxidation of cholesterol and blood clots. Although these studies used vitamin E supplements, foods that contain vitamin E can always help.

Squash

If you just think of winter squash as a decoration for your Thanksgiving table, you're in for a low-calorie, disease-fighting treat. For that matter, summer squash gives you protection, too—just in smaller doses.

Cancer. Winter squash—of any shape and color—is rich in beta-carotene, an important antioxidant that may help stop cancer before it gets started. One study found that it provides protection against lung cancer. One serving (about ½ cup, cubed) of butternut squash gives you more than 3 milligrams of beta-carotene. The same amount of Hubbard squash dishes out almost 2 milligrams of beta-carotene.

As if that weren't enough, researchers have found that something in squash keeps tumors from developing, although they haven't yet identified the substance with this disease-squashing ability.

Heart disease and stroke. Acorn squash dishes up heart protection, too. A ½-cup serving, baked and cubed, gives you about 18 percent of the Daily Value of vitamin C to maintain high levels of beneficial HDL cholesterol. It also reduces levels of the harmful LDL cholesterol that lodges in your arteries and can lay the groundwork for a heart attack or stroke.

Other nutrients, such as folate, magnesium, and potassium, team up to lower levels of LDL cholesterol, raise levels of protective HDL cholesterol, drop high blood pressure, and keep blood from forming those nasty clots that can lead to heart attacks and strokes.

Strawberries

"Strawberry fields forever," sang the Beatles when your kids were growing up. Strawberries will get your immune system humming, too.

Cancer. In one study involving lab animals, researchers found that ellagic acid, found in strawberries, fights cancer of the lung, skin, esophagus, and liver. It also decreases the number of tumors in animals. When applied to the skin of animals, it prevents cancers. Ellagic acid seems to keep carcinogens from damaging the DNA of healthy cells. It's even possible that it eats up substances that carcinogens need to get off the ground.

Glutathione may help boost your cells' ability to divide, thereby launching a strong counterattack against cancer. And the best news for you is that glutathione works best in older folks. You also get 1 gram of insoluble fiber to help protect you from colon and breast cancer.

Heart disease and stroke. One cup of strawberries gives you 247 milligrams of potassium, keeping your blood pressure rosy, and 140 percent of the Daily Value of vitamin C, helping to lower your cholesterol. You also get soluble fiber to help keep cholesterol in check and folate to help keep levels of homocysteine low, preventing blood clots. The magnesium in strawberries helps prevent blood clots and lower blood pressure. Studies show that pantothenic acid, also in strawberries, may lower cholesterol and triglycerides. There is also riboflavin, which lowers your cholesterol.

Sweet Potatoes and Yams

Let's get the confusion cleared up: Sweet potatoes and yams are different critters that belong to different families. And, chances are, you have never seen an actual yam. These giants of the vegetable world hail from Africa and Asia. They can weigh up to 100 pounds. Now, sweet potatoes—that's a whole different story. These vegetables have their roots in the United States and undoubtedly kept more than one family of frontier homesteaders alive. Anytime you go to the grocery store, you're going to come home with sweet potatoes, not yams.

Cancer. One 4-ounce baked sweet potato is a source of 249 percent of the Daily Value of vitamin A, which may help protect you against cancer of the mouth. And the bright orange color tells you that beta-carotene is on board. So is almost half the Daily Value of vitamin C, which strengthens your defenses against cancer of the breast, cervix, esophagus, lung, mouth, pancreas, rectum, and stomach. And a healthy helping of fiber protects against colon cancer. Researchers working with the National Cancer Institute have also discovered that substances in sweet potatoes actually keep cells from mutating, at least in the laboratory.

Heart disease and stroke. There's plenty of beta-carotene, which may help shut out the harmful LDL cholesterol that leads to plaque buildup and clotting in the arteries. A common misconception about soluble fiber is that some of the best sources are tasteless and often involve oats. It doesn't have to be that way, since sweet potatoes are an excellent source of cholesterol-fighting soluble fiber. Vitamin C in sweet potatoes raises HDLs, which protects you from heart disease. It disarms the harmful LDLs and gets rid of triglycerides. Your blood pressure drops, thanks to a lot of potassium—397 milligrams in one 4-ounce baked sweet potato.

Tangerines

They're a lot like oranges, but easier to eat. You don't get as much vitamin C in a tangerine as in an orange—although at 43 percent of the Daily Value, the amount you do get in a tangerine is nothing to sneeze at.

Cancer. Substances in tangerines keep cells from mutating. Other components strengthen the production of enzymes that make carcinogens more water-soluble so that the body can get rid of them quickly. And others may keep nitrates in the stomach from being converted into dangerous nitrosamines, naturally occurring carcinogens.

In one tangerine you also get more than 43 percent of your Daily Value of vitamin C to help prevent cancer of the breast, cervix, esophagus, lung, mouth, pancreas, rectum, and stomach. Its vitamin B_6 beefs up your immune system, and its fiber lowers your risk of colon cancer.

Heart disease and stroke. Tangerines are a source of vitamin C and vitamin A, which may knock down the levels of the dangerous LDL cholesterol and raise the levels of the good stuff, HDL. Vitamin C also lowers mild high blood pressure, providing an added benefit to tangerines. Potassium in tangerines also helps lower your blood pressure.

Tea

The American colonists started a war by dumping a load of tea into Boston Harbor. If they had known about its disease-preventing properties, they might have selected something else to throw overboard.

Cancer. Whether it's green, black, or decaf, tea protects. Substances in tea help enzymes neutralize cancer-causing agents and may repair damaged DNA. One study showed that tea drinkers have a lower risk of breast and stomach cancer. In other studies substances in tea block skin cancer.

Heart disease and stroke. Drink tea and cut your risk of heart disease: Black, green, or even decaf varieties are rich in flavonoids, substances that protect your heart and lower your risk of heart disease. In a Dutch study, researchers found that the antioxidant quercetin, found in tea, lowers the risk of stroke by one-third. The effects of tea were reportedly most beneficial to older folks. You get the most benefit from bagged tea because the leaves are more thoroughly crushed.

Tomatoes

Until the 1800s people believed that tomatoes were poisonous. After all, it is a relative of the nightshade family of plants known for poisonous leaves, berries, flowers, and fruit. But researchers found that tomatoes protect, whether on a pizza, in a sauce, or fresh off the vine.

Cancer. Substances in tomatoes fight cell mutation. Tomatoes also arm your defenses with glutathione, which may reduce the risk of oral and throat cancer and makes your immune system work better. You also get the powerful cancer fighter lycopene. Other substances in tomatoes battle nitrosamines, substances produced in our bodies that can lead to cancer.

Heart disease and stroke. One ripe tomato offers a generous 399 milligrams of potassium to lower blood pressure, and 57 percent of the Daily Value of vitamin C, which helps control bad LDL cholesterol. You also get vitamin B_6, which may help reduce the incidence of blood clots.

Trout

Weave all the tales you like about the one that got away. When it comes to trout on your plate, opt for the smaller size—it will contain less fat.

Cancer. Your immune system gets a boost with 17 percent of the Daily Value of vitamin B_6. You also get more than 5 percent of the Daily Value of folate, which is known to reduce the risk of developing cancer of the cervix, colon, rectum, lung, and possibly the esophagus.

Heart disease and stroke. Some researchers have zeroed in on fish as an easy way to help your heart. In one study people who ate one serving of fatty fish a week lowered their risk of heart attack by 50 percent. Another study reported that people who eat ⅔ ounce of any type of fish a day can cut their risk of stroke in half. In a 3-ounce serving of baked trout, you'll also get heart protection from calcium, folate, magnesium, riboflavin, thiamin, vitamin B_{12}, and vitamin B_6. An impressive 375 milligrams of potassium will help lower mild high blood pressure.

Tuna

Pop quiz: Name the most-consumed fish in America. Yes, tuna. But not all tuna is equal. Look for fresh bluefin or canned albacore.

Cancer. A 3-ounce serving of baked, fresh bluefin tuna is a source of almost 43 percent of the Daily Value of vitamin A, which in some studies has been shown to reduce the risk of cancer. Compare that figure to just over 1 percent of the Daily Value of vitamin A from the same amount of the canned tuna. You also get more than 22 percent of the Daily Value of vitamin B_6 to build up your immunity—that's 4 more milligrams than the canned tuna. Canned tuna contains about 8 milligrams of copper, however, compared to fresh bluefin's 4.

Heart disease and stroke. Bluefin tuna provides a rich source of the omega-3 fatty acids that may help lower your cholesterol and protect you from heart disease. Albacore, or white tuna, also gives you a good helping of protection from omega-3's.

A heart-healthy helping of magnesium lowers your blood's tendency to clot and reduces your risk of a heart attack or stroke. Magnesium also reduces high blood pressure. The assortment of B vitamins in tuna also is a champion in the heart-protection department. Three ounces of fresh baked bluefin tuna provides more than 15 percent of the Daily Value of riboflavin, a B vitamin that helps other heart-saving nutrients work harder and more efficiently. Even better, you get more than 154 percent of the Daily Value for vitamin B_{12}, another important heart protector, and 274 milligrams of potassium to help lower your blood pressure.

Turkey

Ben Franklin had such high regard for the turkey that he wanted to make it the official bird of the United States. But no, we have the eagle on our coins and the turkey on our table, which is good for you, since eating turkey cuts your risk of heart disease, cancer, and stroke.

Cancer. Turkey's a rich old bird—at least in terms of disease protection. A 3-ounce serving is low in fat (2 grams) and cholesterol (30 milligrams); it's the leanest of all meats. And that's important to reduce your risk of cancer. Plus, it gives you more than 8 percent of your Daily Value for zinc, a mineral that's important to your immune system. You also boost your immune system with 9 percent of the Daily Value of vitamin B_6.

Heart disease and stroke. Turkey provides an assortment of heart-protecting B vitamins: pantothenic acid, riboflavin, vitamin B_{12}, and vitamin B_6. Working together, they lower your risk of heart disease. They increase the HDL cholesterol that protects your arteries from plaque buildup and lower the levels of homocysteine. You'll also benefit from potassium, which protects you from deadly high blood pressure.

Turnips

Ever want to step back in history? Eat what the ancients ate? Well, you can do that with turnips, the food of choice in ancient Rome and medieval Europe. And it probably protected as well then as it does today. Don't ignore the leaves—turnip greens protect you, too.

Cancer. In the laboratory, substances in turnip greens keep tumors from developing and cells from mutating, meaning that cancers can't get a foothold as easily. Chemicals such as indoles, isothiocyanates, and sulforaphane give carcinogens a run for their money. Researchers believe that sulforaphane activates an enzyme that collars cancerous agents and removes them from your body's cells.

One-half cup of mashed turnips, gives you almost 5 grams of insoluble fiber, an important protector against colon cancer.

Heart disease and stroke. More than 2.5 grams of soluble fiber makes turnips a top pick for heart protection. You also get 22 percent of your Daily Value of vitamin C to help lower levels of harmful LDL cholesterol and raise levels of the protective HDL cholesterol.

Walnuts

You could also call them the royal nuts. In ancient Rome, for instance, they were consumed by royalty and dedicated to the god Jupiter. They're good for us commoners, too. Crack some nuts to crack down on your cancer risk.

Cancer. Walnuts are rich in ellagic acid. In lab animals, this substance fights cancer of the lung, skin, esophagus, and liver. The same tests determined that it decreases the number of tumors. When ellagic acid was applied to the skin of mice, it kept cancers from forming.

Researchers at Ohio State University believe that ellagic acid keeps cancerous substances from starting the process of DNA damage. It may also neutralize cancer-causing substances before they do damage. These researchers also believe that ellagic acid may actually beat cancerous substances to the punch—taking in substances they need in order to do their damage.

Heart disease and stroke. Don't like fish but want to get the potential benefits of the omega-3 fatty acids found in fish? Eat English or black walnuts and you may be taking steps to help lower your cholesterol levels and protect your heart. While ⅓ cup of walnuts will load you up with almost 25 grams of fat, the nuts contain no cholesterol. Walnuts also give you other important health helpers: folate and vitamin B_6—B vitamins that lower your risk of heart disease. One-third cup of walnuts gives you 201 milligrams of potassium to help lower high blood pressure.

Watercress

Upon finding this green leafy vegetable in her salad, a character in the 1939 film *The Women* exclaimed, "Watercress! I'd just as soon eat my way across a front lawn." Well, obviously she had never tried it or she would have learned to relish the tangy taste. If she had been able to predict the science of the last few years, she would also treasure watercress for its disease-preventing possibilities.

Cancer. Watercress contains one particularly powerful naturally occurring chemical substance, PEITC, or phenethyl-isothiocyanate, that blocks lung cancer in animals exposed to tobacco carcinogens. One-half cup of chopped watercress gets you a little beta-carotene, which may help protect you from cancer. You also get insoluble fiber, which has been shown to prevent colon cancer.

Heart disease and stroke. One-half cup of chopped watercress is a source of almost 16 percent of the Daily Value for vitamin A, which may block the harmful LDL cholesterol that can put you at risk for a heart attack or stroke.

Vitamin C in watercress lowers LDL and triglyceride levels as well as your risk of plaque buildup in your arteries. You also get a little calcium, which may lower blood pressure, and soluble fiber, which fights bad LDL cholesterol.

Watermelon

Isn't it nice—the watermelon that's such a treat on a hot summer day is also great for disease protection? Beyond nutrients, watermelon gives you a lot of—what else?—water, which also is vital to your health.

Cancer. You get a lot of glutathione from watermelon. Researchers at Emory University in Atlanta found that this substance may function as an anticarcinogen to reduce your risk of oral and throat cancer by up to 50 percent. A lab study at Tufts University in Boston found that glutathione helps white blood cells in a test tube fight off invaders—and that means it could possibly make your immune system work as well as that of a much younger person. When you consider that people over age 60 have blood levels of glutathione about 17 percent lower than people under 40, it's easy to see why you should head for foods that provide a lot.

Heart disease. One-half cup of watermelon gives you more than 12 percent of your Daily Value of vitamin C, helping to lower your levels of harmful LDL cholesterol, which can become a permanent and hazardous fixture on your artery walls. You get a healthy helping of vitamin B_6, which helps deactivate your blood's clotting system. Watermelon is also a source of beta-carotene and vitamin A, which some studies show helps fight heart disease.

Wheat Germ

Wheat germ is the part of the wheatberry that is cast off when flour is refined from whole wheat to white. What a waste.

Cancer. Wheat germ gives you vitamin E, which helps your immune system work better by strengthening the T cells that protect you from disease. It also reduces prostaglandin E_2, which interferes with your immune system as you get older. People who get a lot of vitamin E also have a lower risk of stomach cancer.

Heart disease and stroke. Several studies have shown that supplemental vitamin E slows down the progress of heart disease. It helps prevent the oxidation of cholesterol and helps prevent clumping of platelets in blood vessels. These studies used vitamin E supplements, but foods that contain vitamin E are a good bet, too. In people who've had a heart attack, vitamin E reduces the risk of a second attack.

When you eat ¼ cup of toasted wheat germ, you take in 25 percent of the Daily Value of folate. Researchers believe that this nutrient can help prevent heart attacks and strokes because it reduces levels of an amino acid called homocysteine. In a study of 536 men, researchers found that those people with the highest levels of homocysteine had a slightly elevated risk for stroke. Homocysteine injures the walls of your arteries.

Yogurt

It's really just curdled milk mixed with bacteria, all of which sounds pretty awful until you think about how much good yogurt can do for you.

Beyond the nutritional protection it gives, yogurt works as a substitute for less healthy foods. For example, cheese made from low-fat yogurt (basically, yogurt with some of the liquid removed) can substitute for the high-fat kind of cheese and still give you the calcium that you need.

Cancer. An 8-ounce or 1-cup serving of plain low-fat yogurt gives you almost 42 percent of your Daily Value of calcium, which may help guard you against colon cancer. You get folate, which is important to help protect DNA's genetic codes so that they're able to divide and replicate properly, keeping cancer at bay. Folate may also protect against cancer of the cervix, colon, rectum, lung, and possibly the esophagus. Yogurt provides more than 13 percent of your Daily Value of zinc, which helps keep your immune system strong.

Heart disease and stroke. The B vitamins—folate, riboflavin, vitamin B_{12} and vitamin B_6—protect your heart. People who get a lot of folate and vitamins B_6 and B_{12} in their diets may have up to 25 percent lower risk of heart disease. One 8-ounce serving of low-fat yogurt gives you almost 29 percent of your Daily Value of riboflavin, more than 21 percent of vitamin B_{12}, and more than 6 percent of your Daily Value for folate. In addition, its 264 milligrams of potassium helps lower high blood pressure.

Prescription for Prevention

When you get right down to it, your best recipe for prevention of heart disease, cancer, and stroke—next to quitting smoking, of course—is right in your own kitchen: in foods you can buy cheaply and prepare easily.
Here is what you can do to lower your risk.

Do:

- *Eat foods from plants. Fruits, vegetables, grains, nuts, and seeds are low in cholesterol and high in natural substances that fight disease.*

- *Eat a variety of healthy foods. You'll get a wide assortment of protective substances from a diversified diet.*

- *Emphasize fresh, not processed foods. You'll get more nutrients that way.*

Don't:

- *Overcook your vegetables. While some protective compounds are impervious to heat, others aren't.*

- *Overindulge in nuts and other foods that are high in protective substances but also high in calories.*

Chapter 5

Super Supplements

Gain a Nutritional Edge from Vitamins and Minerals

S troll down the vitamin and supplement aisle at your local super-market, drugstore, or health food store. You'll find neat rows of products—everything from multivitamins to Geritol, garlic to hawthorn, assortments of antioxidants, and bottles upon bottles of specific vitamins, minerals, and herbs. Contents measured in RDAs, DVs, IUs, milligrams, and micrograms.

Whew. Sorting through all this stuff is a lot like trying to do your taxes without the instruction book (or, for that matter, with the book). The names and numbers are all there, but how do you put it all together? How can you concoct a regimen that puts all the B_6s, B_{12}s, coenzymes, and a lot of things you've never heard of into a protective package to reduce your risk of heart disease, cancer, and stroke?

Over-60 Supplements

"Some studies suggest that specific vitamin and mineral supplements can help reduce your risk of heart disease by up to 30 to 40 percent and even slow the disease's progress," says Jeffrey Blumberg, M.D., associate director and chief of the Antioxidants Research Laboratory at the U.S. Department of Agriculture Human Nutrition Research Center on Aging in Boston.

It involves nothing more fancy than over-the-counter supplements. They're relatively inexpensive, and some of them may go a long way toward cutting high blood pressure and stopping the blood clots that lead to strokes.

Vitamins can boost the immune system, which is important in battling cancer cells. The bottom line: "Older people who take vitamin and mineral supplements have stronger immune systems," says John Bogden, Ph.D., professor of preventive medicine and community health at the New Jersey Medical School in Newark. "Generally, the immune system starts to decline around age 50 and may already be compromised by age 60." If your immune system can't protect you, the door is wide open for cancer and other diseases.

But it doesn't have to be this way. When researchers in Italy looked at healthy 100-year-olds, they made a surprising discovery—immune systems so strong that they could easily have belonged to people 80 years younger. "That's probably why these people got to be 100-plus. Their immune systems never deteriorated," says Dr. Bogden.

Supplements will help strengthen the immune system, but they don't work miracles. "While supplements are cheap, easy to take, and—in many cases—beneficial, they're not magic bullets," says Dr. Blumberg. "They're supplements, not substitutes for healthy eating."

You can't do the bacon-and-eggs, burgers-and-fries routine, pop a pill, and think that everything will be fine. Still, researchers estimate that up to one-third of older adults may not be getting enough important vitamins and minerals through diet alone.

Pop a Pill to Prevent Disease

You get the benefits of a vitamin supplement if you are over 55, although your system may not really register the improvement for six months to a year. That's not an excuse to procrastinate. As you get older, getting the nutrients that you need—through a combination of diet and supplements—becomes increasingly important to shore up your body's defenses, says Dr. Bogden. Here's how supplements help.

Keep low-cal eating low-risk. It's a catch-22 situation: Take in too many calories and you don't want to face the bathroom scales, let alone the extra risk of cancer, heart disease, and stroke. But if you try to lose weight (or maintain the weight that you have) by cutting calories, you may end up low on vitamins and minerals and high on risk, especially if you make poor food choices, unless you add key vitamins and minerals through carefully chosen supplements, explains Dr. Bogden.

Dietitians at Utah State University tried to create balanced diets of less than 2,200 calories—probably close to the number of calories you take in. They found it nearly impossible to do that and meet the recommended daily amount of important vitamins and minerals.

Sidestep the slowdowns. As you get older, a lot of your body's systems seem to shift into semi-retirement. They just slow down and work less efficiently. The right supplements help compensate. For instance, you just don't have as much of the beneficial stomach acid that helps your system get what it needs from your food. That means that up to 40 percent of the nutrients you take in may go unused. You're likely to be low in such protective components as vitamins D, B_6, B_{12}, riboflavin, folate (the natural form of the supplement folic acid), and calcium.

Your body's system for storing the nutrients that you take in isn't what it used to be either. That's because your percentage of body fat increases with age, notes Sharon Miller, Ph.D., associate dean of the College of Health and Human Sciences at Northern Illinois University in DeKalb.

Bypass the by-products. "The body's metabolism keeps you alive and healthy, but it also produces harmful by-products. It's very much like the fire that gives you warmth—along with the unpleasant smoke," says Richard Cutler, Ph.D., president, chief executive officer, and scientific research director at Genox in Baltimore, where he specializes in antioxidant research.

The body's "smoke" includes free radicals and other compounds that damage the cells' DNA and lead to many of aging's effects. Your body makes antioxidants to fight off these substances. As you get older, production levels drop, probably because your metabolism slows with time.

It becomes harder and harder to get enough antioxidant protection from food alone. Supplements can make big contributions to the cause.

The Must-Have Micronutrients

Some researchers think that deficiencies in the diet pave the way for heart disease, stroke, and cancer. Many experts believe that an extra dose of key vitamins and minerals—often difficult to get through diet alone—

provides maximum protection from the killers.

Listed below are two kinds of guidelines for vitamin and mineral consumption. The Daily Values are the U.S. government's general guidelines for basic daily nutritional needs. Also listed are recommendations for protection offered by the doctors who were interviewed in this chapter. You can get most of these nutrients in a multivitamin. But you may want to take extra supplements of some vitamins and minerals to promote optimum health, says Dr. Blumberg. Regardless, always keep your doses within the recommended range—some vitamins and minerals are toxic when taken in large doses, he cautions.

Vitamin A/Beta-carotene: For All-Purpose Protection

Daily Values: Vitamin A, 5,000 international units; beta-carotene, no Daily Value

Experts recommend: Keep to the Daily Value of vitamin A. Six to 20 milligrams of beta-carotene.

Is a multivitamin likely to contain enough? Vitamin A, yes; beta-carotene, no

Multivitamins may contain vitamin A, beta-carotene, or a combination of the two. To the body, beta-carotene and vitamin A are one and the same. But experts note that it's safer to take beta-carotene. That's because the body stores beta-carotene and converts it into vitamin A whenever it needs it. Vitamin A stays in the system. Too much can damage your liver. An excess of beta-carotene will turn your skin orange.

You can get the recommended levels by adjusting your diet instead of popping a pill. "You can get the equivalent of the Daily Value of vitamin A just by eating a carrot a day," says James Goodwin, M.D., director of the Center on Aging at the University of Texas Medical Branch in Galveston.

Heart disease. Beta-carotene keeps the harmful low-density lipoprotein (LDL) cholesterol from getting a grip on artery walls.

In the Harvard Physicians' Health Study, doctors with heart disease took 50 milligrams of beta-carotene on alternate days for six years—and had one-half as many fatal heart attacks and angioplasties.

Examine Your Lifestyle Risks

Beyond what you eat, how you live determines your nutritional needs. Check out your lifestyle to see whether you need more than the average amount of some vitamins and minerals.

Sun damage: Are you covered? If you're retired and spend your days at the pool, in the garden, or on the tennis courts, you probably need a supplement. Sunlight gives you beneficial vitamin D, but it also exposes you to cell-damaging substances. Your body's supply of protective antioxidants gets used up fast, notes Richard Cutler, Ph.D., president, chief executive officer, and scientific research director at Genox in Baltimore.

In one study ultraviolet light led to lower levels of important antioxidants. When test subjects spent 15 minutes a day under solar lamps for a two-week period, their infection-fighting T cells became less active, a sign that their immune systems weren't working as well.

Shield yourself (a little) from smoke. Cigarette smoking exposes you to millions of harmful free radicals, lead, mercury, and radioactive materials. As your body battles these invaders, you may end up with lower levels of key vitamins that protect you. One study showed that a smoker needs 250 milligrams of vitamin C to show a blood level comparable to a nonsmoker getting the Daily Value of 60 milligrams.

Although you may reduce some of the risk by taking a multivitamin and additional supplements of vitamin C, vitamin E, and beta-carotene, the best thing to do is to quit smoking altogether, says Jeffrey Blumberg, M.D., associate director and chief of the Antioxidants Research Laboratory at the U.S. Department of Agriculture Human Nutrition Research Center on Aging in Boston.

Daily stresses call for protection. You'll probably need extra vitamins and minerals if you drink even moderately or if you exercise intensely, says Dr. Blumberg.

Some medical problems also increase your needs, such as irritable bowel, chronic diarrhea, constipation, yeast infection, surgery, radiation, chronic stress, and the overuse of prescription drugs.

What about an Antioxidant Supplement?

I recommend that older people take an antioxidant formula, in addition to a multiple vitamin," says James Goodwin, M.D., director of the Center on Aging at the University of Texas Medical Branch in Galveston.

"Pick one with around 200 international units of vitamin E, 250 milligrams of vitamin C, and 30 milligrams or so of beta-carotene, plus 70 to 100 micrograms of selenium. That should give most people all the protection they need," he says.

And, since most multivitamins contain only 200 milligrams of calcium, you'll need an additional supplement for calcium.

Stroke. The Harvard study also showed that the doctors who took beta-carotene had half as many strokes over the six-year period.

Cancer. Vitamin A contributes to the body's first line of defense against bacteria and viruses by maintaining the protective mucous membranes that line the digestive, respiratory, urinary, and reproductive tracts. It also produces the bacteria-fighting chemicals in tears, saliva, and sweat.

In one study smokers with precancerous oral lesions took 30 milligrams of beta-carotene for eight weeks. Seventy percent of their lesions stopped growing or actually got smaller.

In a study conducted in Linxian, China, the diets of 30,000 people ages 40 to 69 were supplemented with either a placebo or different combinations of vitamins and minerals in doses one to two times the U.S. Recommended Dietary Allowances. After five years of daily supplementation, those taking a beta-carotene, vitamin E, and selenium combination saw their rates of cancer death drop by 13 percent.

If you take a supplement. "I want to be alone," said Greta Garbo. Well, beta-carotene doesn't. It needs the company of a little fat to get into your system, since it's a fat-soluble nutrient. Take it with a meal or snack.

Monitor Your Medications

If you are on medication, check with your doctor about whether you should take supplements. Some vitamins and minerals can interfere with your body's ability to use certain medicines, says Jeffrey Blumberg, M.D., associate director and chief of the Antioxidants Research Laboratory at U.S. Department of Agriculture Human Nutrition Research Center on Aging in Boston.

This clash can work in reverse, too. Some drugs may make vitamins pass through your system more quickly than they should—or stick around too long.

So if you're taking medicine, especially those listed below, ask your doctor whether you need to increase or decrease your intake of vitamins and minerals, advises Dr. Blumberg.

Drug	Interferes with
Alcohol	Folic acid, Niacin Thiamin Vitamin B$_6$, Zinc
Aluminum hydroxide (antacids)	Vitamin A, Calcium Phosphate
Amphetamines	Vitamin C
Anticonvulsants	Folic acid, Vitamin D Calcium
Antidepressants	Vitamin C
Antihypertensives (treat high blood pressure)	All nutrients
Calcitonin (treats Paget's disease)	Calcium
Chelating agents (treat metal poisoning)	Vitamin B$_6$
Cholestyramine (reduces cholesterol)	Folic acid, Vitamin A Vitamin B$_{12}$, Vitamin D Vitamin E, Vitamin K Calcium

Drug	Interferes with
Colchicine (treats gout)	Vitamin B_{12}
Corticosteroids (steroids such as cortisone)	Calcium
Cycloserine (fights tuberculosis)	Vitamin B_6
Estrogen	Folic acid, Calcium
Hydralazine (fights high blood pressure)	Vitamin B_6
Isoniazid (prevents and treats tuberculosis)	Vitamin B_6
Laxatives containing phosphate	Calcium
Levodopa or L-DOPA (treats Parkinson's disease)	Vitamin B_6
Methotrexate (treats psoriasis, rheumatoid arthritis)	Folic acid, Vitamin B_{12}
Mineral oil (a component of many drugs)	Vitamin A, Vitamin D Vitamin E, Calcium Phosphorus
Neomycin (treats infections)	Vitamin B_6, Vitamin B_{12} Iron
Phenobarbital (relieves anxiety and tension)	Folic acid, Vitamin B_6 Vitamin B_{12}, Vitamin D
Phenytoin (prevents seizures)	Folic acid, Vitamin B_6 Vitamin D
Sulfasalazine (treats inflammatory bowel disease)	Folic acid
Sulfonamides (antibiotics)	Vitamin C
Theophylline (treats bronchial asthma, emphysema)	Vitamin B_6
Triamterene (diuretic)	Folic acid, Potassium
Warfarin (anticoagulant)	Vitamin A, Vitamin E Vitamin K

The B Vitamins: Key Players for Protection

Daily Values: Vitamin B_6, 2 milligrams; vitamin B_{12}, 6 micrograms; folic acid, 400 micrograms; niacin, 20 milligrams; riboflavin, 1.7 milligrams; pantothenic acid, 10 milligrams

Experts recommend: Vitamin B_6, 2 to 10 milligrams; vitamin B_{12}, 2 to 10 micrograms; folic acid, 400 to 800 micrograms (some experts maintain that 400 or more micrograms of folic acid can interfere with your body's ability to use zinc). Stick to the Daily Value levels for niacin, riboflavin, and pantothenic acid.

Is a multivitamin likely to contain enough? Yes.

Getting older usually means ending up with lower levels of the protective B vitamins. It just becomes harder for the body to get them in and use them. If you're a vegetarian, you're probably particularly low on vitamin B_{12}, since it's found primarily in animal products.

Heart disease. "We see evidence that folic acid and vitamins B_6 and B_{12} reduce heart disease by 10 to 25 percent, and since heart disease is a major disease of aging, it's important that older people get enough," says Dr. Blumberg.

Low levels of the B vitamins could saddle you with high blood levels of homocysteine, increasing your risk for heart disease and heart attack. "The relationship of high homocysteine levels to low levels of the B vitamins, particularly folic acid, is quite clear," says Dr. Blumberg. Homocysteine is also poisonous to your cells.

Riboflavin powers up folic acid and vitamin B_6. Niacin probably protects against heart disease, but experts caution against taking more than the Daily Value. In experiments, very high amounts of niacin raise the beneficial high-density lipoprotein (HDL) cholesterol levels, but they can also cause liver damage and worsen stomach ulcers, diabetes, and arthritis.

Cancer. Studies of older adults show that low levels of vitamin B_6 depress the immune system. Fortunately, the system gets back in gear when it gets more B_6.

The high levels of folic acid can protect you against cervical and colon cancer, possibly by keeping both tissue growth and DNA (your cells' genetic material) production normal and healthy.

If you take a supplement. Don't exceed recommended levels. Mega-doses of vitamin B$_6$ can cause nerve damage.

Vitamin C: See a Longer Life

Daily Value: 60 milligrams
Experts recommend: 250 to 1,000 milligrams
Is a multivitamin likely to contain enough? No.

Some researchers believe that the added boost from vitamin C supplements can give men six more years of life and women an additional two years.

You can get protective levels of vitamin C from foods or supplements. One 8-ounce glass of orange juice, for example, contains 100 milligrams.

Studies show that as you get older you absorb vitamin C less easily. To counteract this, Dr. Blumberg says that it is advisable to take vitamin C at doses higher than the Daily Value. Men probably need at least 125 milligrams a day and women around 75 to 80 milligrams a day.

Heart disease. High levels of vitamin C generally accompany highs in the beneficial HDL cholesterol levels and lows in the harmful LDL cholesterol and triglyceride levels. In a 10-year study men who consumed 300 milligrams of vitamin C per day (partly from supplements) had almost half the death rate from heart disease as those who took less than 50 milligrams a day.

Stroke. Since vitamin C helps keep arteries clear of the LDL that clogs and narrows them, it leaves you less vulnerable to strokes.

Cancer. Vitamin C seems to prevent cancer-causing agents from getting down to business. It keeps certain cells from mutating and scarfs up free radicals.

If you take a supplement. You can lose the benefits of vitamin C if you smoke or breathe in secondhand smoke. You'll need at least 100 milligrams of vitamin C a day to help replenish your supply.

Both natural and synthetic vitamin C are equally effective, though chewable vitamin C may damage your tooth enamel.

Don't over-supplement; you may end up with diarrhea. Taking too much could lead to kidney problems. Plus, very large doses may keep your body from absorbing copper, an important immune-system protector.

Vitamin D: Direct from the Sun

Daily Value: 400 international units (10 micrograms)
Experts recommend: 400 international units (10 micrograms)
Is a multivitamin likely to contain enough? Yes.

To get vitamin D, you need to go outdoors and get into the light—both window glass and sunscreen block the signals that tell your system to start the production of vitamin D. As you get older, your skin becomes less able to synthesize vitamin D from sunlight. And it is harder for your body to convert vitamin D into its active form. Some studies suggest that between one-half and three-fourths of all older people get less vitamin D than what they need.

You can also stock up on vitamin D with fortified milk (especially during the winter months if you stay indoors).

But don't overdo it if you're taking supplements. High levels of vitamin D can be toxic, and anything over 400 international units should be taken only with a doctor's supervision.

Vitamin E: Leader of the Pack

Daily Value: 30 international units
Experts recommend: 100 to 400 international units
Is a multivitamin likely to contain enough? No.

Vitamin E is emerging as the quarterback in the game of protection, but few Americans get more than 6 to 12 international units in their diets, well below the Daily Value. "It's incredibly difficult to get enough vitamin E. The biggest source in the American diet is mayonnaise, followed by potato chips—foods that you want to stay away from," says Dr. Goodwin.

You get the most vitamin E from eggs and oils, also troublesome foods in today's low-fat world.

Heart disease. In study after study, vitamin E protects against heart disease, partly because it seems to go with the flow, traveling alongside the LDL cholesterol in the bloodstream to help ambush it before it can clog arteries.

In one study, researchers looked at the diets of more than 87,000 nurses between the ages of 34 and 59 and followed their eating habits for eight years. They found that those who took at least 100 international units of vitamin E a day for two years had 36 percent fewer heart attacks than those who did not supplement their diets. Scientists have also found that vitamin E actually helps slow the development of heart disease in cardiac patients by reducing the size of lesions.

Stroke. Vitamin E can help keep your blood from clotting and sticking to artery walls. In an East Carolina University Medical School study, 52 people who had experienced small strokes, or transient ischemic attacks, took aspirin (the standard treatment) plus 400 international units of vitamin E. After two years, it turned out that this group had 25 percent fewer strokes than people in a control group who just took aspirin.

Cancer. Some researchers theorize that, as you get older, your body produces prostaglandin E$_2$ (PGE$_2$), which interferes with the infection-fighting T cells. Vitamin E reduces PGE$_2$ levels and jump-starts the immune system.

At the U.S. Department of Agriculture Human Nutrition Research Center on Aging at Tufts University in Boston, people ages 62 to 70 took 800 international units of vitamin E for 30 days—and ended up with improved immune responsiveness.

In addition, vitamin E probably protects cells, particularly their membranes, making it harder for cancer-causing substances to get a toehold. In a study of 35,215 women, researchers found that those who took in more than 66 international units of vitamin E had a 68 percent lower risk of developing colon cancer. In another study the likelihood of a common skin cancer dropped by 70 percent in people who took 100 international units of vitamin E daily.

Choosing and Using a Multivitamin

The better the immune system works, the longer you live. Older people who take a quality over-the-counter multivitamin show improved immune systems," says John Bogden, Ph.D., professor of preventive medicine and community health at the New Jersey Medical School in Newark.

In one of his studies, Dr. Bogden used skin tests to show the strength of the immune system. Study participants took a common brand-name multivitamin—and ended up with stronger immune systems. "Most of the people in the program were getting close to the Daily Values of most vitamins through their diets. We weren't using the multivitamins to correct big deficiencies. It's possible that, for immunity, the vitamin requirements are higher than the Daily Values. Diet plus a supplement seems the best protection."

When you shop for a multivitamin, choose one with close to the Daily Value of copper, because it's a key nutrient for the immune system. Pick one with an equal percentage of zinc to make sure that you get the benefit of the copper, advises Dr. Bogden.

"Stick with the major brands," says Richard Cutler, Ph.D., president, chief executive officer, and scientific research director at Genox in Baltimore, who works extensively with antioxidants.

If you take a supplement. "The fact that vitamin E is safe and potentially effective against a variety of chronic diseases is good enough reason to consider taking a supplement," says Dr. Blumberg.

But don't give yourself megadoses—one report suggests that very high levels of vitamin E ingested over a long period of time may activate latent immune and autoimmune diseases.

Because vitamin E is fat-soluble, take it with a meal to get the most benefit, advises Dr. Blumberg. Most low-fat meals will still contain the amount of fat that you need.

Once you choose a multivitamin, here's how to get the most out of it.

Time it yourself. Avoid multivitamins with time-release formulas. They may release nutrients far down the intestinal tract, where absorption is poor. A better approach is to divide the dose so that you take in nutrients several times a day, says Dr. Bogden.

Store safely. Some experts suggest storing your multivitamins with the spices. Keep the bottle away from hot or humid places such as the bathroom, a sunny windowsill, or near the sink or stove, suggests Dr. Bogden.

Take it with a meal. Some nutrients are only released with fat. Jeffrey Blumberg, M.D., associate director and chief of the Antioxidants Research Laboratory at the U.S. Department of Agriculture Human Nutrition Research Center on Aging in Boston, says that you need to take in some dietary fat with your multivitamin to get the benefits of key protectors. But there is no need to make a special effort to consume fat, explains Dr. Blumberg. You would even get the amount of fat needed from a low-fat meal.

Use it or lose it. Buying a bucket-size container of vitamins may not be the bargain it first seemed. Make sure that you have time to use up the entire bottle before the product's expiration date. Otherwise, those vitamins may lose their punch, notes Dr. Bogden.

Calcium: Benefits Beyond Bone

Daily Value: 1,000 milligrams

Experts recommend: 1,500 milligrams for women over age 50 and men over age 65; 1,000 milligrams for men under age 65

Is a multivitamin likely to contain enough? No.

Calcium does a lot more than ward off osteoporosis. And few people get enough for protection. "Everybody has bought the cholesterol phobia and avoids dairy products—which are high in calcium—like the plaque," says Dr. Goodwin. "In one study, we found that healthy women past menopause get only about 350 milligrams of calcium from their diets."

Heart disease. Calcium may also help cut high blood pressure as well as LDL levels. In one study men who took 1,800 milligrams of a calcium supplement had an 11 percent drop in LDLs—and a 20 percent lower risk of having a heart attack. Calcium also keeps the levels of harmful triglycerides in the body low, unlike some cholesterol-lowering medications.

If you take a supplement. Each 8-ounce serving of milk, yogurt, or calcium-fortified orange juice or 1½-ounce serving of cheese contains about 300 milligrams of calcium. Figure out how much extra you need by deducting the amount that you get in your diet from your goal of 1,500 milligrams a day.

Some experts prefer calcium citrate because it's easily absorbed by the body, can be taken on an empty stomach, and seldom causes gas or constipation. Take the other form of calcium—calcium carbonate—with meals for better absorption.

Caution: Supplements made from bonemeal, dolomite, or oyster shells may contain high amounts of lead.

Take 500 milligrams of a calcium supplement at a time. That's probably as much as your body can absorb, says Dr. Goodwin.

Since calcium interferes with your body's ability to use other substances (zinc, for example), don't take your calcium and multivitamin supplement together, says Ananda S. Prasad, M.D., Ph.D., professor of medicine at Wayne State University School of Medicine in Detroit.

Calcium also blocks your body's ability to use tetracycline. More important, remember that the reverse is also true, cautions Dr. Blumberg. Tetracycline inhibits calcium function in the body.

Fiber keeps your body from absorbing calcium, so don't take your calcium supplement with high-fiber foods, suggests Dr. Goodwin. If, for example, you take your supplement along with a high-fiber wheat-bran cereal (containing 10 grams or more of fiber), your body will get 25 percent less calcium than it would otherwise.

You might also try chewable calcium products, citrus-flavored drinkable supplements, and calcium-fortified orange juice.

Chromium: A Classic Risk-Cutter

Daily Value: 120 micrograms
Experts recommend: 50 to 200 micrograms
Is a multivitamin likely to contain enough? No.

Most people don't get enough, although you get chromium in a wide range of foods, including meats, whole grains, broccoli, black pepper, brewer's yeast, and barbecue sauce.

Heart disease. Low levels of chromium are linked to glucose intolerance, a risk factor for heart disease. Chromium may also help increase the beneficial HDL cholesterol levels. In one study 76 heart disease patients took 250 micrograms of chromium a day for 7 to 16 months. Their HDL levels increased to potentially give them a 30 percent reduction in heart disease risk.

Copper: To Build Immunity

Daily Value: 2 milligrams
Experts recommend: 2 milligrams
Is a multivitamin likely to contain enough? Yes.

Most people don't come close to the Daily Value through diet alone, say experts. You get copper in foods such as nuts, cocoa, shellfish, mushrooms, and gelatin.

Heart disease. Copper is part of the protective antioxidant enzyme system and helps kill destructive free radicals.

Cancer. Scientists believe that copper may play an important part in keeping the immune system healthy.

If you take a supplement. Match your copper and zinc intakes. If you use a product that contains 75 percent of the Daily Value of zinc, get 75 percent of the Daily Value of copper, too, says David B. Milne, Ph.D., research chemist at the U.S. Department of Agriculture Grand Forks Human Nutrition Research Center in Grand Forks, North Dakota. Otherwise, you won't get the full benefits of these nutrients.

Future Science: Home Testing

You can test your blood pressure and cholesterol levels with home kits, so why can't you test your levels of protective antioxidants?

Well, emerging products may allow you to do just that. Researchers are busy working on perfecting inexpensive take-home tests that you can buy at the grocery store to get a reading of your body's levels of important antioxidants. If you're low, a change in diet may bring up your protective levels. If necessary, a made-to-order supplemental package can be concocted to meet your specific needs.

"We're working on that now," says Richard Cutler, Ph.D., president, chief executive officer, and scientific research director at Genox in Baltimore. "You'll get the most protection that way because you're taking in exactly what you need. If you repeat the test periodically, you can also tell that the supplements you take are actually benefiting your body by raising the levels of important protective substances."

Iron: Less Is Better

Daily Value: 18 milligrams
Experts recommend: 10 milligrams or less
Is a multivitamin likely to contain enough? Yes.

Choose a supplement that either doesn't contain iron or contains no more than half the Daily Value, recommends Dr. Bogden. Regardless of your gender, avoid "women's supplements" because of high iron content.

As you age, your body stores more iron. Some studies show that high levels of iron increase heart attack risk, but the evidence is not conclusive. There's some evidence that extra iron means added risk of cancer, too.

Magnesium: From a Multitude of Sources

Daily Value: 400 milligrams
Experts recommend: 400 milligrams
Is a multivitamin likely to contain enough? Yes.

You get magnesium from a variety of sources, including foods and hard drinking water.

People with kidney disease or who have kidney problems and who consume a lot of products that contain magnesium, such as combined antacid/anti-gas drugs (like Maalox Antacid Plus Anti-Gas or Mylanta), some laxatives (like Correctol), and some pain relievers (like Arthritis Strength Bufferin), can develop magnesium poisoning. Products that slow the digestive system, including some antidepressants, can also leave you with too much magnesium.

Heart disease. Magnesium helps lower blood pressure and may improve insulin sensitivity. Researchers note that people who drink hard water—which is rich in magnesium—have lower rates of sudden, fatal heart attacks.

Stroke. Researchers believe that magnesium helps prevent the clotting that leads to strokes.

Potassium: Taking the Pressure Off

Daily Value: 3,500 milligrams
Experts recommend: 3,500 milligrams
Is a multivitamin likely to contain enough? No.

You get this mineral in a variety of fruits, vegetables, and meats, and, according to Dr. Blumberg, supplementing potassium is unnecessary. Some drugs lower potassium levels, including diuretics, digitalis, and steroids.

Heart disease. Potassium helps lower blood pressure, so it's not surprising that people with high blood pressure often have low levels of potassium (as well as calcium and magnesium).

If you're using medications such as diuretics, check with your doctor before taking more than the Daily Value.

Selenium: Shooting Down Cancer Risk

Daily Value: 70 micrograms
Experts recommend: 70 to 100 micrograms
Is a multivitamin likely to contain enough? Yes.

"Some antioxidant supplements contain a little extra selenium for protection. That's fine," says Dr. Bogden. But the mineral is toxic at levels higher than 1 milligram per day.

Heart disease. Selenium may play a role in lowering heart disease risk. In Italy, deaths from heart disease rose dramatically among residents of a village whose public water supply was changed from wells high in selenium to water with a lower selenium content.

Cancer. Evidence indicates that getting enough selenium may cut your risk of most cancers, including lung, skin, breast, and prostate cancer. A study in the Netherlands found that people with high levels of selenium had half the rate of lung cancer compared to those with low selenium levels.

Zinc: Get Immunity

Daily Value: 15 milligrams
Experts recommend: 15 milligrams
Is a multivitamin likely to contain enough? Yes.

"A significant number of older people have zinc deficiency," says Dr. Prasad. If you're low in this mineral, you may have a loss of taste or smell. Sometimes zinc deficiency also results in loss of appetite.

Cancer. Studies show that zinc supplements improved signs of immune function. But some studies suggest that too much zinc can also weaken your immune system.

Prescription for Prevention

While supplements aren't a substitute for healthy eating, they can reduce your risk of heart disease by 30 to 40 percent. They also strengthen your immune system, which is particularly important as it becomes less efficient with age.

Do:

- *Choose a high-quality multivitamin.*

- *Check the expiration date to make sure that you'll use up the vitamins before that date arrives.*

- *Add an antioxidant supplement containing 100 to 400 international units of vitamin E, 250 to 1,000 milligrams of vitamin C, 6 to 20 milligrams of beta-carotene, plus 70 to 100 micrograms of selenium.*

- *Add a calcium supplement or get enough calcium through your diet. For women over 50 and men over 65, take in a total of 1,500 milligrams per day (1,000 milligrams a day for men ages 60 to 65).*

- *Buy a product that contains equal percentages of the Daily Value for copper and zinc.*

- *Choose a multivitamin that contains half or less the Daily Value of iron.*

- *Take your multivitamin and antioxidant supplement with meals or low-fat snacks to get the full benefit of fat-soluble and water-soluble vitamins.*

- *Buy dairy products fortified with vitamin D.*

Don't:

- *Take larger than expert-recommended doses of any vitamin or mineral without approval from your doctor. Some can be dangerous at high levels.*

- *Take calcium and your multivitamin supplement together.*

- *Take calcium without checking with your doctor if you're on tetracycline.*

- *Over-consume magnesium products such as certain laxatives, antacid/anti-gas combination drugs, and pain relievers if you have kidney problems.*

- *Increase your current consumption of supplements without checking with your doctor, especially if you're on medications.*

Chapter 6

Weight Control

Trim Down to Trim Your Disease Risk

When he wasn't acting or directing classic films like *Citizen Kane*, Orson Welles ate. Reportedly, it wasn't uncommon for him to eat four to five large portions of caviar a day, and three huge steaks and mounds of rich desserts for dinner. His lifetime of gluttony weakened his heart and dangerously elevated his blood pressure. Welles died at age 70 of a massive heart attack.

"To my mind, Orson Welles's health was the antithesis of what you want to experience as you get older," says Michael Klaper, M.D., director of the Institute of Nutrition Education and Research in Manhattan Beach, California.

"I would rather be a lean older person than an obese one because when it comes to heart disease, stroke, and cancer, it's clear that being overweight puts you at high risk for these diseases," Dr. Klaper says. "Overweight people in their sixties or seventies concern me because they're really setting themselves up for many of the same problems that Welles had."

While most of us certainly don't overindulge as much that Welles did, the pounds do seem to creep up on us and threaten to erode our health as we age. But it doesn't have to be this way.

"Even if you go into your sixties a bit overweight and inactive, you definitely haven't written yourself a death sentence," Dr. Klaper says. "I've seen some people at these ages who have made dramatic turnabouts in their weights. If you begin eating a good diet and become leaner and more active in your sixties or seventies, there's a good chance that you'll still be that way when you hit 90 or even 100."

Where Did These Extra Pounds Come From?

As a person strides toward 60, the amount of muscle in the body naturally drops and fat begins to account for a greater percentage of weight. So even if you didn't gain a pound, you would still have more body fat at 70 than you did at age 30.

At the same time, metabolism—the rate at which your body burns calories—slows down. Many people also get less exercise as they age, yet continue eating the same amount of food as they did when they were younger. The result is more pounds. In fact, many people gain about a pound a year after age 35.

By age 60, roughly 40 percent of American men and women are overweight. After age 75, the number of people who are overweight dips to 30 percent because many people who are extremely overweight have died. Furthermore, most of us who survive into our eighties naturally begin shedding pounds because of diminished appetites, says Artemis Simopoulos, M.D., president of the Center for Genetics, Nutrition, and Health in Washington, D.C.

Although excess weight is one of the primary causes of premature death after age 60, how much of an impact being overweight has on your risk of stroke, heart disease, and cancer in these years is a riddle that scientists are just beginning to probe.

"It's a darn good question that we don't fully have an answer for yet," says Edward Saltzman, M.D., a scientist at the U.S. Department of Agriculture Human Nutrition Research Center on Aging at Tufts University in Boston. "In the past the diseases associated with being extremely overweight would have precluded many people from living into their sixties or seventies. Now that medical technology is getting better at extending life, we're seeing more people who are overweight living longer. So many of the data for these people are relatively new."

The bulk of the emerging evidence suggests that too much body fat—whether it is caused by overeating, a sedentary lifestyle, or the natural reduction of body muscle and buildup of fat as you age—is just as harmful now as it was when you were 40 or 50, says Walter Willett, M.D.,

Age Alters Your Healthy Weight

For years, height and weight charts were based on the assumption that one size fits all, no matter what your age. But researchers are finding that slim and trim takes on a whole new meaning after age 60, says Reubin Andres, M.D., clinical director of the National Institute on Aging Gerontology Research Center in Baltimore.

As we age, a greater percentage of our body weight is fat, and that is something that most height and weight charts don't make allowances for, Dr. Andres says. Using the body mass index (BMI), a calculation of body fat based on height and weight, Dr. Andres has found that people older than 60 have lower death rates at slightly higher BMIs than those who are younger. In other words, even if you are carrying around a few more pounds than you used to, you may still be at a healthy weight for your age.

Based on his calculations, here's what Dr. Andres says are healthy weight ranges for men and women in their sixties. Although re-

Dr.P.H., professor of epidemiology and nutrition and chairman of the Department of Nutrition at the Harvard School of Public Health. Researchers believe that excessive body fat at any age increases the production of sex hormones such as estrogen that promote colon, breast, and endometrial cancer. Increased body fat also drives up blood pressure, forces the heart to work harder, and raises low-density lipoproteins (LDLs)—the bad cholesterol that contributes to the clogging of arteries and increases your risk of stroke and heart disease.

It Isn't As Hard As You Think

Fortunately, losing weight after age 60 is easier than you might suspect. In fact, one study has shown that people in their sixties and seventies who enrolled in a weight-control program were twice as successful in their efforts to lose weight and make lifestyle changes than younger men

searchers haven't calculated the optimal weight after age 69, these weight ranges are probably reasonable for people in their seventies and eighties as well, says William Hazzard, M.D., chairman of the Department of Internal Medicine at Bowman Gray School of Medicine of Wake Forest University in Winston-Salem, North Carolina.

Height	Weight	Height	Weight
4'10"	115–142	5'8"	158–196
4'11"	119–147	5'9"	162–201
5'0"	123–152	5'10"	167–207
5'1"	127–157	5'11"	172–213
5'2"	131–163	6'0"	177–219
5'3"	135–168	6'1"	182–225
5'4"	140–173	6'2"	187–232
5'5"	144–179	6'3"	192–238
5'6"	148–184	6'4"	197–244
5'7"	153–190		

and women, says Eileen Rosendahl, Ph.D., a geriatric psychologist and assistant professor at the Albert Einstein College of Medicine of Yeshiva University in New York City.

That is because you probably have more time to devote to the effort than you did when you were younger, and fat cells on the abdomen, the type that is really harmful, melt away more quickly than fat on the buttocks and thighs, says Lodovico Balducci, M.D., program leader of the senior adult oncology program at the University of South Florida College of Medicine in Tampa.

"You don't have to get down to an ideal body weight to get the benefits of intentional weight loss. I'm starting to believe that losing just a few pounds may be very good for you," says David F. Williamson, Ph.D., a researcher at the Centers for Disease Control and Prevention in Atlanta. One way for an older person to lose those pounds is by improving his level of physical activity, he says.

Overweight? The Shadow Knows

Scientists rely on sophisticated formulas and tests to determine if you're overweight. But Sharon Emmons, R.D., a clinical dietitian and geriatric nutrition specialist at the University of South Alabama College of Medicine in Mobile, often uses a more down-to-earth approach.

"I tell my clients to stand out in the sun and look at their shadows. For men, if your shadow resembles Alfred Hitchcock—your belly protruding out beyond your chest—then you might want to lose a few pounds. For women, if your shadow looks more like a rectangle than an hourglass, then it may be time to lose weight as well," says Emmons.

For a more precise measure, however, Emmons and other weight-control experts turn to body mass index, or BMI—a calculation that takes into account both your height and weight—which has proven to be an excellent predictor of a person's susceptibility to certain diseases like stroke, heart disease, and cancer.

To figure your BMI, multiply your weight in pounds by 700. Divide that number by your height in inches. Then divide by your height again. The result is your BMI. So, for example, if you weigh 150 pounds, multiple that by 700. Then divide that number by your height—let's say 66 inches—twice. The result is 24. A healthy BMI for a man or woman over age 60 is below 29, says Jose Morais, M.D., a gerontologist and nutritionist at Royal Victoria Hospital in Montreal. If you're above that, try some of the weight-loss strategies suggested in this chapter or ask your physician during your next checkup about ways to control your weight.

The Weight of the Evidence

If you're overweight, losing just 10 to 15 pounds (depending on your height) can reduce your risk of life-threatening diseases and improve your overall health. But if you don't make an effort to get your weight under control, you'll be more vulnerable to the big three killers, Dr. Klaper says.

Here's a look at the persuasive arguments that scientists are finding for shedding modest amounts of weight after age 60. Among other things, weight control does the following:

Promotes longevity. In a study of 15,069 overweight women, Dr. Williamson found that those who had lost 20 pounds in the year before the study began were 25 percent less likely to die of heart disease or cancer in the next 12 years than overweight women who didn't lose weight. These women also reduced their overall risk of dying by 20 percent and slashed in half their chances of succumbing to weight-related cancer of the breast, cervix, ovary, and others, as well as reducing their risk of dying with diabetes.

Researchers traced the lives of 19,000 Harvard University alumni men for up to 26 years. Those who weighed 20 percent under the U.S. average for men of similar age and height had the lowest rates of death.

Protects the heart. In the Framingham Heart Study—an ongoing assessment of the health habits of 5,200 people in Massachusetts—researchers showed that men and women in their sixties and seventies who weighed 30 percent more than what is considered a healthy weight were at least twice as likely to develop heart disease.

"I strongly feel that an overweight person who is age 60-plus should lose weight. Excess weight magnifies the risk factors of hypertension, diabetes, and high cholesterol levels that are associated with heart disease. Developing diabetes, for example, increases cardiac risk by more than 100 percent. But all these things are reversible to some extent if you lose those extra pounds," says Robert Di Bianco, M.D., associate clinical professor at Georgetown University School of Medicine and a Washington, D.C., cardiologist.

Slashes stroke risk. In another ongoing phase of the Framingham study, researchers have been tracking the weights and blood pressures of men and women up to age 94 for 30 years. Every pound of excess weight, according to William Kannel, M.D., professor of medicine and public health at Boston University Medical Center, causes you to retain more sodium in your bloodstream, increases your risk of diabetes, and drives your systolic blood pressure (the top number in a blood pressure reading) up 4.5 millimeters. Combined, these weight-related risk factors may quadruple your chances of a heart attack or stroke, Dr. Kannel says.

"Weight control is very important for preventing stroke," says Philip

Body Fat: Where You Have It Matters

Apples are a food to admire. You just don't want to be shaped like one.

Doctors have long known that people who have extra weight around their bellies (apple-shaped bodies) are at greater risk of heart disease, stroke, and cancer than those who are trimmer. The danger increases after age 60 because more men and women develop that shape.

"Body shape—fat distribution—becomes more important as we age because weight, which relects both muscle and fat mass, becomes a less reliable guide to fat stores after age 60," says Walter Willett, M.D., Dr.P.H., professor of epidemiology and nutrition and chairman of the Department of Nutrition at the Harvard School of Public Health.

If you're shaped like a pear—with more fat on your hips and thighs—you still have an increased risk of these diseases, but not as much as an apple-shaped man or woman, says David V. Schapira, M.D., director of the Stanley S. Scott Cancer Center at Louisiana State University Medical Center in New Orleans.

To accurately assess your body fat distribution, measure your waist at its narrowest point and your hips at the widest point (over the buttocks). Divide your waist measurement by the number of inches around your hips. If you're a woman, a number greater than 0.75 suggests that you are at greater risk of health problems. For men, a number higher than 1 is a warning sign.

The best way to diminish an apple shape is through exercise. Even as little as walking 30 minutes a day, three times a week, can be an important beginning, Dr. Willett says.

Wolf, M.D., professor of neurology at Boston University School of Medicine. "Being overweight doesn't seem to be an independent risk factor for stroke. But if you look at the main risk factors for stroke—high blood pressure, high blood sugar, and high cholesterol levels—losing weight will lower every one of them."

Pounds Add to Your Cancer Risk, Too

Although scientists believe that extra pounds have more impact on heart disease than on cancer risk, slimming down may decrease the possibility that you'll develop some tumors, says Rachel Ballard-Barbash, M.D., an epidemiologist at the National Cancer Institute in Bethesda, Maryland. Specifically, avoiding midlife weight gain can help you:

Stifle breast and endometrial cancer. Dr. Barbash has found that women with more upper-body fat, the so-called apple-shaped bodies, are at 70 to 100 percent greater risk of developing breast cancer than women whose fat is on their lower bodies—the so-called pear shape in which fat clings to the hips and thighs.

Other studies involving women up to age 83 have found that the heaviest women who were apple-shaped have a 5 to 6 times greater risk of breast cancer and had 15 times greater incidence of endometrial cancer than women who were trimmer, says David V. Schapira, M.D., director of the Stanley S. Scott Cancer Center at Louisiana State University Medical Center in New Orleans.

"Theoretically, breast cancer risk can be reduced by 45 percent just by losing 10 to 15 pounds," Dr. Schapira says.

In addition, if a woman who weighs 25 percent or more over her ideal weight develops breast cancer, she is 60 percent more likely to have a recurrence of the disease in the next 10 years than does a woman who has her weight under control at diagnosis.

"Weight control is one of the few modifiable lifestyle behaviors that may reduce a woman's risk of diagnosis and death due to breast cancer," says Ruby Senie, Ph.D., associate attending epidemiologist at Memorial Sloan-Kettering Cancer Center in New York City.

Corral cancer of the esophagus. Men in their sixties who are 20 percent over their recommended healthy weight are at three times greater risk of developing adenocarcenoma, a cancer of the esophagus, than men who tip the scales right on, according to researchers at National Cancer Institute who studied 174 men who had the disease and 750 who didn't.

Fight off colon cancer. In a six-year follow-up study of 47,723 male dentists, pharmacists, and other health professionals up to age 74, Harvard University researchers found that men who had waist circumferences of 43 inches or more were 2½ times more likely to develop colon cancer than those whose waists were less than 35 inches.

What's Going On?

Doctors suspect that excessive body fat sparks increased production of sex hormones like estrogen and testosterone that are thought to promote breast and endometrial cancer. At the same time high amounts of body fat slash levels of a protein that binds to these sex hormones and deactivates them. The result is a greater risk of developing these cancers, Dr. Schapira says.

Extra weight also triggers gastric reflux, bathing the esophagus with excessive amounts of acid that may promote precancerous growths, says Linda Morris Brown, an epidemiologist at the National Cancer Institute in Bethesda, Maryland.

Researchers are less certain how excess weight contributes to cancer of the esophagus and colon. They do know, however, that some of the same things that cause excess weight—high-fat foods and lack of exercise—also increase the risk of colon cancer. So being overweight may not directly cause colon cancer, but it could be a potent warning that other aspects of your lifestyle are endangering your health, says Tim Byers, M.D., professor of preventive medicine at the University of Colorado School of Medicine in Denver.

You Can Make a Big Difference Now

For many of us, controlling weight has been like trying to catch a live trout with bare hands. But, as discussed, making another effort even after age 60 can have an immense impact on your health and well-being.

"The safety of being thin is huge. There are 300,000 excess deaths in the non-thin population each year, and we spend $100 billion a year to treat diseases like heart disease, stroke, and cancer that are related to not being thin," says George Blackburn, M.D., Ph.D., associate professor of surgery at Harvard Medical School and chief of the nutrition/metabolism laboratory in the Cancer Research Institute at Beth Israel Deaconess Medical Center West in Boston.

In most cases diet alone won't do the job for you. Your best bet is to use dietary changes as part of a comprehensive effort that includes exercise, Dr. Balducci says.

Remember that the pounds may come off more slowly than in the past, says Sharon Emmons, R.D., a clinical dietitian and geriatric nutrition specialist at the University of South Alabama College of Medicine in Mobile. If you lose a half-pound to a pound a week at this age, you're doing great, she says.

Usually, losing weight at that rate means shaving only 150 calories a day from your menu, Dr. Blackburn says. That's about the equivalent of a slice of cheese pizza, a 12-ounce beer, a ½-cup serving of vanilla ice cream, or five gingersnaps.

Shoot for losing no more than 10 pounds or 5 percent of your body weight (whichever is less) in 12 weeks, Dr. Blackburn says. Then try to maintain that weight loss for three months before attempting to lose more weight. The body, particularly after age 60, is willing to lose weight for about three months, he says. Then it doesn't want to budge for quite a while. If you push yourself too much, you're more likely to start overeating and regain the weight that you have dropped, Dr. Blackburn says. With these goals in mind, here's a look at the nuts and bolts of weight control, beginning with motivation.

Feed Your Head First

Weight control begins in the mind.

"I don't think that you'll seriously be able to get your weight under control without considering what is going on between your ears," says Maurice Larocque, M.D., a bariatric physician in Montreal and author of *Slim Within*, a 21-day, audiocassette weight-loss program. "The thoughts that you plant in your mind will determine if you succeed or fail."

Here are some ways to help you think more positively about weight control so that you can achieve your goal and permanently reduce your

Do You Use Food to Quell Emotions?

Loneliness, frustration, boredom, anger, grief, anxiety, guilt, and other emotions are savage beasts. If you regularly soothe them with food, like many people over 60 do, you may be packing on pounds without really solving the underlying problem. Here is a simple test, developed by Stephen P. Gullo, Ph.D., author of *Thin Tastes Better,* that will help you analyze how emotions affect your eating habits and determine what to do what about it. Rate each of the following statements on a scale of 1 (rarely true) to 5 (always true). Scoring follows.

1. There is no problem that can't be solved by chocolate.

2. I like to treat myself to a nice dinner or some other food treat to celebrate accomplishments.

3. On previous diets I've sometimes cheated because I just felt that I deserved a little treat.

4. When I'm stressed or upset, I feel better after I've eaten.

5. I have a favorite restaurant where my friends and I go to celebrate or just get together.

6. I have a particular food that I always crave when I'm under stress.

7. I always gain weight when I'm under pressure.

8. Whenever I've gone off a diet plan, there was something unpleasant going on in my life.

9. I always overeat when my children or grandchildren visit me.

10. I always overeat after I fight with friends or family.

Scoring: Add up your total. If you scored 21 or less, you're doing pretty well—you may occasionally turn to food for solace, but it isn't your first

risk of stroke, heart disease, and cancer.

Find new reasons to like yourself. "We know that 80 percent of people who are overweight don't like themselves. They can't find any plea-

line of defense. If you scored 22 to 36, you may be using food to pacify your emotions, but you're just as likely to use other ways of dealing with feelings—such as talking it out with friends, taking a bath, or exercising—that are less fattening. If you scored 37 or more, you may be relying too much on food to cope with stress.

Here are alternatives to help relieve emotional strain without resorting to food.

Think, then act. Before you open the refrigerator, ask yourself if eating is really going to relieve your anger, boredom, depression, or other emotional need, says Eileen Rosendahl, Ph.D., a geriatric psychologist and assistant professor at the Albert Einstein College of Medicine of Yeshiva University in New York City. Try to find something else to do—take a walk, garden, or visit an ill friend—that will make you feel gratified or happy instead of guilty.

Beware the "comfort" trap. "I often tell groups of older people, 'Maybe you've lost someone recently and are seeking comfort in food. But keep in mind that your loved ones are at peace and watching over you. So please don't let them down. They only want what is best for you, and being overweight simply isn't healthy,' " says Maria Simonson, Sc.D., Ph.D., director of the Health, Weight, and Stress Clinic at the Johns Hopkins Medical Institutions in Baltimore.

Sneak in a nap instead of a snack. When you're tired, emotions can overwhelm you and tempt you to seek comfort from food, says Edith Howard Hogan, R.D., a spokeswoman for the American Dietetic Association in Washington, D.C. Get at least 6 hours of sleep a day. If you feel an urge to eat, lie down, close your eyes for a few minutes, and the emotional tug to chow down should pass.

sure within themselves that would encourage them to care for their bodies. So you need to learn to love yourself before you can make any progress toward slimness," Dr. Larocque says. Twice a day, take a moment to focus on some aspect of yourself that you like such as your legs, nose, or eyes. As you begin to lose weight, take pride in the features that are improving. Tell yourself, "I'm 70, but look at me. I really like how my belly is trimming down. I'm starting to get back the shape that I had when I was 45."

Write 'em down. Jot down on an index card your three most important motivators for losing weight, such as more stamina, more energy, and lessening your risk of heart disease. Read and think about what those motivators mean to you for 5 minutes when you awaken and just before you go to bed, suggests Peter Miller, Ph.D., executive director of the Hilton Head Health Institute in Hilton Head, South Carolina. Doing that will keep your mind locked on your goal.

Take a picture. Once a month, have a friend or a spouse take pictures of you from front, side, and back views. Focus on the parts of your body where you are making progress, like your shrinking tummy or your strengthening arms and legs. Take a couple of minutes each day to imagine how much better you'll look next month, Dr. Larocque says.

Let go. The more relaxed that you are, the more open you'll be to positive thoughts that will help keep your weight under control, Dr. Larocque says. Try the following relaxation exercise twice a day: Get into a comfortable position—either lying or sitting—in a darkened room. Close your eyes and begin breathing very slowly and deeply. Relax the muscles of your forehead and jaw. Part your lips slightly. Now relax the muscles of your mouth, neck, arms, and legs. Now breathe more deeply, inhale slowly. Then push your shoulders upward until it seems as though they are touching your ears. Hold your breath for a count of five, then exhale slowly and drop your shoulders. Push your shoulders up again and repeat the breathing sequence. Sense yourself beginning to feel relaxed. Your arms are very heavy and limp.

Feel the sun's warmth on your arms. They are getting warmer and warmer. Now let your legs go limp and feel the sun's warmth on them. Repeat the sun imagery with your eyelids, jaw, forehead, and finally with your entire body. Feel the sun's energy inside your whole body. See yourself and smile. You are full of energy, and you use it. You appreciate each step that you are taking on your road to weight control. Now count to three, then open your eyes and get on with your day.

Mirror, mirror on the wall . . . Like the queen in *Snow White,* you can be the fairest one of all. Just use your imagination, says Barbara Morse, an imagery counselor and recreational therapist in San Diego who works with men and women over age 60.

Imagine yourself in a hall of mirrors, each one reflecting a different image of you, Morse says. Try to see as many perspectives in the mirrors as you can. One may make you look short and fat, another tall and skinny. See reflections of yourself as a child, as a person older than you are now, and as you see yourself today. Now look in a mirror and give yourself whatever type of body you would like. Change your hair color or style. Work with the image in the mirror until it reflects you exactly as you would like to be.

Step into that mirror and become that image that you have visualized. When the image fits and you feel comfortable, walk out of the hall of mirrors, taking the magic mirror with you. Ask the mirror what you need to do to maintain this image. Pay attention to the directions and follow them. Wear this new image as if it were an elegant gown or suit perfectly suited for you. Do this visualization twice a day for 5 minutes each, or whenever you feel your motivation to control your weight slipping, Morse says.

Put the scale away. Don't weigh yourself every day, says Maria Simonson, Sc.D., Ph.D., director of the Health, Weight, and Stress Clinic at the Johns Hopkins Medical Institutions in Baltimore. Instead, step onto the scale once a week at the same time of day. It will give a more accurate measure of your progress and be more encouraging than the constant ups and downs of daily weigh-ins.

Lean on a buddy. Sharing your experience with a friend or a support group can help keep you motivated and lessen your temptation to stray. "A lot of people try to lose weight alone and that's difficult, especially after age 60 because the rate of weight loss often is slower than when you were younger, and that can be discouraging," Dr. Rosendahl says.

Discard all-or-nothing thinking. "Surprisingly, a lot of people over age 60 who are overweight are perfectionists," Dr. Larocque says. "They expect to reach 105 percent of their weight goals, and if they only achieve 90 percent of them, they think the whole effort is a failure."

Instead of focusing on your overall goal, set your sights on a modest weight target—like a pound a week—that you can easily achieve. If you don't reach your goal one week, try not to think of it as a failure but as a learning experience. Jot down the things that you did and didn't do that will help you make a better effort in the next seven days.

"You don't have to be perfect, you just have to keep trying," Dr. Larocque says.

Take a day off. "We encourage our patients to take what we call planned holidays," says Patrick O'Neil, Ph.D., director of the weight management center at the Medical University of South Carolina College of Medicine in Charleston. "It's a time when you decide in advance that you're going to give yourself a rest from weight control and have a do-as-you-choose day."

Doing that about once a month helps you learn how to regain control of your eating habits after a lapse and will boost your self-confidence so that you can get back on track after an unplanned slip, Dr. O'Neil says. A day off will also give you something to look forward to as your weight-control effort progresses.

Squelch the Saboteurs

Although positive motivation can help you overcome your own worst enemy—yourself—there are still plenty of well-intentioned friends and family members who can quickly sabotage your weight-control efforts.

"Defeating the saboteurs in your life is very important, particularly after age 60. They're one of the major obstacles that you'll face, and one of the main reasons that people in this age group stop losing weight," Dr. Larocque says.

Jealousy, guilt, envy, and fear are some of the underlying reasons that provoke saboteurs to derail your efforts, he says.

"Often, these people are trying to defend their own reasons for staying fat by attacking you," Dr. Larocque says. "They might tell you, 'Gee, you look so old now that you've lost all that weight. Have you seen your face?

It looks like you have a lot of new wrinkles. Are you sure this weight-loss thing is right for you?'"

To overcome these attacks, realize that the saboteur is probably more concerned about his own feelings than your well-being. So ask yourself, why is this person really saying these things or offering me fattening foods that I shouldn't eat? Once you understand what is motivating the saboteur, it will be easier for you to ignore his temptations or criticisms and focus on the compliments of others, Dr. Larocque says.

Many other techniques can help you subdue these saboteurs: Here is a sampling.

Let them in on it. Sit down with your family and close friends and discuss why you want to lose weight and what they can do to help, Dr. Miller says. You could, for example, ask for their compliments and support but discourage them from tempting you with rich desserts.

If friends or relatives ignore your request, politely remind them that you're trying to make important lifestyle changes for your health and happiness. If they persist, be blunt, Dr. Miller says. Make it clear that you, and only you, will decide what you'll eat, when you'll eat it, and why you'll eat it, and you don't appreciate their attempts to undermine your efforts.

Make a contract. Ask potential saboteurs like your spouse or a close friend to sign a written agreement to support your effort, Dr. Larocque says. In writing, let the person know why you consider being overweight a threat to your health. Point out that any serious attempt to get your weight under control will require changes in habits and attitudes, including those of people close to you. Then list five ways the other person can help you, such as providing cooperation when requested, being attentive and praising even the slightest achievement, not pointing out the occasional slip-up, listening without judgment to your feelings, and providing encouragement to persevere regardless of difficulties. Then ask the person to sign and date two copies. Keep one for yourself and give the other one to the person. Carry your copy with you and, if necessary, pull it out to remind your friend or spouse about your deal.

Help them face their fears. Sometimes friends and loved ones worry that your new weight will ruin your relationship, particularly if their own weight or ailments prevent them from being as active as you are now. Reassure your loved ones that you're still the same inside and that you will always care and be there for them, Dr. Larocque suggests.

Keep binge buddies at bay. Some saboteurs love "eatings" rather than outings. These are the people who ask you out for lunch or dessert all the time. Instead of reluctantly accepting, suggest doing an activity that doesn't involve food, like visiting a museum, says Marilyn Cerino, R.D., coordinator of the weight-management and nutrition programs at the Benjamin Franklin Center for Health in Philadelphia.

Keep playing the same tune. Keep saying no thanks without offering an explanation. "If you give saboteurs a reason, they'll find an in. If you say, 'I can't because I'm trying to lose weight,' they'll say, 'Gee, I don't think that dieting is good for you.' They will come up with something if you let them. So become a broken record and keep saying no thank you until they get the point," says Susan Olson, Ph.D., a Seattle psychologist and weight-control expert in private practice.

Move It to Lose It

You can slash calories to the bone and down all the magic pills, instant liquid shakes, grapefruit, cottage cheese, or diet bars you want, but you really won't get your weight under control until you do one critical thing: exercise.

"I know some older people who are very virtuous eaters who are extremely frustrated with their weight. The trouble is they don't exercise, and unless you exercise, you're not going to lose weight," Dr. Rosendahl says.

In particular, exercise helps you retain muscle and fends off the natural accumulation of body fat as you age, Dr. Blackburn says.

That's important because researchers believe that moderate or mild exercise stimulates the immune system. So if you try to lose weight without exercise, you're going to lose muscle as well as fat. And once weakened this way, your body will sacrifice much of its ability to destroy viruses and abnormal cells that can develop into serious illnesses, says Robert C. Klesges, Ph.D., professor of psychology and preventive medicine at the University of Memphis in Tennessee.

Losing just a few pounds through exercise also may be a beneficial way to reduce your risk of heart disease and stroke, says Robert S. Schwartz, M.D., professor of internal medicine and gerontology at the University of Washington School of Medicine in Seattle.

In his studies of healthy older men up to age 82, Dr. Schwartz has found that a 5-pound weight loss caused by six months of brisk walking and biking can increase levels of the good high-density lipoprotein cholesterol and lower harmful LDL cholesterol by as much as a 20-pound weight loss caused by calorie reduction alone.

"People are more likely to be successful keeping off weight by exercising. You may not lose as much weight or look very different, but metabolically I think exercise produces tremendous improvement," Dr. Schwartz says.

Exercise also is a powerful motivator that can help suppress your appetite and keep you on track for weight control.

"It certainly can help people over 60 stick with a new lifestyle. After they begin exercising, they often feel an increased sense of well-being and accomplishment and develop better self-esteem and a sense of control over their bodies. All of these things feed into helping them eat better and staying with their effort," says Samuel Klein, M.D., director of the Center for Human Nutrition at Washington University School of Medicine in St. Louis.

Although all of the benefits of exercise are discussed elsewhere, here are a few specific approaches to help you control your weight and reduce your risk of the big three killers. Be sure to check with your doctor before beginning any exercise routine.

Lift it off. Resistance training will not only strengthen your muscles but also help you increase your metabolism so that you burn extra fat, says Margarita Treuth, Ph.D., assistant professor at Baylor College of Medicine in Houston.

In a pair of small studies involving 15 men up to age 65 and 15 women ages 60 to 77, Dr. Treuth found that those who worked out with resistance-training equipment three times a week for 16 weeks burned an extra 50 calories a day. Over a year, these workouts—one set (12 to 15 repetitions) of several upper-body exercises like biceps curls and two sets of lower-body strengthening exercises like leg presses—can help burn calories, she says.

"At these ages, it appears that resistance exercise can increase resting metabolism and help control weight," Dr. Treuth says.

To do a simple biceps curl, for instance, stand with your back against a wall and grasp a 1-pound food can in each of your hands. Lower your arms so that they are fully extended at your sides. Turn your palms so that they face forward. Then, slowly lift the cans up so that they touch your shoulders. Lower and repeat 10 to 12 times. (If you feel ambitious, after you lift the cans to your shoulder, pause for a count of five, then extend your arms over your head.)

Do that once a day for three weeks, then add a second set of 10 to 12 repetitions to your daily routine, says Mark Bank, an exercise physiologist at Walter O. Boswell Memorial Hospital in Sun City, Arizona, a retirement community near Phoenix. (For other easy resistance exercises, see page 234.)

Walk a mile toward leanness. Just strolling a mile daily burns 110 calories, Dr. Simonson says. That may not seem like much, but if you stick with it, you can lose up to 11 pounds a year even if you don't go fast. "Never overdo it. Keep it safe, even if it means moving slower," she suggests.

Stop those hunger pangs with yoga. "Yoga is a good exercise for older people trying to lose weight because it energizes their minds, bodies, and spirits and supplies them with a feeling of satisfaction that can replace any desire to eat," says Morse.

And you don't have to twist yourself into a knot to do it. In fact, you can practice many simple yoga techniques while sitting in a chair. Try the yoga sequence on the following pages three times a week while remembering to breathe deeply, evenly, and continuously, suggests Carrie Angus, M.D., director of the Center for Health and Healing at the Himalayan International Institute of Yoga Science and Philosophy in Honesdale, Pennsylvania.

1. DOUBLE SHOULDER ROLLS
Sit tall in a straight-back chair and lift
your shoulders up as far as possible toward the back of your neck. Roll your
shoulders forward and then relax them
down. If you do this correctly, your
shoulders should move in a circular
motion, Dr. Angus says. Repeat this
three to five times.

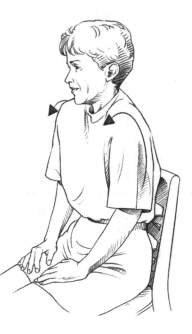

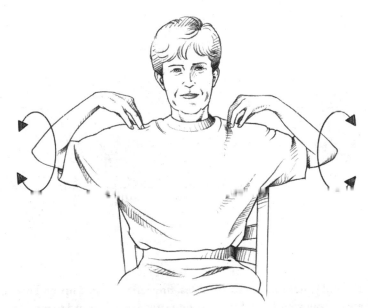

2. ELBOW ROLLS
Put your hands on your shoulders and point each elbow out to the
side. Slowly rotate your elbows in large circles. Do five rotations
forward and five backward.

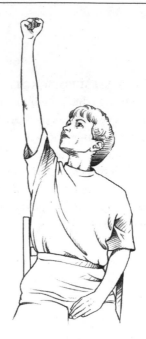

3. ARM REACHES
Lift your right arm up as high as possible, make a fist, and look up at your hand. Hold that position for a count of five, then relax. Do that three to five times with each arm.

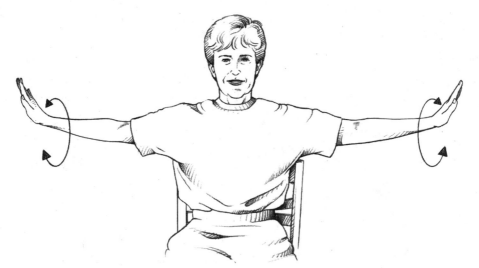

4. ARM ROTATIONS
Extend your arms out to the sides, fingertips turned up, and palms away from your body. Slowly rotate your arms forward in circular motions, 5 to 10 times. To determine how wide a circle to make, start small and increase the size until you feel a gentle stretch. Your circles may be as small as 6 inches or as wide as 2 feet. Repeat the motion in the opposite direction.

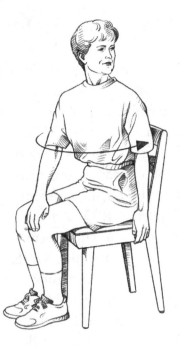

5. SEATED TWISTS
Sitting slightly forward in the chair, take your right hand and put it on your left knee. Place your left hand behind you on the chair seat. Gently twist to your left so that you're looking over your left shoulder (make sure your feet stay flat on the floor, facing forward). Hold this position, breathing gently for a slow count of 10. Relax and repeat this sequence to the right. Do this three times in each direction.

Do it a foot at a time. "You don't have to do all your exercising all at once," Dr. Simonson says. "A person over 60 can easily cover a mile a day by doing errands on foot, walking around the house, cleaning up after herself, or parking a few extra spaces away from the mall."

Do what you can. Maybe you can't always play tennis, walk, or lift weights. But you can still move your body, says Dr. Simonson, who lost nearly 200 pounds in two years. Sit in a chair and kick your feet up in the air, bend over and reach for your toes, pretend you're riding a bicycle and pedal your feet up and down, or play classical music on your stereo and flail your arms like a conductor.

"Every bit of exercise will help you burn calories," says Dr. Simonson,

Your Buffet Survival Guide

Buffets may seem like a deal because they offer a wide selection of foods at a reasonable price. But unless you choose wisely, you could unwittingly load your plate with harmful amounts of calories and fat.

"People who are retired adore buffets. You have to be careful, though, because you can easily eat a meal that is more than 50 percent of calories from fat, because a lot of foods at these places are fried or drenched in butter or oils. But if you have some self-control, you can do well at a buffet," says Cheryl Pingleton, R.D., a dietitian at the Grand Court Lifestyles, a retirement community in Phoenix.

Here are some ways to make the most of the buffet, according to Pingleton and John Foreyt, Ph.D., director of the Nutrition Research Clinic at Baylor College of Medicine in Houston.

Eat something before you go. The worst thing that you can do is to skip breakfast or lunch so that you can chow down at the buffet later in the day. By the time you hit the buffet line, you'll be so hungry that you won't make wise food choices.

Make it a hike. Nab a table as far from the buffet as possible. It will lessen your temptation to graze or go back for seconds.

Serve yourself just once. It's easy to pile on food and turn your plate into a mountain at a buffet, then eat it all and go back for more. Just grab one plate and only go through the line once. Stick with small portions, too. No two foods should overlap each other on your plate.

Make the most of the salad bar. Go for gelatin or plain green salads. Stay away from fat- and calorie-laden creamed or potato salads. If you

who considers herself a senior. "If you don't feel like exercising, just try it for 5 minutes. Even that can make a difference."

Fine-Tune Your Eating Habits

After 60, some people have already given up so much—their teeth, their eyesight, their sex lives—that they don't want to make drastic

insist on using dressing, stick with oil-based ones like Italian or French that have a bit less fat. Even then, take no more than half a ladle full and lightly flavor the salad instead of drenching it.

Go for the grilled. Look for baked, roasted, or grilled entrées like a fish fillet or lean roast beef. Avoid anything that is breaded or fried like fish sticks or chicken. If you must get fried chicken, remove the skin before you eat it.

See through your soup. Pick a broth soup over a creamed one. It will drastically cut the calories in your meal.

Dab oil away. Try dabbing off any visible oils on vegetables like green beans or corn with paper napkins or stick to fresh veggies like tomatoes and carrot sticks. Avoid vegetables served in creamy sauces—they have more calories and fat. Vegetables that look as though they have been cooked in water can be risky, too, because they often are covered with butter.

Ask for a baked potato. Whipped potatoes are fatty because buffets usually add whole milk and butter. Use margarine and chives on your baked potato or eat it plain. Stay away from gravies and sour creams.

Be wary of rolls. Some buffets smear butter-flavored oil on top of their rolls. If a roll appears oily, don't eat it. Look for bread sticks, crackers, or sliced whole-wheat bread instead.

Keep the ending light. For dessert, reach for fresh fruit, sorbet, or frozen yogurt instead of ice cream, muffins, or pies.

changes in their diets in order to control weight, says Edith Howard Hogan, R.D., a spokesperson for the American Dietetic Association in Washington, D.C.

And you don't have to. "Small changes can add up to big differences in weight," Hogan says. "All it takes is a few little daily adjustments that are so easy that you really shouldn't have any problem incorporating them into a winning weight-control effort." Here's a sampling.

Conquer Your Cravings

Cravings are a paradox. If you say no, they just keep coming back again and again. So say yes once in a while. "If you don't give in to cravings occasionally, your weight-control effort is headed for failure, because denying yourself too often sets you up for binges. Once a month or so, let yourself have a couple of spoonfuls of the foods you love," says Maria Simonson, Sc.D., Ph.D., director of the Health, Weight, and Stress Clinic at the Johns Hopkins Medical Institutions in Baltimore.

Wait out the wave. Cravings surge and ebb like waves. So instead of dashing for the kitchen, wait 10 minutes, and the craving will probably subside, Dr. Simonson says.

Get naked. "If you're determined to eat something that you shouldn't, take all of your clothes off and sit in front of a mirror as you eat," Dr. Simonson says. Believe me, you will not be tempted to do it again for a very long time."

Face your tormentor. Schedule a time when you won't be interrupted for 10 to 20 minutes. Then place the food you usually crave in front of you. Look at it, think about why you want it, then eat half of it and throw the rest away, says Peter Miller, Ph.D., executive director of the Hilton Head Health Institute in Hilton Head, South Carolina. Do that three times a week, eating smaller and smaller portions each time.

Feast on imaginary doughnuts. One simple way to fight off a craving is to imagine yourself giving in to it, says Barbara Morse, an imagery counselor and recreational therapist in San Diego. Visualize a doughnut shop, grocery store, or favorite restaurant that has lots of tempting but fattening foods. Now choose one, two, or as many as you would like. Sit down with your doughnuts and eat them bit by bit, savoring each mouthful. Feel the bites going down your throat and into your stomach. Continue to eat doughnuts until you feel full.

Repeat this visualization whenever you feel a craving for your favorite food. Eventually, you should be able to think "doughnut" and immediately feel full and satisfied without having to eat.

Plan your meals. Take a moment just before you go to bed or when you wake in the morning to go over your meal strategy for the day, Dr. Miller says. Jot down when you're going to eat, where you're going to eat, what you're going to eat, and try to stick to it. Imagine yourself making the right food choices throughout the day and feeling good about yourself.

Make your kitchen convenient, not cozy. If your kitchen is too comfortable, you'll be tempted to spend more time there nibbling on snacks and other foods. "Some people have a television, a rocking chair, and a desk in their kitchens. It's the focal point of their homes, and if they have a weight problem, the first thing they need to do is get all of that stuff out of there," Cerino says.

Cancel your membership in the clean plate club. A lot of us in this age group grew up with, "Oh, good for you, you cleaned all the food off of your plate," says Barbara Beahm, R.D., a registered dietitian in Great Bend, Kansas, and a spokesperson for the Kansas Dietetic Association. But as we age, that philosophy can make it harder to keep weight down.

"Breaking away from the clean plate club takes some effort. But one way to do it is to ask yourself, before you eat those last bits of food on your plate, what is more wasteful: To throw something away or to carry unnecessary pounds around on your waist that will add to your risk of stroke, heart disease, cancer, and other medical problems?" Beahm says.

Never say never. "When someone tells me, 'I love cheesecake, but I'm never going to eat it again,' I can guarantee you that she's either going to drop out of our weight-loss group or be one of the few who have gained weight after six weeks," Dr. Klesges says.

If you want to reach your weight goal, strive for moderation, not denial, Dr. Simonson says. Remember that even the experts cheat once in a while.

Become a stove-top eater. Instead of putting foods into serving bowls and placing them on the table, take modest portions—so that they don't overlap on your plate—right from pots and pans in the oven or on the stove, Beahm says. Then quickly wrap up any leftovers and put them away before you eat. You'll be less tempted to go back for seconds, and you'll probably end up with a spare meal in the freezer instead of a spare tire around your belly.

10 Quick Low-Calorie Snacks

Here are 10 snacks—all 100 calories or less—that can satisfy your taste buds and still fit into your weight-control effort. This list was developed by Marilyn Cerino, R.D., coordinator of the weight-management and nutrition programs at the Benjamin Franklin Center for Health in Philadelphia.

- 3 chocolate kisses, 75 calories, 4.5 grams of fat
- 24 fresh grapes, 81 calories, 0 gram of fat
- 1 cup fresh strawberries with 1 tablespoon confectioner's sugar, 86 calories, 0 gram of fat
- $\frac{1}{2}$ cup cranberry juice over ice with club soda and an orange slice, 91 calories, 0 gram of fat
- 5 vanilla wafers, 93 calories, 3 grams of fat
- 19 pieces of candy corn, 95 calories, 1.9 grams of fat
- 2 tablespoons low-fat yogurt topped with $\frac{1}{2}$ cup cherries and 2 teaspoons sliced almonds, 96 calories, 3 grams of fat
- 2 cups warm air-popped popcorn tossed with 1 teaspoon melted margarine and 1 teaspoon honey, 97 calories, 3.8 grams of fat
- $\frac{1}{2}$ cup sugar-free instant pudding with skim milk and $\frac{1}{2}$ teaspoon shaved semi-sweet chocolate, 99 calories, 0.6 grams of fat
- 10 (1-inch) cubes of angel food cake topped with $\frac{1}{4}$ cup frozen raspberries in light syrup, 100 calories, 0 gram of fat

Slow down and chew. Take your time and enjoy eating, Beahm suggests. If you eat too fast, your stomach may be full long before the message to stop chowing down reaches your brain. That is particularly true after age 60 when your digestive tract reacts more leisurely to food. To prevent overeating, allow at least 20 minutes for every meal.

When you're eating, ask yourself if you really tasted and enjoyed that previous bite of food. If the answer is no, then it's time to slow down the conveyor belt from the plate to your mouth, Beahm says.

Put your fork down between bites and chew carefully so that you have time to savor the flavors and textures of the food in your mouth, she says. Glance at the clock before you begin eating. If you're finished within 5 minutes, try to stretch that out to 8 minutes during the next meal. Gradually increase the time it takes you to eat until you reach 20 minutes, Beahm says.

Try downsizing. Use salad plates and smaller serving dishes. It will squelch your appetite and shave calories off your meals, Dr. Simonson says.

In restaurants ask for a child's portion or request that the waiter put half of the entrée into a take-home bag before serving you with the remaining portion, she says.

Lop off fat. Trimming the visible fats off meats can save you about 60 calories per meal, Hogan says. Over a year, that can add up to 21,000 calories. And that's 6½ pounds less fat that you have to worry about gaining. Slashing other fats including cooking oils from your recipes can make another huge dent in your weight. (For more tips on the low-fat lifestyle, see Low-Fat Eating on page 3.)

Fiber up. Fibrous foods like fruits, vegetables, beans, and grains are good for weight control because they are packed with nutrients and usually have few calories. Fiber also adds bulk to your diet, so you'll feel full faster and eat less, Beahm says.

A person over 60 should be eating 25 to 30 grams of fiber a day (one orange has about 3 grams) for weight control and to prevent heart disease and cancer, Beahm says.

Drink water. Have an 8-ounce glass of water about 10 minutes before you eat, Dr. Simonson says. That way, your stomach will already have something in it, and you won't need to eat as much to feel full.

Munch on carbs first. Kick off meals with a food rich in carbohydrates like an angel hair pasta appetizer or bean or noodle soup, Dr. Blackburn says. That should lessen your fat craving 20 minutes into the meal, and you probably won't yearn for calorie-laden, high-fat desserts.

Eat six a day. If you eat smaller meals more frequently, you'll be less likely to overindulge, Hogan says. After breakfast, have a midmorning snack like yogurt or an apple. Have a hearty lunch entrée like stew, baked

How I Did It: An Expert Learns the Hard Way

Unlike some weight-loss experts who have never had to shed a pound in their lives, at age 70-plus, Maria Simonson, Sc.D., Ph.D., knows your struggle all too well.

"I know how you feel. I know how easy it is to psychologically pounce onto an excuse so that you have a reason to hold on to that weight," says Dr. Simonson, director of the Health, Weight, and Stress Clinic at the Johns Hopkins Medical Institutions in Baltimore. Why does she know? Well, after a stroke at age 50 temporarily immobilized her, she ballooned up to 348 pounds.

"I could've gotten out of my wheelchair after six months, but everyone was feeling sorry for me, and I gloried in it. I only got on my feet when the wheelchair got too small," says Dr. Simonson. Then one day when she was preparing to speak about malnutrition to a group of medical interns, she overheard one of them say, "That fat tub is going to lecture about malnutrition? I bet she doesn't even know how to spell it."

That night she took all of her clothes off and stood in front of a mirror. "I thought, 'My God, I have let myself become this. I won't live another five years if I keep on this way.' I made up my mind right then to start anew," Dr. Simonson says.

It was a struggle. In fact, she tried at least four commercial weight-loss programs without success.

"I'd lose 4, 5, or maybe 10 pounds. Then I'd go on a working and traveling binge, eating whatever I could get my hands on," Dr. Simonson says. "Sometimes I'd go to these professional dinner meetings and I'd tell myself, 'Oh, I'm just going to have one more helping of a piece of cake.' That would just blow all of my good resolutions to hell, and the next thing I knew my weight was back up there.

chicken breast, or spaghetti. Then have a late-afternoon snack like cheese and crackers, a small dinner, and a light evening snack like a scoop of nonfat frozen yogurt.

"Finally, I decided that if I really wanted to lose weight, I'd have to do it myself. Reading about it, thinking about it, being told about it were all fine. But it was up to me to follow a program and be consistent."

So Dr. Simonson and her friend, Gwen Campbell, who also was trying to lose weight, decided to develop their own program.

For weight loss, she cut back on what she ate and began walking. For motivation, Dr. Simonson began noticing other people who were overweight and told herself that although she looked like them now, she wouldn't for much longer. And for inspiration, she prayed.

"It may sound old-fashioned, but I asked God to help me, and it made a difference," she says. "I began to realize that it's not just what you eat but how you feel that is important."

Her early success inspired her to co-found the weight-loss clinic at Johns Hopkins, where she continued losing weight along with her patients. Within two years she lost 190 pounds, and she still maintains 158 pounds on her 5-foot-6 frame.

"Losing that weight gave me a better sense of self-esteem. I learned to develop self-discipline and hold on to it," Dr. Simonson says. "Of course, I still have foods that tempt me, like chocolate eclairs. I love them. But if I get a tremendous craving, I'll talk to myself. I'll say, 'Do you really want to wear a size 52 dress again?' Even when I do give in, I'll cut off about a quarter of it for myself and give the rest to my 110-pound housekeeper.

"A friend of mine keeps a reminder on her refrigerator which reads, 'You deserve the best. That means a long, healthy life with your husband, not a piece of cheesecake.' I think it's one of the most practical and self-motivating pieces of advice to remember," says Dr. Simonson. "You are worth the effort. Always bear that in mind."

Eat breakfast. Skipping meals, especially breakfast, puts your body on a starvation alert. So it is more likely to conserve fat instead of shedding it, Emmons says. Eating such foods as toast, cereal, and leftover pasta early in

When Weight Loss Is a Danger Sign

Although being overweight after 60 poses far more health risks than being underweight, an unwanted plunge in weight is worrisome, too, says Maurice Larocque, M.D., a bariatric doctor in Montreal.

"People who are underweight and healthy usually live longer than people who are overweight. So if a person is underweight because they're physically active and don't overeat, that's good," says Dr. Larocque.

But a sudden, unexplained weight loss should be checked out by a physician because it can seriously weaken the heart or be an early warning sign of cancer, says Dr. Larocque.

If you're not ill, but your appetite diminishes, as it often does after age 60, it's important to increase the amount of protein in your diet and keep exercising to help the body retain lean muscle and keep the heart and other muscles working efficiently, Dr. Larocque says.

Once you lose muscle, it's harder to get it back as you get older, he says. And what takes its place? Cancer-promoting and heart disease–inducing body fat.

So if you're eating fewer calories than usual, he recommends having at least 1 gram of protein for every 2 pounds of body weight. If you weight 150 pounds, for instance, you need about 70 grams from kidney

the morning will get you off on the right caloric track for the rest of the day and help you fend off the afternoon munchies.

If you need another incentive, consider that breakfast skippers—no matter their weight—are three times more prone to develop heart disease and stroke-inducing blood clots than people who stop to taste their oatmeal, according to researchers at Memorial University of Newfoundland in St. Johns.

Brown-bag it. Prepare your lunch the night before, even if you're retired, Dr. Larocque says. If you do it right after dinner, you'll be more thoughtful and probably select lower-calorie foods than you might other-

beans; skim milk; low-fat cheese, yogurt, and other dairy products; lean meats like pork tenderloin; tuna fish; potatoes; and other protein-rich foods, Dr. Larocque says. Read nutrition labels to find out how much protein a food contains, he suggests.

To rekindle your appetite, try these ideas.

Have a before-dinner drink. In moderation alcohol stimulates hunger. So if you drink, have no more than a 2-ounce glass of wine or beer about 20 minutes before you're going to eat to prime your digestive tract, says Marilyn Cerino, R.D., coordinator of the weight-management and nutrition programs at the Benjamin Franklin Center for Health in Philadelphia.

Appearance counts. How a meal looks matters to you, especially after age 60 when the senses of taste, smell, and other cues that trigger appetite naturally fade, Cerino says. Use colorful plates and napkins—orange seems to spark hunger pangs best. Try to serve three foods of differing colors, textures, and temperature at each meal, she says.

Keep track of time. Carry a small pocket alarm clock and set it to go off every 3 to 4 hours as a reminder to eat. Even if you only have a piece of bread or fruit, the alarm may help you establish regular eating times and tweak your appetite, Cerino says.

with. Choose the next day when you're famished.

Dine light at night. Eat your smallest meal of the day for dinner, especially if you are going to be watching television, playing bingo, or doing another sedentary activity in the evening, Hogan says. If you eat most of your calories early in the day when you are most active, you'll have more opportunities to burn them off before they turn into fat, she says. So try a tuna salad or lean turkey breast sandwich and a cup of soup instead of a full-course dinner.

Keep a top 10 list. Write down 10 healthy foods such as carrots or fig bars on an index card and carry it with you, Dr. Miller suggests. Then when you have a craving or are tempted by a high-calorie food, you'll have a handy list of alternatives. Update your list once a week so that you'll always have a few new foods to try.

Alternate yellow and green. To ensure that you're getting plenty of nutrients like vitamins A, B, and C after you begin a weight-control effort, eat fresh, low-calorie yellow or orange vegetables like squash, pumpkin, and carrots one day then switch to green vegetables such as fresh spinach, turnip greens, or dark leafy lettuces the next day, says Virginia Stoner, in her seventies, past president of the Dietary Managers Association and a certified dietary manager from Hampstead, Maryland.

Imbibe cautiously. Alcohol is a double-edged sword. It seems to have a beneficial effect on the heart. But one serving of alcohol contains more than 100 calories, and it hinders your body's ability to burn fat, Hogan says.

Alcohol also can stimulate appetite and impair your judgment so that your willpower to control what you're eating collapses. If you insist on indulging, limit yourself to one serving, Cerino suggests. That's one 12-ounce beer, 6 ounces of wine, or one cocktail containing 1 ounce of liquor a day.

Control it with carbs. "I've found in my weight-management classes that people who avoid eating complex carbohydrates like potatoes and bread in the mistaken belief that these foods are fattening, turn instead to chocolate and sweets in the late afternoon," Beahm says.

And instead of filling you up, sugary sweets can actually stimulate your appetite, Dr. Blackburn says.

Eating at least six servings of grains, pastas, and other complex carbohydrates a day can dampen urges for candies, cakes, and other fattening snacks, Beahm says.

Don't touch the finger foods. Most people will eat more with their fingers than they do with a knife and fork. So avoid keeping a large stash of finger foods like nuts, chips, and cookies in your house and stay away from entrées like fried chicken, too. Buy smaller packages and only have one open at a time, Dr. Simonson says.

Pass on the peanuts. A 2-ounce serving of salted peanuts has 328 calories. If you need to nibble on something crunchy, reach for pretzels instead—20 small ones have as little as 80 calories, and most are fat-free.

You can just eat one. If you insist on eating high-fat, high-calorie snacks like peanuts or potato chips, don't eat them right out of the package. Instead, divide the chips into individual servings and store them in plastic sandwich bags for later use. That way, when you reach for these snacks, you'll be less tempted to eat more than you should, Emmons says.

Skip the fried shrimp. Boiled shrimp have about 84 calories per 3-ounce serving compared to 206 calories if they're fried, Dr. Simonson says.

Pick pumpkin pies. If you love pie, stick to pumpkin or fruit types. They're lower in calories, Dr. Simonson says. Pecan pie, for instance, has about 430 calories a slice compared to 240 for pumpkin. You cut another 100 calories off if you don't eat the crust, she says.

Back off bacon. An ounce of bacon (slightly more than four medium slices) has 163 calories. A 1-ounce slice of Canadian bacon is leaner and only has about 57 calories, Dr. Simonson says.

Prescription for Prevention

As we age, metabolism slows and fat begins to account for a greater percentage of body weight. Overall, the average person gains about a pound a year after age 35. This extra body fat can increase the production of sex hormones such as estrogen that promote colon, breast, and endometrial cancer. Increased body fat also drives up blood pressure, forces the heart to work harder, and raises LDL—the bad cholesterol that contributes to the clogging of arteries and in-

Do:

- *Write down your three most important motivators for losing weight. Read and think for 5 minutes twice a day about what those motivators mean to you.*

- *Unwind. Practice a relaxation technique such as guided imagery twice a day. The more relaxed you are, the more open you'll be to positive thoughts that will help keep your weight under control.*

- *Sit down with your family and close friends and discuss why you want to lose weight and what they can do to help.*

- *Exercise regularly. Try walking 30 minutes a day, three times a week.*

- *Serve yourself directly from the stove and immediately put leftovers away. That will discourage overeating.*

- *Eat six smaller meals instead of three large ones.*

- *Use smaller plates and chew slowly.*

Don't:

- *Weigh yourself daily. Small fluctuations can be discouraging. Step on the scale no more than once a week. The results will seem more dramatic.*

- *Be pressured into eating something that you don't want. Keep saying no thank you until the person tempting you gives up.*

- *Make your kitchen too comfortable. You'll be tempted to spend more time there nibbling on snacks and other foods.*

- *Keep a large stash of nuts, chips, and other snacks in your house. Buy smaller packages and only have one open at a time.*

Chapter 7

Exercise

Protective Programs Designed Just for You

You don't want buns of steel. You want to steel your defenses against diseases that kill. And you would like to do it without stressing the bones, joints, and muscles that need more TLC with each passing year.

Yes, physical activity is good for you. But if you're like most people ages 60 and over, you bypass the exercise programs, books, and videos that shout "no pain, no gain." And you have made the smart choice. Research shows that moderate exercise gives you as much—maybe even more—protection from disease as the old grunt-and-groan-and-sweat type of workout.

"Moderate exercise can help you lower your risk of disease and carry on an active lifestyle beyond your eighties," says James M. Rippe, M.D., director of the Center for Clinical and Lifestyle Research at Tufts University School of Medicine in Boston and author of *Fit over Forty*.

Two-Phase Program for Protection

Experts today recommend a two-part exercise program: aerobic exercise (walking or bicycling, for example) to condition your heart and cardiovascular system, and strength-training exercises (calisthenics and high-intensity weight lifting) to build muscle and cut fat. And you need to exercise only two or three times a week.

You can ease into this routine gradually and safely. That's a big plus since "by age 60, just about everyone has some element of osteoarthritis, osteoporosis, joint irritation, or lack of flexibility," says Dr. Rippe. "Light exercise doesn't aggravate these conditions." In fact, exercise usually reduces them.

If you join exercise groups or walking clubs, you reap even more benefits—social activity and new friends. "We like to call this recreation, not exercise," says Gerald Fletcher, M.D., professor of medicine at the Mayo Clinic in Jacksonville, Florida.

Experts note that exercisers enjoy a better quality of life. "Exercisers are more active in the rest of their lives," says Dr. Rippe. "Many of the age-related declines that we see are tied to the expectation that people become more sedentary and uninterested in things around them as they age. It is true that if you're inactive, your metabolism slows, you gain weight, and you become even more inactive. But it doesn't have to be like that."

Stay Young at Heart

Researchers have found that exercise can give your body's systems the capacity to work as well as someone 20 years younger. So it is not surprising that physically active people—regardless of their biological ages—have lower rates of heart disease and are less vulnerable to strokes.

If you haven't exercised for years, don't be put off: "As soon as you start to exercise, your risk of cardiovascular problems drops by 25 percent," says Dr. Fletcher.

"Studies show that even if you start a regular exercise program in your sixties, you lower your risk of heart disease for the rest of your life," says Dr. Rippe. "If you're 60 years old, you may have another 25 years left, so the quality of life during those years is something to think about."

Don't let a heart attack hold you back. "Exercise has been proven to be a great therapy," says Kenneth H. Cooper, M.D., president and founder of the Cooper Clinic and the Cooper Institute for Aerobics in Dallas, who is also known as the father of aerobics. Studies show that people who become involved in an exercise program after their first heart attacks are 20 to 40 percent more likely to be alive seven years later than those who survived a heart attack and then remained totally sedentary.

Exercise is so important that cardiologists often prescribe (not just recommend or suggest) exercise for patients with heart disease, observes Alan Rozanski, M.D., director of nuclear cardiology and cardiac stress testing at St. Luke's Hospital in New York City.

In one study, researchers followed 68 patients who were on a waiting list for heart transplants and who also participated in an exercise program of graded walking. After three to six months, the hearts of 30 patients had improved to the point that they no longer needed new hearts. Two years later, their hearts were still going strong.

How does aerobic exercise perform these miracles? It makes your heart pump more vigorously to carry extra blood and oxygen to hard-working muscles. Over time, the demands of exercise make your heart physically fit—stronger and more efficient. "The heart becomes a bigger, stronger pump that pumps more blood with each beat," says Bryant Stamford, Ph.D., professor of exercise physiology and director of the Health Promotion Center at the University of Louisville in Kentucky.

You get practical payoffs: The well-exercised heart doesn't have to beat as fast when you do something demanding. Even though your body is stressed, your heart isn't. When nonexercisers shovel the sidewalk after a snowstorm, for instance, their likelihood of a heart attack jumps to 107 times their normal risk. Someone who exercises five times a week has a risk that rises to only 2.4 times.

Drive High Blood Pressure Down

Heart attacks and strokes don't come out of the blue. Much of the trouble that leads to these killers starts in the arteries, the tubes that carry the blood and allow it to flow to the body's organs. High blood pressure, a condition that becomes more common with advancing years, often sets the stage for all the other problems. Exercise can help get it down.

When you have high blood pressure, the blood circulates too vigorously under too much force. The pressure tears up the artery walls, which allows the harmful low-density lipoprotein (LDL) cholesterol to attach and form plaque. Over time, this turns arteries that used to be as smooth and efficient as the interstate into the equivalent of one-lane gravel roads.

215

When You Need the Doctor's Okay

It is always a good idea to check with your doctor before you begin an exercise program. But it is a must if you have more than two risk factors for heart disease, says Gerald Fletcher, M.D., professor of medicine at the Mayo Clinic in Jacksonville, Florida.

These risk factors are high cholesterol levels, high blood pressure, diabetes, a smoking habit, or a family history of heart disease.

If you're at risk for heart problems, your doctor probably will want to do an exercise tolerance test to check for cardiovascular disease, custom-design an exercise program to ease you into the swing of things, and monitor your progress.

"High blood pressure wouldn't be such a serious problem if it didn't do so much damage to artery walls," says Dr. Stamford.

"We think exercise lowers blood pressure because it opens up the small vessels and capillaries and helps blood flow into the working muscles that need the extra nourishment," says Dr. Stamford. An added benefit for the muscles: They become better able to absorb oxygen and glucose (blood sugar). Exercisers with high blood pressure often find that exercise lowers it, which in turn allows their doctors to lower or eliminate their medications.

You reap the benefits of exercise long after your workout, even when you are lolling in a recliner with the newspaper. That is because exercise lowers the resting heart rate, which reduces pressure on the whole cardiovascular system, says Dr. Stamford.

If the blood flow gets blocked completely, which becomes more likely as the arteries narrow, you could have a heart attack (if an artery to the heart gets blocked) or stroke (if the blockage occurs in an artery leading to the brain). This happens when the platelets—the tiny disklike structures that help the blood coagulate—stick to each other and to the artery walls to create a clot. Exercise reduces your risk because it keeps the platelets from clustering excessively and damming the flow.

When you exercise, you also protect your artery walls. Studies in Europe suggest that a combination of diet and exercise decreases the soft plaque that gradually builds up and hardens, narrowing the artery.

The Honolulu Heart Program on Oahu, Hawaii, conducted a 22-year study of 5,362 Japanese-American men ages 55 to 68. The researchers found that nonexercisers were four times more likely to experience one type of stroke and three times more likely to experience another type of stroke when compared to more active men.

Get a Grip with the Good Cholesterol

Any time you exercise, your body ends up with more of the high-density lipoproteins, or HDLs. That's the so-called good cholesterol that grabs the harmful LDL cholesterol and carries it out of the bloodstream before it can attach to artery walls. The biggest predictor of future heart disease is an HDL reading below 35, says Dr. Cooper. (That number is a measure of milligrams per deciliter or mg/dl.)

"We used to think that you had to exercise vigorously to raise HDL levels. But now we think that moderate amounts of low-key exercise such as walking can increase HDL levels by about 10 percent," says Dr. Rippe.

Researchers at Stanford University studied men and women ages 50 to 65 who exercised lightly. After two years, an HDL check showed that 52 percent of the exercisers had lowered their risk of heart disease by 10 percent. Another study showed that women who walked a slow 3 miles four or five times a week also upped their HDL levels. And a joint study of postmenopausal women showed that while good cholesterol levels rose with exercise, the amounts of artery-clogging LDL cholesterol dropped.

As you get older, your arteries gradually stiffen, which increases your risk of atherosclerosis, unless you take steps to flex them by exercising your body. Researchers at the Gerontology Research Center in Baltimore evaluated the arteries of 146 older men and women. The arteries of exercisers were up to one-third more flexible than those of couch potatoes.

Build Your Muscles to Block Disease

Strength-training exercises put one of the major risk factors in heart disease, cancer, and stroke into reverse—the otherwise inevitable increase

Exercise: All-Purpose Protection

Beyond combating heart disease, cancer, and stroke, exercise helps fight off or control a lot of other health problems. Here's what else.

Betters your balance. As you age, your risk of falling increases. Studies show that weight lifting or balance training improves overall balance. In healthy community-dwelling elders, tai chi has been shown to decrease fall rates.

Improves your sex life. Researchers have found that physical impotence often results from poor blood circulation to the penis. Since exercise improves circulation on a system-wide basis, doctors speculate that it will help reduce the problem.

Increases mobility. When you work your heart, more blood goes to all parts of your body, including your brain. Those who exercise, studies show, perform better on mental tests and respond faster to stimuli.

Makes more muscle. Strength training also produces larger, stronger muscles. The stress of exercise probably creates microscopic tears in the muscle fibers, according to William J. Evans, Ph.D., a physiology and nutrition researcher at Pennsylvania State University in University Park. In between exercise sessions, the muscles repair and strengthen the fibers and learn to synthesize and use proteins more efficiently. The brain gets into the act, too, putting more muscle cells to work to meet the extra demands.

Improves your mood. "There is no question that exercise has been shown to improve mood and relieve anxiety and depression, although the reasons why are hard to prove in a laboratory setting," says Robert S. Brown, Sr., M.D., Ph.D., clinical professor of psychiatric medicine at the University of Virginia in Charlottesville and a longtime researcher on exercise and its effect on mental health. "I've never treated

of body fat. We're not talking about weight problems here, just the simple fact that as you age, you lose muscle, and it's replaced by fat.

Even if their weight remains unchanged, nonexercisers will probably

a physically fit person with a major depression."

Exercise also produces physiological changes that may elevate mood. "My theory is that exercise—at least to the point of sweating—raises body temperature, which speeds up the metabolism," adds Dr. Brown. "That results in more oxygen going to the brain, optimizing essential chemical reactions." Exercise also releases endorphins, the so-called pleasure chemicals in the brain that can block pain and invoke feelings of well-being—or even euphoria like the much-ballyhooed runner's high experienced by long-distance runners and other athletes.

Controls diabetes. Exercise helps your body produce the insulin that it needs to process glucose (blood sugar) and get it out of the blood and into the cells. "Millions of people are insulin-resistant," says Bryant Stamford, Ph.D., director of the Health Promotion Center at the University of Louisville. Glucose stays in the blood, which creates real problems because it crystallizes. A sugar crystal looks like a medieval mace, a weapon consisting of a ball with spikes on it. It tears up the lining in small blood vessels, which sets the stage for harmful cholesterol to attach to the artery walls and balloon into atherosclerosis, or hardening of the arteries. Exercise can help prevent that.

Strengthens bone. Exercise strengthens bones weakened by osteoporosis because it increases blood flow and helps cells create new, healthier bone. A study at Tufts University in Boston followed 39 women ages 50 to 70 and found that bone mass, muscle mass, strength, and balance all improved with exercise.

Eases joint pain. Because exercise develops the muscles that support your joints, says Dr. Evans, it usually eases the pain of arthritis and other joint ailments.

greet their eightieth birthdays (assuming that they get there) with 30 percent less muscle than they had in their prime.

This alarming ratio makes you older than you have to be. As your

Listen to Your Body

Most exercise-related injuries happen because people try to do more than their bodies can handle. If you're overloading your system, your body will let you know. After exercising, you should be:

Very energetic. Exercise should give you additional energy. "If you're exhausted when you finish exercising, you've overdone it," says fitness pioneer Jack LaLanne. "You should finish a session feeling exhilarated, yet relaxed. That way, you won't do too much and get hurt." If exercise leaves you languid, shorten your walk or lighten your strength-training weights.

If you still haven't recuperated a half-hour after stopping exercise, check with your doctor, says Gerald Fletcher, M.D., professor of medicine at the Mayo Clinic in Jacksonville, Florida.

Clearheaded. A feeling of nausea or faintness lets you know that your efforts are too intense for your body, although these symptoms can also mean that you're not spending enough time on your cooldown exercises. Review your routine. Add or lengthen the cooldown exercises. If that doesn't make a difference, shorten your walk and reduce your weights, says Dr. Fletcher.

Pain-free. Exercise isn't supposed to hurt or leave you feeling stiff (although you may feel some soreness when you begin to exercise). Devote more time to warm-up and cooldown exercises, because they provide maximum protection against aches and pains, says Terri Merritt, a clinical exercise physiologist at the Preventive Medicine Research Institute in Sausalito, California. If problems persist, see your

muscle decreases, stairs feel like a vertical mountain climb. Hefting that can of beans off the kitchen shelf gets harder and harder. And a common sack of groceries feels like an Olympic barbell in your hands. That's not good for your risk of cancer, heart disease, and stroke—and certainly not good if you want to continue to live independently.

One quick encounter with a tape measure will probably give you all

doctor or a fitness expert to rule out underlying problems and to make sure that you are doing exercises correctly.

If you are overweight, your knees may not be strong enough to support you. If they hurt, shorten (or eliminate) your walks and concentrate on strength-training sessions to build up muscles and tendons to take some of the load off the joints, recommends William J. Evans, Ph.D., professor of applied physiology and nutrition and director of the Noll Physiological Research Center at Pennsylvania State University in University Park.

You may experience lower back pain when you start to exercise. That's because, if you have spent a lot of time sitting, your hamstring muscles have shortened. When you walk or exercise, these muscles pull on the buttock muscles which, in turn, yank on the lower back muscles. If your abdominal muscles aren't strong enough to help support the lower back, you'll feel it. Include abdominal-strengthening exercises with your warm-up and cooldown stretches says Merritt.

Remember that warm-up and cooldown exercises protect muscles and tendons as well as the cardiovascular system. Don't try to shorten your workout by omitting them.

Breathing easily. While your breathing rate will increase when you exercise, you should still be able to carry on a conversation. If you can't talk and walk or talk and lift at the same time, your work pace is too intense. Slow down and lighten your weight load, recommends Dr. Fletcher.

the evidence you need that these changes are taking place. Researchers in England have determined that your body's fat level manifests itself in your girth, not just in your weight. You're at the threshold of increased health risk if your waist measures over 31 inches (for most women) or over 37 inches (for most men).

You can't head off the effects of time with diet alone. Researchers

Exercise Danger Signals

When you exercise or do anything strenuous, you put an added burden on your cardiovascular system. If you have any of these symptoms or medical conditions, see your doctor before you start or resume exercise, according to Gerald Fletcher, M.D., professor of medicine at the Mayo Clinic in Jacksonville, Florida.

If you get a headache, cramps, or heart palpitations or if you feel dizzy, faint, or cool while exercising: If you're in the sun, get into the shade or someplace cool.

If you feel any discomfort in your upper body, including your chest, arms, neck, or jaw: You might feel aching, burning, tightness, or a sensation of fullness.

If you start to wheeze: You become very short of breath, or your breathing doesn't return to normal within 5 minutes.

If walking gives you a cramp in one calf that flares up when you walk and simmers down when you rest: This could be a symptom of intermittent claudication, a condition caused by plaque buildup in the arteries of your leg. If that's the case, you may have similar deposits in your coronary arteries.

If you have a substantial infection, such as bronchitis: Put off exercise until all is normal—your temperature, white blood cell count, and cultures. It's okay to exercise if you have a small skin irritation, as long as it is not irritated by exercise.

If you have a cold or the flu: Wait until all symptoms (including fever) have been gone for two days before you exercise again.

think that the changes in your body are connected to age-related alterations in your metabolism and your oxygen intake.

Exercise is your only defense, and it can go a long way toward reversing the loss that leaves you weak and at risk, observes William J. Evans, Ph.D., professor of applied physiology and nutrition and director of the Noll Physiological Research Center at Pennsylvania State University in University Park.

Just how potent are exercise's effects? Healthy men and women ages 56 to 80 participated in a 12-week strength-training program and on average lost 4 pounds of body fat. Their metabolisms increased by 7 percent, which contributed to their needing 15 percent more calories a day just to maintain their weight.

Regular exercise is associated with lower rates of colon cancer, probably because exercise speeds the passage of substances through the gut, according to Dr. Evans. Researchers at the European Institute of Oncology in Milan concluded that exercise might reduce the risk of colon cancer in men by up to one-third.

Laboratory research gives further support to the importance of exercise as a cancer fighter. In one study exercise was tied to increased killer-cell ability to attack tumors in mice. Some studies also suggest that regular exercisers are less likely to develop prostate and breast cancer.

Jump-Start Your Immune System with Exercise

Moderate amounts of exercise not only strengthen you but may also muscle up your immune system, some researchers believe. In fact, when you exercise, your blood platelets and white-blood-cell count go up. During moderate exercise, the body manufactures more natural killer cells, which help keep immunity strong and fight free radicals caused by pollutants. With those two factors on your side, your risk of cancer drops.

Experts believe an immune system strengthened by exercise also may help fight some forms of cancer.

A stronger immune system makes life more pleasant on a day-to-day level, too. "We notice fewer colds, coughs, and bronchitis in people who exercise," says Dr. Fletcher.

Researchers aren't sure how exercise effects the immune system, but Dr. Stamford speculates that "when you exercise, you stress all of your body's systems. The immune system reacts like the body's fire department to take care of the stress."

The rest of the body responds to the stress of exercise by becoming stronger and better able to cope with the next round of demands. It's likely that the immune system muscles in on disease, too.

223

Find the Right Time

It is important to exercise when you can get the maximum benefit without risk. Here is advice from our experts for choosing the right time to work out.

Easy does it, early bird. If you're a morning person, exercise after you have been up and about for at least 10 minutes. While you sleep, fluids sometimes pool throughout your body, even in such important places as the disks in the spinal column, in ligaments, and in muscles, says Richard Birrer, M.D., vice chairman of family medicine at the Catholic Medical Center in New York City. If you get up suddenly and begin to exercise, the accumulated fluids can cause major injuries, such as a herniated disk.

Avoid internal conflicts. Exercising right after eating causes problems because both your intestinal tract and your muscles will need extra blood. The conflicting needs of each system may leave you with cramps or a feeling of nausea or faintness. Give your body 2 hours to complete its digestive chores.

Choose your shots. If you have diabetes, avoid injecting insulin into a muscle that will soon be used for exercise. Working muscles process insulin differently than do nonworking muscles.

Live Easy with Exercise

Okay, you have to make an effort to exercise, but there is a great trade-off. It can make other aspects of your life a lot easier. Here are some of the other things that exercise does to improve your life and battle disease.

Eases sleep. Without good sleep your body is more likely to catch diseases and less able to fight them off. "If you have a low activity level, it's normally hard to sleep," says Richard P. Allen, Ph.D., assistant professor in the Department of Neurology at the Johns Hopkins University Sleep Disorder Center in Baltimore.

A study conducted through Stanford University looked at 43 people ages 50 to 76. Those who exercised four times a week fell asleep faster, slept better and longer, and felt more rested than those who didn't.

Some studies show that exercise helps improve the quality of slow-wave sleep, the phase of rest that produces the strongest sleep experience.

Cuts the fat. Exercise helps the body get rid of triglycerides, a type of fat in the blood linked to an increased risk of heart attacks, generalized atherosclerosis (hardening of the arteries), and other medical problems. Researchers think that exercise enhances an enzyme in the blood and muscles that plucks triglycerides out of the bloodstream.

Trims the pounds. Extra body weight means extra risk for heart disease, cancer, and stroke. If you don't increase your calorie intake and burn at least 700 calories per week (the amount that you would use if you walked for 20 minutes, three times a week), you'll lose weight. Exercise also seems to help your body use the proteins that it takes in more efficiently.

Reduces stress. "It's not stress that kills, per se," says Dr. Cooper. "Rather, it's the way we handle it. And exercise has been shown to help people handle their stress better and thus should lower their incidence of heart disease and other health problems."

Research also suggests that exercise axes thromboxane, a chemical in the blood that promotes clotting and encourages platelets to stick together, which can trigger heart attacks. Nonexercisers with aggressive type A personalities show the highest levels of the chemical.

Lowers the dose. Because exercise helps the heart work better and may speed weight loss, people with heart disease, high blood pressure, or diabetes may show so much improvement that their doctors can lower the dose of their medicines or drop the pills altogether, notes Kaaren Douglas, M.D., director of the program in geriatric medicine at the University of California, Irvine.

Get Off to a Good Start

Here are the guidelines that you'll need to get your total exercise program of aerobic and strength-training exercise off the ground safely.

Get a physical. Exercise works because it stresses your body, which grows stronger as a result. It's important to make sure that your body's systems can handle the extra work, so you'll want to schedule a checkup with your doctor, says Dr. Stamford.

Warm up. Experts recommend 10 to 15 minutes of warm-up activity, which can include stretches, light calisthenics, or slow walking.

As you get older, your body needs to ease into exercise more gradually, according to Richard Birrer, M.D., vice chairman of family medicine at the Catholic Medical Center in New York City. That's because by ages 65 to 70 most physiological systems are down by about a third and take longer to warm up and cool down, notes Dr. Birrer. For example, the pulse rate goes down, he adds.

Break it up . . . or don't. Exercising more than 30 minutes at a time helps you lose weight, if you exercise three to five times a week and follow an appropriate diet, experts say. If you don't need to lose weight, three 10-minute exercise sessions per day will be just as beneficial for disease protection, advises Dr. Stamford.

Set goals. On your first walk or exercise session, you may decide to walk for 10 to 15 minutes and do three repetitions of each exercise.

That may turn out to be too much. Most people don't realize how out of shape they are. "It's not unusual for someone to get halfway around the block and feel winded. You have to start exercising gradually," says Terri Merritt, a clinical exercise physiologist at the Preventive Medicine Research Institute in Sausalito, California, who works closely with Dean Ornish, M.D., whose regimen for reversing heart disease is known the world over.

Don't be discouraged. Says fitness guru and author Jack LaLanne, "Any time you exercise, it's like putting money in the bank. If you can only start with a nickel, that's okay. Eventually, it'll add up. Any exercise is better than no exercise."

"If you haven't walked in 25,000 years, you're going to be winded after a block or two," says comedian Sid Caesar, who started exercising at age 57 to get his life moving toward good health. "But if you keep walking, in another week or two, you won't be."

When you can easily meet your goal, up your efforts. Lengthen your walks or vary the terrain to make the work harder. Increase the number of repetitions for each exercise or add weights to make the exercise more difficult. Don't get carried away, though. Even as you increase the workload, the effort should never be too taxing, according to Merritt.

Time it right. Experts say that you'll be able to stay with your program better if you exercise at the same time each day.

Play it safe. Find a place where you can do the walking phase of your program safely. "Your neighborhood isn't safe if you don't feel safe. If that's the case, look for other locations. Drive to another neighborhood or a public area where you feel comfortable," advises Dr. Douglas.

Mall-walking programs, often operated by hospitals or health centers, provide a haven where you can walk regardless of the weather. Call local malls to find out about programs, suggests Dr. Douglas. She recalls a trip to the Midwest, where "they opened up the mall at 7:00 A.M. just for walkers, and the place was mobbed with people doing laps. There were so many people, they practically knocked me over."

Dress for comfort. Your body has to get rid of the heat produced by exercise, so wear loose-fitting cotton or high-tech fabrics, such as Gore-Tex, that breathe. Use layers of clothing to stay warm and simultaneously dispel perspiration and heat. Use sweat suits only in cold weather when you need to stay warm. In hot weather and in direct sunlight, wear light-colored clothing and a cap to avoid sunburn or overheating, says Merritt.

Wear athletic socks designed to wick perspiration away from your body like acrylic or other breathable materials.

Check the water supply. It's easy to become dehydrated as you exercise. Drink water or juice beforehand to make sure that your system doesn't run dry, especially if the temperature is above 70°F. Bring liquids with you as well. Some experts advise that you take a drink of water every 20 minutes. Avoid excessive coffee, alcohol, and other diuretics that will contribute to dehydration, says Dr. Fletcher.

Cool down. End your session by walking very slowly for 5 minutes or by doing stretching exercises, advises Dr. Fletcher. Don't sit down immediately after exercise; slow movement will help your body cool properly. It will reduce the likelihood of muscle cramps and help the blood circulate. Massaging muscles after your cooldown will also help keep the

Warm Up for Comfort

Before you walk or do strength-training exercises, always ease into the effort by stretching your muscles, which makes them more flexible. If you just jump into vigorous exercise, you could get hurt. "Warm-up exercises that stretch your muscles prevent injury," says William J. Evans, Ph.D., professor of applied physiology and nutrition and director of the Noll Physiological Research Center at Pennsylvania State University in University Park.

"Count up to 30 during most stretches—from the time that you begin the stretch, stretch out, hold the stretch, and return to your normal position," says Richard Birrer, M.D., vice chairman of family medicine at the Catholic Medical Center in New York City.

Some experts recommend about 5 minutes of slow walking, followed by stretching. "I advise older people to go out and walk slowly for the first quarter mile or so, just to warm up their muscles a little, and then stretch," says Kenneth H. Cooper, M.D., president and founder of the Cooper Clinic and the Cooper Institute for Aerobics in Dallas.

While just about any warm-up exercise loosens tense muscles and makes you feel good, concentrate on exercises that work the muscles in your lower body. "They're the most important for mobility, so it's important to stretch, limber, and strengthen those muscles," explains Dr. Evans.

For warm-up exercises, Dr. Evans recommends the modified squats and knee extensions described in this chapter, as well as the following step-ups.

blood moving, according to the American Medical Association.

In hot weather, wearing sweaty clothes after exercise will help your body cool. In cold weather, change wet clothes to help keep warm. Hot showers slow the cooling process, so wait about 45 minutes until your body temperature has returned to normal before you indulge.

Keep tabs on medication. Some medications, even common over-the-

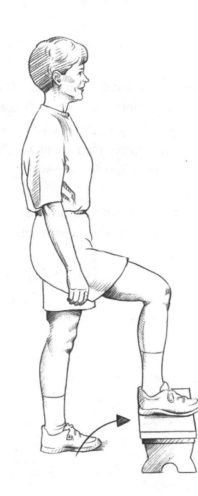

STEP-UPS

For this exercise you will need a step stool, roughly 8 to 10 inches high. Stand with both feet on the floor. Slowly raise your right leg and place your foot on the stool. Using the muscles in your right leg, lift yourself to a standing position on the stool. Hold on to something for support if you have balance problems. Now reverse that motion: Step off the stool, again making sure that your right leg does all the work. Repeat 10 to 15 times. Then repeat the exercise with the left leg.

counter medicines such as decongestants, raise your rate and blood pressure. Dr. Fletcher suggests that you decrease exercise if you're on medication.

One word of caution: We haven't suggested that you take your pulse because, if you're on medication, your readings may not accurately reflect the stress of exercise to your system. To keep from overdoing it, make a habit of methodically estimating your level of exertion. If you want to take your pulse anyway, don't take it by pressing on the artery in your neck. That can cause a stroke. You can safely take your pulse by pressing your wrist, says Dr. Fletcher.

Walk toward Longevity

Ideally, half of your exercise program should consist of aerobic exercise. And to many experts, walking is the aerobic exercise of choice, especially for people age 60 and over. That's because when you walk, the pressure on your joints never rises above 1.5 times your body weight. Jogging or dance or step aerobic exercise can put a lot more pressure—4 times your weight or more—on your bones.

Start slowly and gradually increase the length and difficulty of your walks, says Dr. Rippe. Here's how to strengthen your heart without overtaxing your system.

Try airport aerobics. To get the most benefit, walk briskly—imagine that you're walking through the airport to catch a plane, suggests Dr. Stamford. But don't overdo it. Start your walking program with a goal of 10 to 15 minutes, advises Dr. Douglas.

If you are really out of shape and concerned that you may get too tired to make it back home, wear a watch. Check the time when you start to walk and keep walking around the block until you get a little tired. Glance at your watch to see how long you have walked. That's the length that your walks should be for the next week or two, explains Dr. Douglas.

"If you get tired on the way home, stop, rest, then walk some more," advises Dr. Douglas. Some days you may tire more easily or the work may seem too much. Just shorten your session.

Once you're comfortable, you can gradually increase the length of your walks by about 10 percent every two weeks, according to Dr. Fletcher.

Keep it constant. Try to maintain the same level of exertion for your entire walk. That way, you'll ask your heart to work hard (but not too hard) for your entire session. Your heart gets the biggest benefit from a sustained workout.

You may want to use walking as part of your warm-up. If that's the case, make this phase of your routine slower and more relaxed, says Dr. Fletcher.

Slow for hills. If you come to a hill, forget the heroics. Slow your pace to maintain the same level of exertion that you had on level ground.

Track the temperature. Your work will seem harder if it's hot or humid. Adjust your speed and intensity so that you stay at the right exertion level. If the temperature soars—say, over 95°F with 80 percent humidity—don't exercise outside for more than 30 to 45 minutes, advises Dr. Fletcher. If you have heart problems, reduce your time in the heat by at least 25 percent.

Get More Health from Your Walks

Once you get into a regular walking program and can keep up a set pace, vary it. "If you do the same thing over and over, your muscles aren't challenged and they don't respond as well—and you can get bored. I change my program every three to four weeks," says LaLanne. Here are ways to keep a little pep in your step.

Step lively. Take a tip from racewalkers. They take short steps and get their speed by packing a lot of steps into each minute, says Dr. Stamford.

Weigh it down. Weighted belts are popular. If your condition permits it, the belt will add extra resistance, according to Dr. Evans. Or you can load a knapsack with plastic jars full of water or sand, starting at 2 to 3 pounds and then gradually working up to heavier weights. (Weigh yourself on a bathroom scale—with and without the containers—so that you'll know how heavy your homemade weights are.) When you walk with weight on your back, you'll expend more effort, he adds.

Walk with a swing. The more you move around, the more intense your workout. Swing your arms vigorously. Raise them and punch at the sky, first with one arm and then with the other. "You can get a great cardiovascular workout in 12 to 17 minutes if your exercise is vigorous," says LaLanne.

Beef Up Your Muscles to Pummel Disease

Toning your muscles isn't just an exercise in vanity. When you build muscle, the ratio of body muscle to body fat tips a little more in your favor.

Test Your Rate of Perceived Exertion

The Rate of Perceived Exertion (or Borg) scale lets you decide whether you're exercising hard enough, not hard enough, or going beyond your limits, without taking your pulse. It's easy to use, and you can do it yourself.

First, make a mental scale.

The exertion or Borg scale uses a 6 to represent the least difficult activity—lying down and doing nothing. Twenty—the upper end of the scale—means that you would be working so hard that you couldn't take another step.

Exercise that's very light rates a 7, fairly light gets an 11, and work that is just plain hard gets a 15.

Until your body gets used to the work, keep your exercise between 11 (fairly light) and 14 (somewhat hard). Don't exercise above 15, says Gerald Fletcher, M.D., professor of medicine at the Mayo Clinic in Jacksonville, Florida.

If you wish to increase your fitness level, gradually increase your level (no faster than one level every week or two) until you reach 15. At this point you will begin to get short of breath and feel that you can't go much longer, says Terri Merritt, a clinical exercise physiologist at the Preventive Medicine Research Institute in Sausalito, California.

She explains that you don't have to increase levels or work up the scale if you are just trying to maintain your fitness.

Within the range of 11 to 15, you will be working at between 50 percent and 85 percent of your peak heart rate, where you will get the maximum benefit to your circulatory system.

As you get more accustomed to exercise, you can vary the intensity and the duration. A long walk at a low level of activity, perhaps 11, will give you just as much benefit as a shorter workout at a more intense exertion level of 14.

As you become more fit, you will also find that you have to work longer to get the same degree of exertion.

This lowers your risk of cancer, heart disease, and stroke.

Here's how to get started with a calisthenics program, in which you use your body's own weight to work your muscles. You'll need to work some muscle groups with light weight-lifting exercises using weights that you make or buy.

Use these basic guidelines from Dr. Evans to get the most out of all your exercises.

Keep it slow. Perform all exercises slowly. Unless otherwise noted, spend 2 seconds in the lifting phase of the exercise and 4 to 6 seconds in the lowering part. If you move too quickly, you won't get the muscle-strengthening benefits and you could hurt yourself.

Remember the ins and outs of breathing. Always inhale before you lift, exhale as you lift, and inhale as you lower the weight for maximum benefit.

Pick and choose. Pick several exercises for your upper body and several for your lower body from the resistance and weight-lifting categories. You can switch to different exercises anytime you feel like it.

Up the ante. Unless otherwise noted, work up to the point where you can do three sets of exercises. In each set do 5 to 15 repetitions of the exercise. (Don't rest within the sets. You can rest briefly between each set.) When the work becomes easy, add weights or increase the amount you do.

Get rhythm. If you have trouble establishing a rhythm to your exercise routine so that you perform each repetition within a set with the same gusto, Dr. Evans suggests that you listen to triumphal march music as you exercise.

Give Yourself a Lift

Ever want to feel like a kid again? Well, maybe you remember calisthenics from grade school, those exercises that use the body's own weight to build and tone muscles. They're not complicated, and they require no special equipment. Dr. Evans recommends the following three exercises.

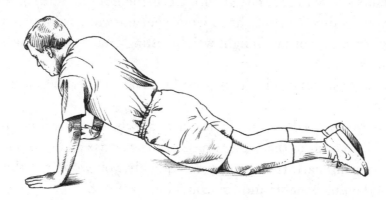

BENT-KNEE PUSH-UPS

Lie on the floor facedown, feet together, knees and palms against the floor. Keeping your knees against the floor, push your body up with your arms. Keep your back as flat as possible. Return to starting position.

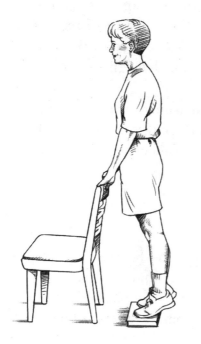

CALF RAISES

Use a chair or wall for support, if necessary. Stand with the balls of your feet on a 2-inch-thick book or board, your heels off the edge. Push yourself up onto your toes, then slowly lower your heels as far as you can.

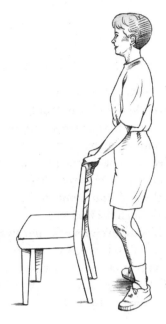

MODIFIED SQUATS
Stand behind a chair, holding the back of the chair for support. With your feet flat on the floor, point your toes outward. Bend your knees slightly while keeping your back straight and feet on the floor. Return to starting position.

Stay Clear of Cramps

You're just strolling merrily along the sidewalk, when suddenly—ouch!—a muscle cramp cripples one of your legs. To avoid cramps, stretch and strengthen your leg muscles with these three exercises recommended by Gary Gordon, D.P.M., director of the Running and Walking Clinic at the Joseph Torg Sports Medicine Center at Allegheny University of the Health Sciences in Philadelphia.

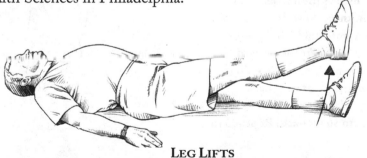

LEG LIFTS
Lie on the floor. Tighten the thigh muscles of one leg and then lift it 12 inches off the ground without bending your knee. Hold your leg in this position for 10 seconds. Then lower the leg and repeat with the opposite leg. Repeat the exercise, alternating legs. Work up to the point where you can do 30 lifts with each leg. When this becomes easy, strap on leg weights to add 1 to 2 pounds to your ankles and work your way up to 30 lifts again.

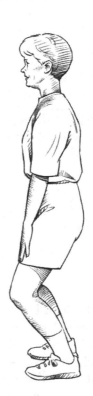

CALF STRETCHES

Stand with heels apart and toes pointing in, with your arms straight out in front of you, palms touching a wall. Keep your back straight and bend your arms, then move your chest toward the wall. You should feel a stretch through the backs of your calves. If you don't, move farther away from the wall and try again. If your calves hurt too much, move closer to the wall. Hold the stretch for 10 to 30 seconds. Repeat 5 to 10 times.

KNEE AND ANKLE BENDS

Stand with your feet about 6 inches apart. With your back straight and your feet on the ground, bend your ankles and knees, lowering your body as far as is comfortable. Keep your hands on your thighs for support. The movement should be coming from your knees, not your back, according to Dr. Gordon. Hold the pose for 10 to 30 seconds. Repeat 5 to 10 times.

Give Your Cancer Defenses a Lift

You don't have to work out like Arnold Schwarzenegger. Even a little weight lifting provides a mighty defense against cancer.

You'll need some weights for the weight-lifting exercises that follow. You can either buy free weights—dumbbells or barbells—or use plastic bottles or milk jugs filled with water or sand. You'll probably want to buy inexpensive weights that you can attach to your ankles.

Finding the best weight for you takes trial and error, says Dr. Evans. The weights should be heavy enough that your muscles benefit, but not so heavy that your muscles can't handle the stress. Find the heaviest weight that you can lift five times and work with that weight. The goal is to do three sets of five repetitions of each exercise. Choose two or three for your upper body and two or three for your lower body, he recommends. Dr. Evans suggests the following exercises.

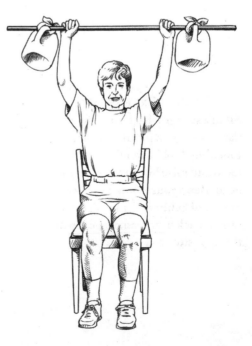

MILITARY PRESSES
Use a barbell or secure a weighted milk jug on each end of a broomstick. Hold the bar behind your head, arms bent. Slowly raise your arms up until they are straight. Return to starting position.

SHOULDER RAISES

Sit in a chair with your feet flat on the floor. Hold a weight in one hand, resting at your side, palm facing in. Keep your elbow straight but not locked as you slowly bring your arm forward and up, until it is fully extended above your head. Return to starting position. Repeat for one set, then switch to the opposite side.

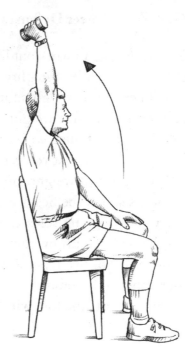

TRICEPS EXTENSIONS

Sit in a straight-back chair, feet flat on the floor, parallel but not touching. Hold a weight in each hand and raise both arms over your head. Bend your elbow and lower one hand behind your head, then raise it back overhead. Repeat with the opposite arm.

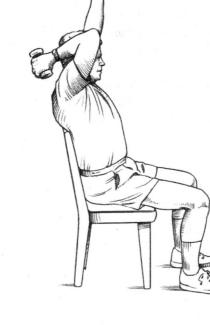

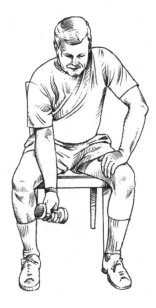
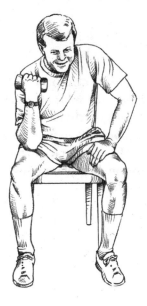

Biceps Curls

Sit in a chair with your legs apart, feet flat on the floor, and one hand on your thigh. Holding a weight in your other hand, extend that arm straight down, while resting your elbow against your inner thigh.

Flex your arm and slowly curl the weight to shoulder level. Return to original position. Repeat for one set, then switch arms.

Knee Extensions

Sit on a chair, with a weight strapped to the ankle of one leg, foot on the floor. Slowly straighten the leg. (Don't point your toe—keep your foot at about a 90-degree angle to your leg.) Then lower the leg to the starting position. Repeat for one set, then switch sides.

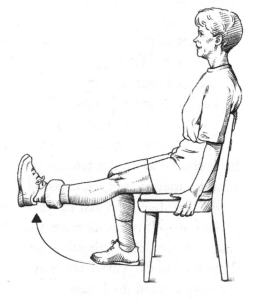

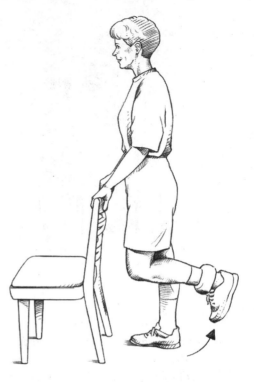

KNEE FLEXIONS
Strap a weight to the ankle of one leg.
Stand and hold on to the back of a chair
for support. Slowly lift your heel toward
your buttock. Lower your leg to the
starting position. Repeat for one set,
then switch sides.

Be Sweet to Your Feet

Exercise in shoes that are designed for the job—otherwise, you're issuing an open invitation to aches, pains, and even stress fractures in your feet and legs.

"A lot of people just put on any old shoe—and they get hurt," notes Dr. Gordon. Walking or running shoes absorb the shock of your stride, thanks to a slightly elevated heel that also helps prevent injuries to the legs' muscles and tendons.

Other types of athletic shoes, such as tennis shoes, take the impact of sideways movement and quick turns. Women who normally wear high heels should avoid flat tennis-type shoes because the sudden shift in foot position may cause a strain, says Dr. Gordon.

While shoes may last for years, their shock absorption lasts for only a few months. If you walk fewer than 25 miles a week, Dr. Gordon suggests that you get a new pair every four to six months. If you walk more than 25 miles a week, replace shoes every two to three months. Use the castoffs for work around the house.

How I Did It: Life Begins at 78

Al Markstein started exercising at age 78, spurred on by his high school buddy and World War II Navy roommate Jack LaLanne, the fitness guru. (They also share the same birthday.)

"Jack kept telling me I had to exercise. I made excuses," says the Orinda, California, resident who is now in his eighties. Then one day LaLanne stopped listening and simply told his friend that he was all signed up for an exercise program at a nearby gym. LaLanne followed up every two weeks to make sure that Markstein followed through. "If he hadn't, I probably would have dropped out. When I started, I could barely pick up a 5-pound barbell," he recalls. "Now I'm doing 27 pounds."

Of his pre-exercise life the retired businessman notes, "When I owned my own company, I was always the first person there and the last to leave. But after I retired, I used to just sit down and be ready to fall asleep. People would ask me to play a game of golf or go to a ball game. I'd make arrangements, but when the day arrived, I'd find an excuse not to go."

Today, Markstein has more go than the Energizer Bunny. When asked what an average day is like, he replies, "Today, I exercised for 2 hours. I'm about to participate in a charity golf tournament. I'll stay at the club for dinner and a raffle. You name it, I'm ready to do it."

While the thought of going to a gym might seem intimidating at first, Markstein finds that the one he frequents has "a real mix of ages. Some people are older than I am. You meet all kinds of people, and there's always some funny guy with a joke or two. It certainly helps make the day go by."

If you already have a pair of shoes made for walking or running, examine the tread. Get a new pair if the bottom tread has worn off, which means there has been enough wear to interfere with shock absorption.

If you need new shoes, follow this advice when shopping for a replacement pair.

How I Did It: Caesar Conquers Addiction

Comedian Sid Caesar began exercising at age 57. The star of stage, screen, and TV suffered bouts with alcohol and sleeping pills that put his career in jeopardy. "I have an addictive personality," says Caesar, now in his seventies. "Finally, I thought, 'Why are you acting like a crazy man? The only one you're hurting is yourself.'"

Caesar looked around for ways to change his life and put that addictive personality to a positive use. And one of those changes meant developing a regular exercise program.

"I started out with a chinning bar because I could carry it with me on the road. I did sit-ups and push-ups. I probably started with 10 or so—if that—and built up little by little."

He scoffs at the no-pain, no-gain theory of exercise. "That stuff is baloney—it's for teenagers. When you're older, you have to take it a little at a time and just do what your body can manage. If it takes you 50 years to get in bad shape, you're not going to get out of it in 2 minutes."

Caesar spent years building up from his low-key start to the iron-man routine for which he is famous. These days, he starts with 15 minutes of stretching followed by a 1½-hour walk that includes the steep slopes near his house in Beverly Hills. After that comes 200 to 300 sit-ups, 40 to 50 push-ups, 20 to 40 chin-ups and, if the weather is nice, 10 to 15 laps in the pool.

What has exercise done for him? "I felt better from the moment that I started—I wouldn't have kept doing it all these years if it didn't make me feel good. When you take care of your body, you have done something for yourself, and that means you have accomplished something."

Examine the patterns. Bring a well-worn pair of everyday shoes with you when you shop for walking shoes. Your wear patterns, particularly in the heels, may help the salesperson pick out the best pair for your feet, advises Merritt.

Help it fit. To get the best fit while fitting new athletic shoes, wear the same kind of socks that you'll exercise in. Shop in the afternoon in case your feet swell during the day. Plan to try on lots of shoes to identify the ones that are most comfortable.

Thumbnail the toe. There is enough toe room if, when you stand, you can fit your thumbnail (about a half-inch) in the space between the end of your big toe and the end of the shoe, says Dr. Gordon. If you have a long thumbnail, of course, stick to the half-inch rule, he advises.

Check the width. A shoe is too wide if the eyelets meet when you lace them up. Your foot will slip around inside the shoe, and you won't get enough support. You may end up with blisters, says Dr. Gordon. A too-narrow shoe will be hard to tie because the eyelets are too far apart.

Some people think they need a wide shoe because their little toe flares out. Ask for a normal-width, curve-lasted model that won't give your little toe a pinched-in feeling, advises Jim Stewart, a registered professional shoe fitter and owner of the Finish Line Running Store, a store specializing in athletic footwear in Allentown, Pennsylvania.

Keep an upright heel. Put the shoe on and have someone look at it from behind, says Stewart. The heel counter, the extra-firm section of the shoe that cradles your heel, should be perpendicular to the ground. If it isn't, you're not getting the heel support that you need from the shoe.

Get enough stiffness. In some shoe models, the shock-absorbing layer of sole is rigid; in others it is more pliable. If you weigh more than 190 pounds, you need the rigid model just to get enough shock absorption, says Dr. Gordon. If you weigh 100 pounds or less, the rigid construction may make your foot work too hard, straining the arch or calf muscles. If you are between 100 and 190 pounds, you may wear a shoe with either a rigid or pliable sole. Unfortunately, you can't easily tell the difference. Ask salespeople at quality athletic shoe stores for recommendations.

Add an insert. You can get additional shock absorption through over-the-counter shoe inserts such as Spenco (which also prevents friction and blisters). This won't help your shoes last longer but will increase your shock absorption protection, says Dr. Gordon.

How I Did It: A Comeback from Heart Attack

In 1991 Alice Ann Hamilton began attending exercise classes at Emory University in Atlanta at age 60. "I started two months after my heart attack," she says. "I had never done any organized exercise."

Hamilton never thought that she had suffered a heart attack. "You never believe that anything like a heart attack is going to happen to you. Now I wonder why my heart attack didn't happen earlier."

Her high-pressure job as assistant superintendent for personnel in the DeKalb County, Georgia, school system took its toll. "When I came home after long hours, I didn't feel like doing much of anything. After I retired, I wanted to take it easy." Yet, she reflects that she had some warning signals. "Not long before my heart attack, I went on a trip to New York with some friends and was surprised at how tired I got after a day of walking around. I had thought I was in better shape."

Once she made the commitment to a comeback, she worried about measuring up. "When I first started at Emory, I worried that I wouldn't be able to do the program," Hamilton says. The heart attack had left her exhausted, her energy level set on low.

She started out with stretching exercises—for instance, trying to touch her toes. She then walked a quarter mile on the track and rode on the stationary bicycle for a few minutes. She recalls that she "also met people who live right around the corner—but I had never known them."

The program gradually became more demanding. "I had to walk faster around the track and do more exercises," Hamilton says. Now, she has graduated to a high-powered step aerobics program.

"I feel great. I have a lot more energy and have been doing volunteer work with the Decatur Emergency Assistance Ministry. I help people in the community. For example, if people in trouble can't pay their utilities, we make arrangements to take care of the bills."

Leave Inactivity Behind

The exercise clothes are ready to go. The new pair of shoes wait by the door. Weights, present and accounted for. But, if you're like most people, it is still hard to take that final step and, as they say in the ad, "just do it."

Odds are, this isn't the first time that you have tried to set up an exercise routine, and you know how important it is to silence that little voice from within that says, "I'll 'just do it'—tomorrow." Here's how to get on the fast track to disease prevention.

Share the load. "Get someone to go with you," advises Merritt. "You may not want to walk or do strength-training exercises because it's too cold or you just feel lazy. When you depend on someone and they depend on you, it makes it easier for both of you."

In fact, a study conducted by the University of Southern California showed that people who exercise with friends at a health club and socialize with them outside the club work out more frequently and enjoy it more.

Adds LaLanne, "When people work out together, they encourage each other and make sure that they are doing the exercises correctly. They also get competitive and, as a result, they both get a more intense workout than they'd get if they worked alone."

Plug in for pleasure. Some experts recommend using the beat of the music to energize your workouts. Try picking something with a faster tempo for your actual workout and then something slower for your warm-up and cooldown. Choose a rhythm that's comfortable for you, Merritt advises. Listen to your body, not the music, to lessen the chances of overexertion.

Keep a record. If you measure your progress, you'll find it easier to stay motivated. Write down in a calendar or a notebook the number of minutes you walk and the number of exercises you do. You'll be surprised at how quickly you're able to do more.

Everyday Exercise

Some experts believe that everyday activities may be just as effective in preventing heart disease, cancer, and stroke as formal exercise routines—and a lot more appealing. Here's what you can do to get off the couch.

Make it meaningful. "Older people have a commonsense view of physical activity—possibly because they've lived through the Depression, when life was more difficult and physical activity translated into something meaningful, not just sweat," says Bryant Stamford, Ph.D., professor of exercise physiology and director of the Health Promotion Center at the University of Louisville. He suggests that, while a regular exercise program will benefit everyone, some people may be happier—and more willing to exercise—if they simply do more of the things that they enjoy.

"If you like to garden, figure out a way to turn that into 30 minutes a day of vigorous activity. It'll help you ward off lethal diseases," he advises.

The Centers for Disease Control and Prevention in Atlanta and the American College of Sports Medicine, which is headquartered in Indianapolis, suggest activities such as walking up the stairs (rather than taking the elevator), walking instead of driving short distances, doing housework, raking leaves, and dancing. In fact, a report issued by these groups states that your risk of coronary heart disease increases as your level of activity goes down.

Take the hard road. "Make things more difficult, not easier," suggests Dr. Stamford. "Usually, if you have trouble getting up the stairs, everyone suggests that you move into a one-story house. But in reality the stairs give you trouble because you have become weaker. If you stop doing stairs, soon you won't be able to get up them at all. Do more of what's difficult, not less."

Prescription for Prevention

A two-part exercise program protects you from cancer, heart disease, and stroke: Aerobic exercise (walking or bicycling, for example) conditions your heart and cardiovascular system; strength-training exercises (calisthenics and weight lifting) build muscle and cut fat to reduce your cancer risk.

Do:

- *Warm up with stretches, light calisthenics, or slow walking before you exercise.*

- *Exercise for more than 30 minutes per session if you want to lose weight. Otherwise, three 10-minute sessions per day will protect against disease.*

- *Wear loose-fitting clothing that breathes. Use layers of clothing to stay warm and, simultaneously, dispel perspiration and heat. Wear athletic socks designed to wick perspiration away from your feet. Make sure your shoes fit and support your feet.*

- *Cool down by slow walking or stretches.*

Don't:

- *Become dehydrated.*

- *Drink coffee, alcohol, or other diuretics before or while you exercise.*

- *Exercise so vigorously that you can't talk and exercise at the same time.*

Chapter 8

Positive Feelings

The Mind's Gift to Your Immune System

Maud Morgan has beaten the odds. In her nineties, the legendary Boston oil painter, whose works adorn galleries nationwide, including the Metropolitan Museum of Art in New York City, is spry, mentally alert, and eager to begin each day. And while age has brought some health concerns and slowed her pace and energy level somewhat, Morgan has never had a heart attack, stroke, or cancer, unlike many people her age.

Good genes? Maybe. Healthy diet and lifestyle? Perhaps.

Optimism? Absolutely, Morgan says. "I've always instinctively seen the optimistic side of everything, and I think that helps keep me healthy," she says. "When you're optimistic, that usually leads to action, and anything that keeps you alive and active increases your health."

If you don't believe it, just ask George Blackburn, M.D., Ph.D., associate professor of surgery at Harvard Medical School and chief of the nutrition/metabolism laboratory in the Cancer Research Institute at Beth Israel Deaconess Medical Center West in Boston, who has known Morgan for years.

"Without a shadow of a doubt, her philosophy of life has had an impact on her survival. When you look at her risk factors from a statistical standpoint, she should have been gone long ago. She confounds all predictions because like many in her generation she abused cigarettes and everything else that we now know isn't good for you," says Dr. Blackburn, who owns a dozen of Morgan's paintings. "There is no Western medicine that I practice that can explain her."

Attitude Matters

As with the fabled Fountain of Youth and mythical Atlantis, the search for the connection between mind and body has been an elusive one. But researchers are discovering that the link between positive feelings and health is neither a fable nor a myth. Compelling research is beginning to show that a positive outlook on life can magnify the health-protecting powers of diet and exercise and can help dampen a multitude of ailments, including heart disease, stroke, and cancer. Even if you develop one of these three diseases, experts say joy, hope, and optimism can improve the quality of your life and enhance your chances of recovery.

"Most illnesses have a lot of psychological underpinnings. A person's lifestyle, character, and the way they cope with life have a big influence on what diseases they get, how long they live, and how they survive in their older years," says Roger Thies, Ph.D., professor of physiology at the University of Oklahoma Health Sciences Center in Oklahoma City.

Unraveling the Mystery

Although physicians and researchers had long suspected that negative emotions influenced our health, it was the late Norman Cousins, the former editor of the *Saturday Review,* who created a sensation when he claimed that laughter helped him overcome a heart attack and a rare life-threatening collagen disease—an illness of the fibrous tissue that binds cells together.

"A patient's attitude is very important," Cousins said. "If he approaches the illness with confidence and purpose—if he remains committed to a high quality of life—then he can enhance the effects of his medical treatment."

What's going on? No one is quite sure yet. In fact, your doctor probably would have an easier time explaining why your golf partner insists on wearing a polka-dot shirt, plaid pants, and fluorescent orange shoes than describing precisely how emotions affect your health.

"Positive moods, optimism, and good mental health are underrated

249

How Optimistic Are You?

Cheer up," a wit said in the 1920s, "the worst is yet to come."

An optimist? A pessimist? Maybe a little of both?

It depends on what he said next, says Christopher Peterson, Ph.D., professor of psychology at the University of Michigan in Ann Arbor and author of *Health and Optimism.*

Generally, optimists have a better sense of control over their lives—at any age—than pessimists, Dr. Peterson says. "An optimist would say, 'I expect good things to happen in the future because I can make them happen,' while a pessimist might say, 'I expect bad things to happen in the future because I'm powerless to do anything about them happening,'" he says.

Unlike pessimists, optimists seem to have an internal break that somehow helps them stop worrying about what they can't change (like the weather) and focus on what they can do (build a fire to keep the house warm, for instance), Dr. Peterson says.

So which are you? To find out, answer the following questions on a scale of 1 (I agree a lot) to 5 (I disagree a lot) as honestly and accurately as you can. Remember that there are no correct or incorrect answers and that this is merely a rough estimate of your optimism or pessimism. Scoring follows. This profile was developed by Charles Carver, Ph.D., professor of psychology at the University of Miami in Coral

and under-studied as a helpful factor in health, particularly in terms of cancer prevention and treatment," says Karl Goodkin, M.D., Ph.D., associate professor of psychiatry, neurology, and psychology at the University of Miami School of Medicine.

Many researchers believe that positive feelings indirectly help to prevent heart disease, stroke, and cancer. Healthy people in their sixties, seventies, and eighties who are optimists, for instance, likely took better care of their bodies when they were younger and continue to exercise regularly,

Gables, Florida, and Michael Scheier, Ph.D., professor of psychology at Carnegie Mellon University in Pittsburgh.

1. In uncertain times, I usually expect the best.

2. If something can go wrong for me, it will.

3. I always look on the bright side of things.

4. I'm always optimistic about my future.

5. I hardly ever expect things to go my way.

6. Things never work out the way I expect them.

7. I'm a believer that every cloud has a silver lining.

8. I rarely count on good things happening to me.

9. Overall, I expect more good things to happen to me than bad.

Add up your score on group A—questions 1, 3, 4, 7, and 9—and group B—questions 2, 5, 6, and 8—separately. Low scores in group A (5 to 10) and high scores in group B (16 to 20) suggest that you are nurturing a healthy optimism. Conversely, if you have high scores in group A (16 or more) and low scores in group B (less than 6), you may want to find more reasons to let a smile be your umbrella.

eat a balanced, low-fat diet, avoid smoking, and drink moderately, says Christopher Peterson, Ph.D., professor of psychology at the University of Michigan in Ann Arbor and author of *Health and Optimism*.

How the Mind Heals

The physiological aspects of emotions themselves—beyond prompting people to be more active—are more uncertain. Some researchers suspect that a small portion of the brain called the insular cortex may be the key. The insular cortex regulates the autonomic nervous system, which controls such automatic functions as breathing, heartbeat, and blood pressure. But it also has a role in higher functions of the brain and helps process emotions like anger, fear, joy, happiness, and sexual arousal.

Could this be where emotions merge with the body's physiology and ultimately affect health? Maybe, says Stephen Oppenheimer, M.D., assistant professor of neurology and cardiology at Johns Hopkins University School of Medicine in Baltimore. In a long-running series of experiments on rats, Dr. Oppenheimer determined that stimulating the insular cortex for hours at a time causes damage to the heart muscle that is strikingly similar to that found in people who succumb to sudden cardiac death.

In other experiments involving people with epilepsy who were undergoing brain surgery that exposed the insular cortex, Dr. Oppenheimer found that stimulating the area with mild electrical pulses changed the person's heart rate and blood pressure.

So years or decades of persistent sorrow, hostility, and other negative emotions may cause a malfunction of the insular cortex and subject an aging body to a steady stream of stress hormones, such as cortisol and norepinephrine, that constrict blood vessels, raise blood pressure, suppress the immune system, and may increase vulnerability to stroke, heart disease, and cancer, Dr. Oppenheimer speculates.

But whatever happens in the brain, many doctors believe that optimism, glee, laughter, love, and other positive emotions can counteract many of these harmful effects—even in your sixties, seventies, and eighties—by triggering the release of hormones such as endorphins that relax the cardiovascular system and cytokines that make the immune system more vigilant for abnormal cells like cancer cells.

"We don't know for a fact that what I call born-again optimism will help keep you healthy in your later years, but there is every reason to believe that would be the case. It certainly wouldn't hurt and will clearly improve your quality, if not the quantity, of the years you have left," Dr. Peterson says.

But it's important to remember that positive feelings are just one of many factors that hinder the development of cancer, stroke, and heart disease. If you rarely exercise and are overweight, smoke, drink heavily, or eat high-fat foods, your risk of these three diseases will still be considerable, no matter how optimistic or hopeful you are, Dr. Peterson warns. With that in mind, here's a glimpse of what influence just a few common feelings can have on your risk of the big three killers and what you can do to cultivate positive emotions and tame negative ones.

Happy Days Are Here Again

We face down death by daring to hope, according to poet Maya Angelou. And, in fact, several studies suggest that people who cling to faith, optimism, and hope—particularly after age 60—may be less susceptible to the big three killers than those who feel hopeless, pessimistic, or depressed.

After analyzing the moods of 2,400 Finnish men ranging from ages 42 to 60, for instance, and following their health for the next six years, researchers at the Western Consortium for Public Health in Berkeley, California, found that those who said they were hopeful were two times less prone to heart attacks than men who were frequently depressed.

"I can't say that depression or hopelessness causes heart disease. But evidence is accumulating that suggests something is going on," says Robert Anda, M.D., a medical epidemiologist at the Centers for Disease Control and Prevention in Atlanta.

In Canada, researchers at the Montreal Heart Institute tracked 222 men and women ages 24 to 88 who had had heart attacks. They found that those who had the most symptoms of depression during hospitalization, such as sadness, apathy, and appetite and sleep disturbances, were at greater risk of dying of heart problems.

Depression may increase the likelihood of heart-damaging clots forming in the arteries, speculates Nancy Frasure-Smith, Ph.D., associate professor of psychiatry at McGill University in Montreal. It's also possible that depressed people are less motivated to stick with preventive treatments. "They may be more inclined to go back to smoking and avoid making other lifestyle changes," she says.

Hang On to Hope

The blues also may be linked to cancer. In a study of the same group of 2,400 Finnish men mentioned earlier, those who strongly agreed with the statements, "The future seems hopeless to me, and I can't believe it will change for the better" and "I feel that it is impossible to reach the goals that I would like to strive for," were about $2\frac{1}{2}$ times more likely to die of cancer than men who were upbeat.

Johns Hopkins University epidemiologists, in a study that included 360 men and women age 65 and older, found that nonsmokers who were relatively cheerful were $2\frac{1}{2}$ to $4\frac{1}{2}$ times less likely to develop cancer than depressed people who smoked more than 15 cigarettes a day.

"Although further research needs to be done to confirm this finding, it makes sense that both quitting smoking and getting out of your depression would be good for you," says George W. Comstock, M.D., professor of epidemiology at Johns Hopkins University School of Hygiene and Public Health in Baltimore, and co-author of the study.

Among 208 women up to age 65 at the University of Miami School of Medicine, researchers found that women who felt hopeful and optimistic or coped well with stressful situations like divorce, retirement, or unemployment were up to two times less likely to have precancerous growths in the cervix than those who felt stressed out or hopeless. Stress, depression, pessimism, and hopelessness also may promote several types of leukemia and other lymphatic cancers, malignant melanomas, and breast and prostate cancer among men and women in their sixties, seventies, and eighties, Dr. Goodkin says.

Smile When You Say Longevity

Other positive emotions also may contribute to disease resistance and longevity. Since 1921, for example, researchers at the University of California, Riverside, have been following the aging process of 1,528 people who were preteens when the study began. With those study subjects, the researchers concluded that positive attributes such as dependability, trust, agreeableness, and open-mindedness were associated with a two- to four-year increase in life expectancy.

"Although common wisdom might argue that a selfish, self-indulgent boor may prosper by stepping on others, this does not seem to be the case. Nor do we find a triumph of the lazy, pampered dropout. In terms of the rush toward death, the encouraging news may be that good guys finish last," according to Howard Friedman, Ph.D., professor of psychology at the university.

Here are some tips for developing a happier vision of the world.

Listen to yourself. Many of us have habitually put ourselves down since childhood. Over a lifetime, those negative messages can turn you into a pessimist and ultimately may affect your health, says Mike Magee, M.D., a motivational speaker and professor of surgery at Jefferson Medical College of Thomas Jefferson University in Philadelphia.

For a week, write down the phrases that you say to yourself like "I'm too old to do that anymore," or "I'm such a jerk." You'll probably end up with a list of 5 to 10 phrases that you repeat over and over again. Now practice stopping those thoughts and replacing them with something more positive. So if you find yourself saying, "I'm too old to dance like that anymore," cut off that thought and replace it with something like, "I'm older now, but I can still dance if I allow for plenty of rest between songs."

Write a letter to yourself. Writing about how you feel can help resolve problems and subdue negative feelings, says James Pennebaker, Ph.D., psychology professor at Southern Methodist University in Dallas.

"If the issue isn't resolved, your body is essentially reliving that experience every time you think about it," Dr. Pennebaker says. "That's very stressful on the body because it constricts blood vessels, raises blood pressure, depresses the immune system, and could exacerbate your risk of stroke, heart disease, and cancer."

Set aside 20 minutes a day for four days and write about how you feel. Don't worry about grammar or spelling. Once you begin writing, don't stop until time is up. That will encourage you to have a free flow of thoughts and feelings. If you like, throw out the paper at the end of each day, Dr. Pennebaker says.

"Writing will help you organize your thoughts and help you get them out of your system," he says. "By the end of the fourth day, most people feel a lot better about themselves."

Check out a miracle. Religious texts are filled with miraculous feats, but there are plenty in modern life to ignite your hope, says Alan Epstein, Ph.D., a relationship counselor in Rome, Italy, and author of *How to Be Happier Day by Day.* Dr. Epstein, for instance, lost a valued ring on three separate occasions six years apart, only to find it each time when it seemed certain to vanish forever.

Investigate something that has happened in your lifetime that seems to defy logic and piques your interest such as a man falling off a 100-foot cliff without breaking a bone. Write it down and carry it with you in your purse or wallet. When you feel despair, pull it out and look at it for inspiration, Dr. Epstein says.

Seek new challenges. "I have new projects ahead of me all of the time," says Margaret Rawson, in her nineties, a Frederick, Maryland, educator and an internationally recognized dyslexia researcher. "There's a lot that I want to do and find out about, so I guess I'll just have to live another 100 years.

She took up flying at age 72, learned to use a computer at 80, published her third book on dyslexia in 1995, and is working on her autobiography.

"I'm not my age, I'm myself," Rawson says. "If you have a negative attitude, you're apt to say, 'No, I can't do that.' But if you have a positive attitude, you say, 'This is something that interests me, and I really want to try it. How can I do it?' " she adds.

Try to do at least one new thing a month. Go to a museum, sneak into a lecture at a local college, eat at a new restaurant, or walk through a different neighborhood. The bottom line is that monotony destroys optimism and your health, says David Bouda, M.D., assistant professor of oncology at the University of Nebraska College of Medicine in Omaha.

"If you don't use your brain and body in different ways occasionally, then you will get old very quickly," Dr. Bouda says.

Look for the end of the rainbow. Spend a moment each day to take a fresh look at something in nature and marvel at it. "When you look at a rainbow, I've never heard anyone say, 'Gee, I wish it had more blue and a little less red,' " Dr. Bouda says. Observing nature will help you get in touch with your spirituality—that you are part of a larger whole—and can spark hope for the future.

Find the hope within you. Meditation or prayer can help you release from your body anxiety, hopelessness, depression, and other negative emotions associated with heart disease, stroke, and cancer, says Patricia Norris, Ph.D., a psychophysiologic psychotherapist at the Life Sciences Institute of Mind-Body Health in Topeka, Kansas.

To try a simple meditation, sit in a comfortable chair and take several deep breaths to help you relax, Dr. Norris says. When you feel serene, close your eyes and slowly repeat, "Let my heart be like the sun and shine without judgment on everyone." Be sure to include yourself. If your mind starts to wander off to concerns like whether your Social Security check will arrive today, focus your concentrations back on the phrase. Do that for 5 minutes at least twice a day or at times when you feel bitter, angry, or sad. It's not to repress the sadness but to hold it out to the sun's light, she says.

"The sun is a symbol. When you go outside, the sun doesn't ask, 'Are you good enough to receive my light today?' It just shines on everyone no matter who you are or how you feel. That's how I think we should envision ourselves," Dr. Norris says.

Find an abundance of happiness. Keep a journal and write down at least 50 wonderful things that happen to you every day, says Susan Jeffers, Ph.D., a 60-year-old Los Angeles–based psychologist and author of *End the Struggle and Dance with Life*. Include even small things like finding a quarter on the sidewalk or watching a gorgeous sunrise. "Make the ordinary extraordinary. After awhile, you'll realize that most things that happen are positive and you don't have to dwell on the negative," says Dr. Jeffers, who credits positive thinking with helping her to survive breast cancer 14 years ago.

Plant hopes in a garden. Houseplants make people feel calmer and more optimistic, says Bruno Cortis, M.D., a Chicago cardiologist in private practice and author of *Heart and Soul,* a psychological and spiritual guide to preventing and healing heart disease. In addition, Dr. Cortis says that at least one study has shown that hospital patients whose windows

257

faced a garden recovered more quickly than those who faced a wall. So starting a garden or tending to a houseplant may help you forget problems and improve your health, he says.

Pamper a pet. "For many people over 60, a cat, dog, or other pet truly can mean the difference between life and death. Studies show that people in this age group who have pets live longer and have stronger immune systems. There is always some animal that people can connect with," says Dennis Gersten, M.D., a San Diego psychiatrist in private practice and publisher of *Atlantis: The Imagery Newsletter*.

Cherish those compliments. If someone shows appreciation for you, don't let go of it. Take a 3- by 5-inch card, write down the date, who the person was, and what they said about you. Put that in a place like the bathroom mirror where you'll see it at least once a day. It will help you fend off negative feelings about yourself, Dr. Magee says. You also may want to keep a list of inspirational quotes from famous people like Abraham Lincoln, Will Rogers, or Helen Keller that are meaningful to you.

Go ahead: Gripe. Surprisingly, an optimist may be the loudest complainer in your neighborhood.

"If you passively go along with everything, you have absolutely no sense of control, and that would foster pessimism. So the person who is moaning, complaining, and demanding might not be very pleasant to be around, but they may be optimistic," Dr. Peterson says. "They believe that everything they are saying is going to make a difference, and it probably does have an effect since they probably get attention."

So if you feel strongly about a problem and truly believe that complaining will make a difference, don't hold your feelings in—let someone know about it, Dr. Peterson urges.

Imagine your joy. Using your imagination to stimulate your inner-healing resources can help boost your self-esteem, happiness, and cancer-fighting immunity, says Dr. Gersten.

This process, called guided imagery, is a powerful tool that can help prevent and alleviate many diseases, Dr. Gersten says. To try it, take a couple of deep breaths, then picture yourself as the spiritual elder of a clan or tribe. You are revered by all of your fellow tribe people for your knowledge and life experiences. You are useful and have a great deal to give to your tribe and the world. See yourself as being much happier now than you were at any other time of your life because you can share your wisdom and joy with others.

Do that once or twice a day for 5 minutes, Dr. Gersten suggests.

Eat smart. It's hard to keep your emotions in balance if you're not eating right, Dr. Gersten says. Although no specific foods will boost your mood, he recommends eating a balanced diet that includes at least six servings of fruits and vegetables and five servings of grains a day to help fend off depression and other unwanted emotions.

Make Me Laugh

He who laughs, lasts.

"You don't stop laughing because you grow old. You grow old because you stop laughing. It's that simple," says Lila Green, in her sixties, speaker, author of *Making Sense of Humor,* and a guest lecturer at the University of Michigan Medical School in Ann Arbor. She speaks on the topic of light-hearted physician-patient communication styles.

Although the evidence isn't conclusive, scientists are discovering that Green may be right: Laughter is the best medicine, particularly after age 60.

When 33 men and women, ages 66 to 101, for example, were asked to compare their sense of humor with siblings who had died of natural causes, researchers at the University of Akron found that the survivors recalled laughing more in their youth than their decreased brothers and sisters.

"It doesn't hurt to laugh. This study supports the prevailing consensus that people who enjoy humor and get a kick out of things may live longer," says Richard Haude, Ph.D., associate professor of psychology at the University of Akron in Ohio.

Laughter strengthens the immune system, decreases the production of stress-related hormones, relaxes tense muscles, keeps your mind engaged, and boosts oxygen flow and blood circulation to all parts of the body, says psychiatrist William Fry, M.D., associate clinical professor emeritus at Stanford University School of Medicine.

How I Did It: An Insurance Agent Keeps His Faith

Luther Hahs wanted to pray, but he couldn't remember how to do it.

Hahs, a 79-year-old retired insurance agent in Cape Girardeau, Missouri, had a stroke while undergoing coronary bypass surgery in 1973 that paralyzed his right arm and leg. For weeks, he lay mumbling incoherently in a Memphis hospital.

Grimly, from his standpoint, the stroke also destroyed his ability to pray.

"I was very despondent. I couldn't pray because I had lost the words," he says. "I sat there looking at the cross, and I just cried. To me, that was my religion, but I couldn't get it out. It seemed hopeless. I had so much brain damage that the doctors didn't think I'd walk or talk again."

But hope and faith would help Hahs through the next few years. Hahs began physical and speech therapy. At first, a speech therapist told him they could only understand three of every ten words he spoke. The rest was unintelligible.

By Christmas he could call his wife, Catherine, "Mommy." On

"The relationship between humor and cancer, stroke, and heart disease is still questionable, but all indications are that they must be linked somehow," Dr. Fry says.

Here are some quick ways to hone your funny bone.

Make farce a habit. Mundane routines can kill laughter, but doing something wildly different can be joyous, Green says. Sit in the bath the opposite way that you normally would, reverse the way you hang toilet paper, wear a funny mask to a friend's house, or serve dessert first at dinner. "You can't cope with change in this fast-paced world unless you're a little bit silly or zany. This will help you do that," she says.

Create a humorous spot. Instead of cluttering your refrigerator or bulletin board with reminders of doctor's appointments and meetings, reserve a spot for cartoons, funny pictures, or sayings, Green suggests.

Easter Sunday, 1974, he managed to utter a three-word prayer.

"I got up, looked at the cross and said, 'God.' Then I looked at my wife and said, 'Mommy.' Then I said, 'Amen.' That was my first prayer," Hahs says.

His speech improved, and he gradually regained some use of his right arm. He also learned how to walk and even drive a car. He still has difficulty reading and writing—it takes him more than 30 minutes to jot three to four sentences in his journal each day. But he has produced a book called *God, Mommy, Amen,* which describes his comeback. The book is available by writing to Southeast Bookstore, 388 North Henderson Street, Cape Girardeau, MO 63701.

"I attribute all of my recovery to my faith and determination. God, my wife, and family mean everything to me," Hahs says. "My advice to others is be an optimist, have faith, ask for help if you need it, and keep trying different ways of doing things if something doesn't work out for you."

Think like a comic. If you have had a particularly rough day, imagine how your favorite comedian would describe it, Green says. It will help you laugh it off.

Learn to laugh at yourself. "When you laugh at yourself, you don't break—you bend," Green says. "It gives you new perspectives about yourself. It helps keep your mind flexible and prevents what I call hardening of the attitudes." Instead of getting angry or embarrassed, laugh with others, and you'll probably feel better about yourself.

Grief: Let It Out, But Don't Let It Linger

"Grief is a totally normal part of life. It's as important to survival as eating and breathing," Dr. Gersten says. "If you block dealing with a

How I Did It: The Tax Man Stares Down Death

When Richard Bloch found out he had lung cancer, he didn't dwell on death and taxes. He clung to hope.

Given 90 days to live, Bloch, the co-founder and former chairman of the board of H & R Block—the nation's largest preparer of income tax returns—decided to fight back.

"The doctor took my hope away, and for five days I lived without hope. It was the worst week of my life, but I wasn't about to quit," Bloch says.

That was nearly 20 years ago, and the tax guru, now in his seventies, credits much of his recovery to his attitude. He sought out a second opinion, began radiation and chemotherapy but also never gave up on life. "Terminal is a place where you go to catch a bus," he says. "I had too much to live for to die."

In addition to traditional cancer treatments, Bloch practiced deep breathing and other relaxation techniques. He also used visual imagery to picture his body fighting off the cancer. Humor helped, too.

"Laughter has always been a big part of my life, and I had heard that humor helps activate the immune system. So while I was receiving treatment, I watched funny videos and listened to recordings of old radio programs like 'Fibber McGee and Molly,'" Bloch says.

Within two months his "inoperable" tumor had shrunk enough that it could be surgically removed. Throughout the ordeal, Bloch's wife, Annette, kept him focused on the future.

"She was always planning something for us to do—vacations with the kids, going out to dinner," he says.

Today, Bloch operates a nonprofit organization that distributes free cancer-treatment information. For more information, write to R. A. Bloch Cancer Foundation, 4400 Main Street, Kansas City, MO 64111.

"Doctors don't cure cancer; patients cure themselves with the help of their doctors. That I believe in fully," Bloch says. "You can't cure a person of cancer who believes that he's going to die."

death, your emotional life dies, and that can affect your physical well-being. So don't run away from the pain of grief. Realize that it is okay to be sad. You don't have to tough it out. In fact, if you try to fight it off, your grief may last forever."

Some acutely bereaved people age 60-plus who lost a loved one 35 years ago have levels of complicated grief that are as high as a person who lost someone two months ago, says Holly Prigerson, Ph.D., a researcher and assistant professor of psychiatry at the University of Pittsburgh School of Medicine. In her studies Dr. Prigerson is discovering that the grief of loss can result in considerable health problems.

For two years, she tracked the health of 150 men and women in their sixties, seventies, and eighties after the death of a spouse. Dr. Prigerson concluded that those who mourned the most severely were more suscep-tible to lingering nightmares, insomnia, feelings of profound guilt, hallu-cinations involving the deceased, and other symptoms similar to post-traumatic stress disorder—a condition that often affects soldiers, fire-fighters, and police officers after a catastrophe.

Significantly, these men and women were up to seven times more prone to develop cancer and five times more likely to have heart problems. Although only two people had strokes, Dr. Prigerson suspects deeply rooted grief may be a contributing factor to that disease as well.

"Most people who have these complicated grief reactions describe their marriages as wonderful. We suspect that part of the problem is that they may have been overly dependent on their spouses," Dr. Prigerson says. "So they need to start thinking about their own personal needs apart from the spouse and begin to establish a new life."

Here are some ways to mourn your loss and re-establish a positive and healthy lifestyle.

Take time to relax. Progressive relaxation and other relaxation tech-niques such as deep breathing may help to elevate your mood and give your immune system a vital boost while you are coping with grief, ac-cording to researchers at the University of Pennsylvania School of Nursing in Philadelphia.

In a preliminary study of nine grieving widows up to 70 years old

Wise Words for a Brighter Day

Here are some uplifting quotes to help you start your own list of inspirational sayings.

"Nothing is worth more than this day."
—**Johann Wolfgang von Goethe,** German author

"My hopes are not always realized, but I always hope."
—**Ovid,** Roman poet

"Although the world is full of suffering, it is also full of overcoming it."
—**Helen Keller,** blind and deaf lecturer

"No matter what happens, keep on beginning and failing. Each time you fail, start all over again, and you will grow stronger until you find that you have accomplished a purpose—not the one you began with perhaps, but one you will be glad to remember."
—**Anne Sullivan,** teacher of Helen Keller

"A clown is like aspirin, only he works twice as fast."
—**Groucho Marx,** comedian

"Frame your mind to mirth and merriment, which bar a thousand harms and lengthen life."
—**William Shakespeare,** poet and playwright

"To laugh often and much, to win the respect of intelligent people and the affection of children . . . to leave the world a bit better . . . to know one life breathed easier because you have lived, that is to have succeeded."
—**Ralph Waldo Emerson,** American essayist and poet

"It is something to be able to paint a particular picture or to carve a statue. . . but it is far more glorious to carve and paint the very atmosphere and medium through which we look, which we morally can do. To affect the quality of the day, that is the highest of the arts."
—**Henry David Thoreau,** American philosopher

"I keep my ideals, because in spite of everything I still believe that people are really good at heart."
—**Anne Frank,** from *Diary of Anne Frank*

whose husbands had died in the previous two months, the researchers found that the women who practiced progressive relaxation three or four times a day for four weeks had increases in immune cell activity, which may be beneficial in maintaining health.

"Relaxation is one of many very valuable skills that you can use to deal with grief," says Arlene Houldin, R.N., Ph.D., associate professor of psychosocial oncology at the University of Pennsylvania School of Nursing. Practice the following technique at least three times a day, 10 to 15 minutes a session, she suggests.

Get into a comfortable position, close your eyes, and concentrate on the rhythmic and natural flow of your breathing, Dr. Houldin says. Inhale and exhale slowly, feeling yourself becoming more and more calm and relaxed. Gradually allow yourself to become aware of the muscles in your forehead and scalp. Feel the muscle fibers uncoil and relax, more deeply and fully with each breath. Slowly let that relaxation flow down from your forehead across your temples, through your eyelids, cheeks, nose, lips, chin, and jaw. As the relaxation gently drifts through the rest of your body, follow the same instructions for your neck, arms, elbows, hands, lungs, heart, thighs, calves, feet, and toes. Before you open your eyes, say slowly to yourself five times, "I am alert, refreshed, yet deeply relaxed." Now slowly count to five, open your eyes, and take a couple of deep breaths before resuming your day.

Keep it at arm's length. Try this: Close one eye and hold an arm out in front of you. Then slowly move your thumb toward your open eye. What happens? The thumb dominates your view and you can't see around it. The same thing can happen with grief. If you become overly consumed by grief, you'll stop seeing the joys of life, says Michael A. Zevon, Ph.D., a psychologist at the Roswell Park Cancer Institute in Buffalo, New York.

"People who can still find meaning and joy in life when they are grieving do better than those who focus all of their attention on their loss," he says.

Get back into your normal routine as soon as it feels comfortable and give yourself a break from your grief every day, Dr. Zevon says. Spend time doing things you enjoy, like playing with your grandchildren, working in the garden, or walking in a park just marveling at the beauty around you.

Reach Out and Touch Someone

Sharing your thoughts with others may have a positive impact on quality of life and your chances of survival, says Elizabeth Maunsell, Ph.D., an epidemiologist at Hôpital du St. Sacrement in Quebec City.

In her study of 224 women with breast cancer—the majority over age 50—Dr. Maunsell found that those who confided in one or more people within three months of treatment were 40 percent less likely to die in the next seven years.

Ask yourself a few questions such as: Who would listen to me no matter what? Who notices my health? Who would come to me in the middle of the night just to talk? If you're not satisfied with those answers, you may need to seek out more social contact, says Bruno Cortis, M.D., a Chicago cardiologist in private practice and author of the book, *Heart and Soul.*

"It's important for 60-plus people to know that they can dare to connect, because there are a lot of others in the same situation," says Susan Jeffers, Ph.D., a Los Angeles–based psychologist and author of *End the Struggle and Dance with Life.*

At a party, recreation center, or other gathering place, focus on making other people feel good about themselves. Introduce yourself to someone and consciously make an effort to keep the conversation focused on that person's interests. The result? You'll probably feel better about yourself and may make a new friend, Dr. Jeffers says. If you have difficulty getting out, call your local geriatric social service agency and ask for a list of others who are interested in developing a network of phone pals.

Talk it out. Sharing your feelings will help you accept the loss, says Mark Berman, Ph.D., a Phoenix psychologist in private practice who specializes in issues of the aging. It also will give others a chance to reassure you that your reactions are normal or suggest that you seek grief counseling.

Get some help. After six months, if you are still grieving and also have a noticeable deterioration of personal hygiene, depression, chronic fatigue, insomnia, weight loss, or feel withdrawn and isolated, consult a psychiatrist, grief counselor, or other mental health care professional, Dr. Gersten suggests.

Alleviate the Anger, Heal the Hostility

Most of us have heard of the type A personality—driven, fast-talking, competitive, distrustful, impatient, aggressive. For a long time, researchers thought that all of those traits combined to increase the risk of heart disease and other killers. But while those characteristics aren't particularly charming, scientists now consider most of them fairly harmless. Instead, researchers are zeroing in on what may be the real dangers of being type A: hostility and anger.

"We know that people, including those over 60, who have negative feelings in their relationships are less healthy. In terms of the killers like heart disease, stroke, and cancer, the mortality rates are higher among those who say that they get angry frequently," says Redford Williams, M.D., director of the Behavioral Medicine Research Center at Duke University Medical Center in Durham, North Carolina, and author of *Anger Kills*.

In fact, it is becoming clearer that comic Woody Allen was brushing up against the truth when his character in the movie *Manhattan* quipped, "I can't get angry. . . . I grow a tumor instead."

In a preliminary study, for instance, researchers at the Institute of HeartMath in Boulder Creek, California, a biomedical research center that examines mind-body connections, asked 30 men and women to think for 5 minutes of either a compassionate moment in their lives or a time when they were upset or angry.

"We found that simply recalling one episode of anger depresses the immune system for up to 7 hours—and that's pretty interesting considering how many times the average person gets upset in a typical day. But one episode of feeling compassion or caring enhances the immune system for about the same amount of time," says Jerry Kaiser, the Institute's director of health services. Since the immune system is the body's first line of defense against emerging cancers, a finding of this type may be an important step toward understanding the possible role of the mind-body connection in the development of tumors, Dr. Williams says.

After following 972 medical students for up to 40 years—many now in their sixties and seventies—researchers at Johns Hopkins University found that those students who were considered loners who suppressed their emotions beneath a bland exterior were 16 times more likely to develop cancer than a group that vented their feelings.

At Cedars-Sinai Medical Center in Los Angeles, researchers examined 70 men and women in their sixties and seventies. Researchers concluded that not only were those people who had high levels of hostility, anger, and frustration also more likely to have myocardial ischemia (reduced blood flow to the heart that can cause angina or a heart attack) but also their episodes lasted longer than in people who were less easily provoked.

After studying 1,871 male employees at Western Electric Company in Chicago for more than 25 years—until the youngest men were 65—researchers concluded that cynicism can elevate the risk of heart disease by 40 to 60 percent, says Richard Shekelle, Ph.D., former professor of epidemiology at the University of Texas Health Sciences Center in Houston and co-author of the study.

Japanese researchers who examined negative emotions in 34 men and women concluded that anger and aggression were associated with stroke because these hostile characteristics lead to increased plaque formation and narrowing of the carotid artery, the main artery leading to the brain.

In some cases, anger and hostility associated with type A personality naturally diminishes a bit after age 60, but it still can be a problem for many people in this age group, says Bart Sparagon, M.D., director of the Meyer Friedman Institute, a type A treatment center in San Francisco.

Make it your best day. Pretend that the world will end tomorrow. What would you do? Get angry and seek revenge against your enemies? "I know of no one who has ever done this exercise who said they'd go out and do nasty things," Dr. Williams says. "People usually say they'd go out and smell the roses or get in touch with family and friends. It's always something positive and upbeat."

Now take a step further, write down what you would do, and then do it. You'll probably do something constructive with your day, be more tolerant of others, and have a more hopeful outlook on life, Dr. Williams says.

Talk yourself out of it. Listen to what you're telling yourself about a situation. If, for instance, the fellow at the front of the buffet line seems to be holding up everyone else, is your inner voice allowing you to objectively analyze the facts—he must be hungry—or is it leading you to jump to conclusions—he's doing this on purpose? Then reason with yourself, Dr. Williams says, even if you think your anger is justified. Ask yourself why you are making a big deal out of a short delay. After all, there is still plenty of food left. Once you take control of your feelings, your anger will probably subside.

Counter it with curiosity. If you're in a situation that normally triggers rage, like standing in a long line at the grocery store, take a time-out. Practice observing other people or read a magazine rather than focusing on your anger. You can also recollect a very pleasant event that made you feel calm or peaceful, Dr. Sparagon suggests.

Make time a friend. At the beginning of each week, write down what is the most precious thing that you want to accomplish in the next seven days. That way, if you accomplish nothing else, you can feel good about yourself because you did that one precious thing. You'll also be less apt to see time as an enemy and get upset that you didn't complete everything that you set out to do, says Meyer Friedman, M.D., a pioneering researcher of type A behavior and founder of the Meyer Friedman Institute.

Be Your Own Best Friend

Although experts can suggest many paths to happiness, ultimately, hope and optimism come from within you, says Frosty Westering, Ed.D., a 69-year-old educational psychologist and head football coach at Pacific Lutheran University in Tacoma, Washington.

"The biggest opponent you have in life is yourself. You're either your own opponent or your own friend," says Dr. Westering, author of *Make the Big Time Where You Are*. "So be the best friend that you can be to yourself. So many people put themselves down. They're constantly telling themselves what they can't do or how bad they are. That forces them to jump through hurdles that they really don't need to.

"After games, for instance, we never talk about what we didn't do as a team. We always talk about the things that are good about this team. So win or lose, we leave the field feeling upbeat about ourselves. That's a lesson we all can learn at any age. It is what's inside that counts. If you feel good about yourself, if you feel young at heart, if you feel as if you're the best you can be every day, then that can make all the difference in the world in your mental and physical well-being."

Prescription for Prevention

Joy, hope, and optimism can improve the quality of your life at any age, doctors say. Intriguing research indicates that positive feelings can enhance the health-protective powers of diet and exercise and can help suppress many diseases, including heart disease, cancer, and stroke.

Do:

- *Jot down at least 50 terrific things that happen to you daily.*

- *Laugh often. It heals both the mind and the body.*

- *Find one new challenge each month. Try new projects and hobbies. Fulfill a lifelong ambition.*

- *Meditate for 5 minutes, twice a day. It will help you purge depression, anxiety, and other negative feelings from your body.*

Don't:

- *Dwell on negative thoughts. If your mind is saturated with glum feelings, write down those feelings and find positive thoughts to replace them.*

- *Neglect good foods. Your emotions can spiral downward if you don't eat right. Eating a balanced diet that includes at least six servings of fruits and vegetables like apples and carrots can help fend off depression and other unwanted emotions.*

Chapter 9

Smoking

It's Never Too Late to Snuff Out This Major Risk

Long before all of the illusions about tobacco evaporated like a stale smoke ring, lighting up was the thing to do. In the Sunday comics, joltin' Joe DiMaggio, the pride of the New York Yankees, told young baseball fans, "They don't get your wind.... So mild, athletes smoke as many as they please." Betty Grable, who would eventually die of lung cancer, was a popular World War II pinup girl and cigarette smoker. In the 1950s a cigarette dangling from James Dean's lips defined coolness for an entire generation.

But not only was smoking hip, manufacturers claimed that it also was healthy. It steadied nerves, increased energy, and suppressed appetite, they said.

In fact, for several years one tobacco company proclaimed that more doctors smoked its brand than any other. Attractive young women from tobacco firms regularly visited doctors' offices to replenish the supply of free cigarettes available in waiting rooms for patients.

So when you were enticed to begin puffing—along with a lot of other unsuspecting men and women—the powerfully addictive nature of smoking and its devastating effects on the body were virtually unknown.

But now that you know better, can quitting after even decades of smoking really make a difference? You bet. The evidence is unimpeachable: Stamping out your last cigarette at 60, 70, or even 80 can halt many of the worst effects of smoking.

"Quitting will significantly reduce your risk of stroke, heart disease, and cancer regardless of your age and improve your quality of life," says

Light Cigarettes: An Unwise Switch

Switching to low-tar, low-nicotine cigarettes may seem like a logical way to slash your risk of debilitating diseases, but doctors say there are still plenty of perils.

"Light" and "ultra-light" cigarettes still contain dangerous amounts of nicotine, carbon monoxide, and tar—the gaseous residues of more than 4,700 chemicals.

"Smoking a low-tar cigarette is like jumping off a 20-story building instead of a 30-story one. There simply is no such thing as a safe, safer, or safest cigarette," says Alan Blum, M.D., assistant professor of family medicine at Baylor College of Medicine in Houston.

Thomas Brandon, Ph.D., associate professor of psychology at the State University of New York at Binghamton and a smoking-cessation expert.

Who Is the Older Smoker?

If you are like the typical male smoker in his sixties or seventies, you began at age 17 and have smoked about 27 cigarettes a day for 51 years. If you are a woman in the same age range, you probably first lit up at about age 24 and have been smoking 20 cigarettes a day for 45 years.

And like about 80 percent of the people who smoke, you have probably tried to quit at least once. But 46 percent of the older smokers doubt that smoking is very harmful or that the benefits of quitting are really worthwhile.

If you're among those people, ponder these facts: Within 8 hours of quitting, your pulse rate and blood pressure drop, and oxygen levels in your body rise. Within 24 hours your risk of a heart attack dips. At around a month your circulation improves, your energy levels surge, and your lung function expands by up to 30 percent. By 1 year your risk of heart disease is half that of someone who continues to smoke. In 5 years, your stroke risk begins to slide; and in 10 years, your chances of getting lung cancer are the same as that of someone who has never smoked.

"I've had 75-year-old patients tell me that the day they quit smoking, in their thirties and forties, was the greatest day of their lives. The feeling of finding something that you had thought you had lost—your health—is better than if you had never lost it at all. And to know that your risk of sudden death from smoking-related heart disease has dramatically decreased—is tremendous," says Alan Blum, M.D., assistant professor of family medicine at Baylor College of Medicine in Houston.

Each Puff Is Harmful

With each puff a smoker inhales more than 4,700 chemicals that have a wide-reaching effect throughout the body.

Some of the milder effects include accelerated wrinkling of the skin, yellowing of the teeth and fingers, and slow wound-healing. Smoking also increases the risk of osteoporosis, hip fractures, cataracts, diabetes, tooth loss, and emphysema.

Then there is smoking's real downside. Every day, 1,147 Americans die of smoking-related causes. That adds up to more than 418,000 lives annually, making smoking the most preventable cause of death in the United States. Nearly 80 percent of those deaths are caused by cardiovascular disease and cancer. Specifically, 29 percent of all smoking-related deaths are attributed to lung cancer.

Here is a quick look at how smoking magnifies the impact of certain diseases and how quitting can slash your risk of developing them.

Smoking Breaks Your Heart

The chemicals in tobacco smoke, including nicotine and carbon monoxide—the same gas found in automobile exhaust—raise blood pressure, constrict blood vessels, and starve the heart of oxygen, forcing it to work harder. At the same time, smoking increases the stickiness of blood platelets so that they are more likely to form dangerous blood clots. It also raises total and low-density lipoprotein (the so-called bad cholesterol), lowers levels of high-density lipoprotein (the good cholesterol), and accelerates the accumulation of plaque in arteries causing ath-

273

erosclerosis, also known as hardening of the arteries.

People age 64 and over who smoke have arteries clogged with about the same levels of plaque as people a decade older who have never smoked, according to researchers at Bowman Gray School of Medicine of Wake Forest University in Winston-Salem, North Carolina.

The bottom line is that a person who smokes is three times more likely to develop heart disease and has four times the risk of having a stroke as a nonsmoker. In addition, one in every four deaths is linked to smoking.

If you quit, your risk of a heart attack is sliced by 50 percent in one year, and after about five years your chances of having a stroke can be slashed to virtually the same risk as someone who never smoked.

Cancer: Smoking Tops the List

Smoking is linked to one in three cancer deaths and nearly 90 percent of all lung cancers. Smoking is associated with cancer of the mouth, throat, esophagus, bladder, pancreas, kidneys, and 30 percent of cervical cancer.

"If it weren't for smoking, these cancers would barely exist," says Andrea LaCroix, Ph.D., associate professor of epidemiology at the University of Washington School of Public Health and Community Medicine in Seattle.

Tobacco smoke contains at least 43 cancer-causing substances that can scramble a cell's genetic code, causing it to reproduce abnormally. Constant exposure to the toxic compounds in smoke can cause these abnormal cells to gradually transform into cancer.

But if you quit—even at age 65—your risk of developing lung cancer by age 75 is less than half that of someone who continues to smoke, according to researchers at the University of Michigan. The risk of developing many other cancers—including those affecting the mouth, kidney, and pancreas—begins to diminish within 10 years of quitting.

"The time to quit smoking is when you still feel fine, because by the time you develop cancer and it is detected, it may be too late to cure it," says Teresa Hayes, M.D., an oncologist at Baylor College of Medicine in Houston. "If you quit smoking, not only will you stop adding to your risk, but if you do develop cancer, your chances of survival will be better because your body will be in better shape and you'll be able to tolerate whatever therapy is needed better than someone who continues to smoke."

Quitting Is Easier Than You Think

Like four of every five smokers, you may want to quit and may have tried several times only to be lured back to tobacco. But don't blame yourself. It's not a sign of weakness, smoking-cessation experts say. Nicotine, the prime ingredient in tobacco, is one of the most addictive drugs known. Once you're in its grasp, it takes a determined effort to break free, particularly if you have been smoking for many years. But you can do it.

"Many older people have smoked for so long that they don't think they can overcome it. But I've helped people who have smoked for 50 years quit successfully," says Gary DeNelsky, Ph.D., director of the smoking-cessation program at the Cleveland Clinic. "Quitting isn't easy, but it isn't like climbing Mount Everest either."

In fact, of the people over age 65 who have ever smoked, 77 percent have stopped, according to the Office of Smoking and Health at the Centers for Disease Control and Prevention in Atlanta. That still adds up to nearly 16 million people who continue to smoke after age 65.

How to Become Smoke-Free

About 1.3 million Americans break free of tobacco's hold each year and become nonsmokers. Most quit on their own using a variety of techniques ranging from Nicotine Anonymous to nutrition.

Remember that the first 7 to 10 days of any effort to quit smoking are the toughest because you'll go through withdrawal symptoms—such as upset stomach, difficulty concentrating, drowsiness, insomnia, and irritability—as your body adjusts to the lack of nicotine, Dr. Brandon says.

Once nicotine is flushed out of your body, your cravings should gradually subside. But you still may be tempted to smoke for months or even years afterward. (Eleven years after he quit, President Dwight Eisenhower scribbled, "God, I wish I had a cigarette," on a memo pad during a tense meeting with Soviet Premier Nikita Khrushchev.) But the longer you go

What Are You Really Smoking?

When tobacco giant Philip Morris announced an unprecedented recall of 8 billion defective cigarettes a few years ago, a young woman smoking in New York told a newspaper reporter, "At least it's not cyanide."

Wrong.

Not only does tobacco smoke contain hydrogen cyanide—a deadly poison used in prison gas chambers—it also harbors 4,700 other chemicals and toxins, including at least 43 cancer-causing substances. Here's just a sampling of what a typical smoker inhales with each puff. Uses or a description for each chemical are listed in parentheses.

Acetone (paint stripper)
Ammonia (floor cleaner)
Arsenic (ant poison)
Butane (lighter fluid)
Cadmium (car battery component)
Carbon monoxide (car exhaust)
Formaldehyde (morgue preservative)
Methanol (antifreeze)
Naphthalene (mothballs)
Nicotine (insecticide)
Polonium 210 (radioactive substance)
Toluene (industrial solvent)

without smoking, the more likely you will be able to resist the urge.

"Everybody needs to find his own way to quit. That's the key. You have to be motivated to quit and be creative in finding ways not to smoke," says Mitchell Nides, Ph.D., a psychologist at the University of California, Los Angeles.

But no matter how you choose to quit, smoking-cessation experts say there are a few fundamentals to keep in mind.

Set a quit date. People who designate a definite day to quit and stick to it are more likely to stop smoking than those who don't, Dr. Brandon says. Avoid picking stressful holidays like New Year's Day or Thanksgiving, and don't select a date that is weeks or months away. Chances are that your resolve to quit will melt away by then. Instead, once you decide to stop, choose a day that falls within the next two weeks.

Go cold turkey. President Eisenhower began smoking when he was a cadet at West Point. By World War II Ike was up to four packs a day. In 1949 doctors advised him to cut back on his smoking. He tried it for a few days then decided that rationing his cigarettes was worse than not smoking at all. So he quit cold turkey and never had another cigarette in his life, says Stephen Ambrose, Ph.D., author of *Eisenhower: Soldier and President*.

All that he did was put smoking out of his mind and developed "a scornful attitude toward those weaklings who did not have the willpower to break their enslavement to nicotine," Dr. Ambrose says.

It worked for Ike, and it can work for you.

"If you quit cold turkey, you'll probably have a week to 10 days of withdrawal, but then you'll be almost over it. Most people find it a lot easier to quit cold turkey than to gradually reduce their smoking," Dr. Brandon says.

Toss 'em overboard. On your quit date, throw out all of your tobacco products. Don't hold back. If you have any hidden in places like sweaters, pockets, and glove compartments, toss those as well, says C. Tracy Orleans, Ph.D., director of Tobacco Control Research at Fox Chase Cancer Center in Philadelphia and principal creator of Clear Horizons, a self-help smoking-cessation program for people age 50 and older. Be sure to get rid of lighters, matches, and ashtrays.

Banish the booze. Alcohol dissolves your resolve and makes it easier for you to light up again, says Thomas Cooper, D.D.S., a nicotine dependency researcher and professor of oral health sciences at the University of Kentucky College of Dentistry in Lexington. Avoid drinking for at least a month after you quit.

One is never enough. Nicotine is a lifelong addiction, so smoking just one cigarette—even after years of abstinence—can lead to another and another.

"'Smoking one won't hurt me,' has probably been the downfall of more smokers who are trying to quit than any other single thing," says Dr.

How We Did It: A Couple Douses Their Deadly Habit

Tracy Gibson doesn't remember his last cigarette. But neither he nor his wife, Bernice, will ever forget what happened next.

Gibson, a two-pack-a-day smoker since his teens, had just lit a cigarette after a July 21, 1993, swim at Rehoboth Beach, Delaware. Seconds later, his heart stopped beating, and he slumped over the back of a beach chair. For the next 11 minutes lifeguards, volunteer firefighters, and paramedics desperately performed cardiopulmonary resuscitation and administered electroshocks to his heart. In the hospital emergency room his heart was shocked more than 14 times to keep it beating. After he regained consciousness, he couldn't recall much of that eventful day.

"My heart failure was caused by hardening of the arteries due to smoking and a fast-food diet," says the former gas station owner, who is now in his sixties. "I had always enjoyed smoking and never really gave much thought to quitting until after that day. But having something like that happen was like going through a very advanced stop-smoking clinic. I've never really had a desire for a cigarette again. I feel better, I breathe better, food tastes better, my clothes don't stink. I'm very thankful to be alive."

For Bernice, watching her husband's near-death experience was

Cooper, who smoked for 36 years before quitting in 1984.

Psychologically, smoking just one often makes people who have quit feel bad about themselves. And to cope with those bad feelings, they will smoke more cigarettes and quickly tumble back into the habit, Dr. Nides says.

If you're severely tempted, get away from the situation or call a supportive friend who can help talk you out of it, Dr. Nides suggests.

Behavior Modification: Change Is Good

When you wake up, you smoke. Take out the garbage, you smoke. Go bowling, you smoke.

enough to make her ditch her own two-pack-a-day habit. On the day he came home from the hospital, she got rid of her favorite lighter and the remaining cigarettes.

"I didn't want to tempt him," says Bernice, who is also in her sixties. He wasn't tempted, but she was.

"My toughest times were after dinner or after I ate because I was used to having a cigarette then," Bernice says. Her solution? She changed her routine.

"I sat in a different spot at the table than I normally would," she says. "After I was finished eating, I would get right up and start doing the dishes. Sometimes when I was doing the dishes, I'd scream, 'I need a cigarette! I need a cigarette!' But everyone would realize that I was just releasing tension and ignore me. After about 30 seconds of that, the urge would pass."

Within a couple of months, her desire to smoke had virtually faded. Three years afterward, the couple was walking three miles a day, eating a low-fat, high-fiber diet, and never lighting up.

"Our kids tell me, 'Mom, you don't look like a smoker anymore.' And I really don't feel like a smoker. It's great," Bernice says.

The urge to have a cigarette is often triggered by everyday tasks and routines. But if you change your behavior, you can become a nonsmoker, doctors say. These self-help techniques, used alone or in combination, will help.

Write an instruction book. Every time you smoke, jot down the time of day and what you were doing. Then describe the step-by-step process of lighting up. A description of an after-dinner cigarette, for example, might read: "I push my chair back from the table. I take a deep breath. I reach into my pocket and grab the package. I tap the package on the table. I slip out a cigarette and twiddle it in my right hand. I put the cigarette in my mouth and reach for my lighter. I light the cigarette and take my first puff."

Outsmarting Your Favorite Smoke of the Day

All cigarettes aren't created equal. If you smoke, you probably have one special time of day when lighting up gives you the greatest pleasure.

In a survey of 5,051 men and women who smoke, 44 percent said that they would miss an after-dinner cigarette the most if they quit smoking, according to researchers at Stanford University and the West Los Angeles Veterans Affairs Hospital. One in three said that the first cigarette in the morning would be the hardest to forgo, followed by the last one of the day and lighting up when drinking alcoholic beverages.

"For most smokers, the after-dinner cigarette seems to be almost irresistible," says Murray Jarvik, M.D., professor of psychiatry at the University of California, Los Angeles, School of Medicine. Why? Eating a big meal like dinner slightly reduces the amount of nicotine in the blood, and that may trigger physical cravings. You also can develop a strong psychological urge to smoke if you associate finishing a meal with lighting up an after-dinner cigarette.

This record keeping is an important starting point for later changes, because it helps you become aware of your smoking patterns and the complex rituals that you have created for lighting up, says Dennis Gersten, M.D., a San Diego psychiatrist in private practice and publisher of *Atlantis: The Imagery Newsletter.*

Switch hands. Once you are aware of your smoking rituals, try to break up that routine somehow.

"You can try to break the pattern any way you want, but I find that switching hands makes people very uncomfortable, which turns out to be a good thing. I had a patient who had been smoking for 40 years. He simply switched from smoking with his right hand to his left, and that was the end of his smoking. It broke the pattern right on the spot," Dr. Gersten says.

But no matter when you are used to smoking your favorite cigarette, a key part of quitting is getting past that moment without taking a puff. The best strategy is changing your routine, says Michael Cummings, Ph.D., senior research scientist and director of the smoking cessation clinic at Roswell Park Cancer Institute in Buffalo, New York. Instead of smoking after a meal, go for a walk or do the dishes. Try munching on a low-fat dessert like fresh fruit in a room where you normally don't eat. Avoid eating any food that seems to bolster your craving for tobacco.

If you really enjoy a smoke first thing in the morning, get up and shower, dress, eat breakfast, and then vigorously plunge into your daily activities. To ensure that you'll have a busy morning, Dr. Cummings suggests that you make appointments for early in the day, then sleep in for an extra few minutes so that you must rush to get ready and won't have time to smoke. Keep a distraction nearby during the day— like a small ball, a pencil, a pen, chewing gum, or hard candies. Then you will have something to do with your hands and mouth.

Short-circuit stress. "A lot of people smoke to cope with stress. So when you quit, you have to come up with some new coping devices," says Michael Cummings, Ph.D., senior research scientist and director of the smoking-cessation clinic at Roswell Park Cancer Institute in Buffalo, New York. For starters, try deep breathing, meditation, squeezing a rubber ball, or pushing your tongue into the roof of your mouth for 10 to 15 seconds.

Quit early in the week. "We suggest that our patients try to quit on a Monday or a Tuesday of a busy week," Dr. Cooper says. "You don't want to quit smoking when you have a lot of time on your hands to think about it."

Dive into the smoke-free world. Plan out your day so that you'll be less tempted to smoke. Browse in a smoke-free shopping mall, eat in a

Tobacco: There's No Safety Valve

Pipes, cigars, and chewing tobacco can be just as deadly as cigarettes. Here's a quick list of the hazards.

- Pipe and cigar smoke contains the same number of toxic compounds as cigarette smoke.
- If you smoke a pipe and cigars and don't inhale, you still have a higher risk for developing cancers of the mouth and lips than a nonsmoker.
- A former cigarette smoker is more likely to inhale pipe and cigar smoke, and if you do inhale, you have the same risk of developing lung cancer and heart disease as cigarette smoker.
- A person who uses chewing tobacco can achieve blood nicotine levels comparable to someone who smokes cigarettes.
- Nitrosamine, a potent cancer-causing agent, is present in chewing tobacco products at levels up to 100 times higher than those allowed in bacon, beer, and other foods.
- Users of chewing tobacco are twice as likely to die of heart disease than those who don't smoke or chew. The constant flow of nicotine from this type of tobacco increases heart rate and blood pressure and can lead to an increased stroke risk.

Here are some of the chemicals found in chewing tobacco.

Arsenic (ant poison)
Benzene (toxic gasoline ingredient)
Cadium (car battery component)
Cyanide (poison)
Formaldehyde (morgue preservative)

Lead (nerve poison)
Nicotine (insecticide)
N-Nitrosamine (cancer-causing agent)
Polonium 210 (radioactive substance)

smoke-free restaurant, or go to a movie or museum where smoking is prohibited, suggests Dr. Nides.

Give yourself daily pep talks. Every morning and at bedtime, write down all the reasons why you want to quit. It will reinforce your resolve to stop smoking. "It's easy to forget why you're trying to quit when you're going through nicotine withdrawal. So reminders are an important way to keep yourself on track," Dr. Brandon says.

You also might try jotting down something you did that day—like walking a mile—that you weren't able to do when you smoked, Dr. Nides says.

Let's make a deal. Sign a contract with yourself, Dr. Brandon suggests. Every day that you go without a cigarette, reward yourself—buy a magazine, sleep in for an extra 30 minutes or take a long stroll.

If you smoke, punish yourself with an activity you detest, like cleaning out the refrigerator or washing out the gutters, Dr. Brandon says.

Give to your least favorite charity. In the first two weeks after you quit, every time you give in to the urge to smoke, pledge a dollar to an organization that you absolutely despise, Dr. Brandon says. It should be such a detestable group that it will make you think twice before lighting up. At the end of each day, give the money to a friend or spouse and insist that they send it off.

"Some people have told me that this particular technique helped stop them from smoking for those critical first few days," Dr. Brandon says.

Save those dollars. Put the money that you would normally spend on cigarettes into a clear container so that you can see it add up. After six months, use that money for a big reward, like a dream vacation, Dr. Brandon suggests.

Stall for time. When an urge hits, if you can delay lighting up for just a minute or two it may pass, Dr. Cummings says. Carry a picture of your grandchildren or other loved ones and pull it out every time an urge strikes. Write down the reasons why you want to quit and keep the list handy for these moments, too.

Nutrition: Eat Well, Stay Smoke-Free

If you start eating like a nonsmoker eats, you may even become one, says William McCarthy, Ph.D., director of science at the Pritikin

---

Medical Advances Ease Quitting

It's only a few inches around and doesn't look impressive, but the transdermal nicotine patch is rapidly becoming a formidable weapon in the struggle to quit smoking.

When worn on the skin, the patch releases tiny amounts of nicotine into the bloodstream for up to 24 hours. That eases withdrawal symptoms and makes it easier for a person to quit. Over several weeks, the dosage of the patch is gradually reduced to wean the person off the drug.

Of 1,070 male and female patch users ages 65 to 74, nearly 30 percent were still smoke-free six months later, says C. Tracy Orleans, Ph.D., director of Tobacco Control Research at Fox Chase Cancer Center in Philadelphia. Most of those who had tried to quit before said that the patch made quitting easier.

"The patch is the state of the art. It increases quit rates two to three times. We're recommending it for anyone who has had trouble dealing with withdrawal symptoms in the past," Dr. Orleans says.

Nicotine gum, another form of nicotine replacement, also has helped many people quit. Both the patch and gum are readily available over the counter, but be sure to check with your doctor to see if either would be appropriate for you.

Longevity Center in Santa Monica, California.

In fact, dietary changes when used in conjunction with other smoking-cessation methods can be a potent ally in your effort to quit, Dr. McCarthy says.

"Dietary changes are a way of moving away from the smoker lifestyle," Dr. McCarthy says. "If you simply extinguish the cigarette and do nothing else about your lifestyle habits, you will still be acting and living like a typical smoker."

Smokers tend to eat more meat, drink more coffee and alcohol, eat fewer fruits and vegetables, consume fewer cereals and grains, and are more likely than nonsmokers to be deficient in vitamins A, C, E, and minerals like calcium, selenium, and zinc.

Smokers who begin eating a typical nonsmoker's diet are more likely to be smoke-free a year later than those who attempt to quit without dietary changes, Dr. McCarthy says.

Dietary changes—particularly cutting fats and adding fruits and vegetables like oranges, apricots, carrots, and sweet potatoes, which are loaded with antioxidants—can help offset some of the ill effects of smoking and reduce your risk of stroke, heart disease, and cancer, says James Scala, Ph.D., a nutritional biochemist and author of *If You Can't/Won't Stop Smoking*. Antioxidants like vitamin C help block or reverse some of the harm done by free radicals, which are unstable molecules that damage cells and tissues. "Research indicates that it is sensible to take up to 1,000 milligrams of vitamin C daily and about 400 international units of vitamin E to reverse some of the bad influences of smoking," says Dr. Scala.

A good diet also will help you cope with some of the challenges of quitting, such as weight gain, Dr. Scala says.

Fear of gaining weight is an imposing barrier for many smokers who are trying to quit. In a survey of 1,234 people who smoked, ages 50 to 74, nearly half believed that gaining 20 pounds is more harmful than smoking. "Actually, you would probably have to gain at least 100 pounds to equal the health risks of continued smoking," says Robert C. Klesges, Ph.D., professor of psychology and preventive medicine at the University of Memphis in Tennessee.

In reality, about half of all people who quit smoking don't gain weight, and those who do put on about 10 pounds. The weight gain only occurs shortly after you quit smoking, and you do not continue to gain weight any faster than someone who had never smoked.

The following dietary changes may help prevent excessive weight gain after you quit. But Dr. McCarthy suggests that you alter your diet long before you stop smoking, because waiting until the day you quit may make it too difficult to make major changes in your diet at the same time that you have to cope with nicotine withdrawal. So adjust your diet first. Then, when you feel comfortable with your new eating habits, quit smoking.

Nicotine Anonymous: No Names, but Lots of Support

Nicotine Anonymous, a 12-step program similar to Alcoholics Anonymous, offers support to those who want to become and remain nicotine-free—although no formal studies of its effectiveness have been conducted.

The organization, founded in 1982, has about 500 chapters world-wide. Members acknowledge that nicotine is an addictive drug and they cannot control their use of it. They say that the meetings offer mutual support for staying smoke-free. The only requirement for membership is the desire to abstain from nicotine.

"I heard things in meetings from others who had quit before me, and I thought, 'Oh my God, I'm going through that, too.' I just realized that what I was experiencing was normal," says Lynn H., a Chicago woman who smoked for 34 years before quitting in her sixties.

"There is something in those meetings that grabs you. There is a lot of caring, friendship, and support," she says. "I still go to remind myself what it was like because it's so easy to forget. And I know that if I forget and decide I can smoke socially, I'll end up right back where I started."

For more information, write to: Nicotine Anonymous World Service Office, Department R, P. O. Box 591777, San Francisco, CA 94159-1777. Be sure to enclose a stamped, self-addressed envelope.

Balance the pyramid. If you follow the basic U.S. Department of Agriculture food pyramid guidelines, you'll be eating more like a non-smoker and may be less tempted to light up again, Dr. McCarthy says. That means 2 to 4 servings of fruits; 3 to 5 servings of vegetables a day; 2 to 3 servings of dairy products like milk and cheese; 6 to 11 servings of breads, rice, and cereals; and no more than one 3-ounce serving of meat, poultry, or fish or 2 to 3 servings of beans, eggs whites, and nuts.

Sip on OJ. Tobacco smoke destroys vitamin C. Replenish your supply by drinking two 8-ounce glasses of orange juice daily, particularly in the first few days after you quit, Dr. Scala says.

Orange juice will also help flush nicotine out of your body and help you become nicotine-free faster, Dr. Cooper says. Avoid orange juice, however, if you're using the nicotine patch or gum, because you want that nicotine to stay in your body to help avoid withdrawal symptoms.

Cap the caffeine. Laying off tobacco increases the stimulating effects of caffeine. So if you drink coffee, you may feel more jittery and might start craving a smoke, Dr. Brandon says. Switch to decaffeinated coffee and drink no more than two 8-ounce cups a day, he suggests.

Stay fluid. Carry a squeeze bottle of water around with you. Whenever you feel the urge for a smoke, take a swig of water instead, Dr. Cummings says. Water helps flush nicotine and other tobacco toxins out of the body and speeds withdrawal. In addition to the normal amount that you drink, he recommends having another six to eight glasses daily when you're trying to quit.

Eat breakfast. People who smoke often use a cigarette to elevate blood sugars and suppress appetite, Dr. Cooper says. It's important to replace your early-morning smoke with an energizing low-fat breakfast like a bran muffin and a glass of apple juice.

Be Johnny Appleseed. Snacking on an apple twice daily for the first 90 days after you quit will help get you past the midmorning and midafternoon slumps without reaching for a cigarette, Dr. Cooper says.

Try new foods. Avoid eating or drinking any foods that you link with smoking, Dr. Brandon says. So if you have always had a cup of coffee and a muffin for breakfast followed by a cigarette, try a glass of milk and a piece of raisin toast instead. The change can dampen your urge to smoke.

Make food work for you. In the first few days after quitting, keep low-fat foods like breadsticks, crackers, carrots, celery, and popcorn handy to toss into your mouth whenever you feel the urge to smoke. If you need something to do with your hands, try eating foods that require peeling, such as oranges, sunflower seeds, tangerines, nuts in the shell, or artichokes, suggests C. Barr Taylor, M.D., professor of psychiatry at Stanford University School of Medicine and author of *The Facts about Smoking*.

Indulge your sweet tooth. If eating a sweet will prevent you from smoking, do it, Dr. Taylor says. If possible, avoid high-fat sweets like cake, ice cream, and chocolate. Instead, pick alternatives that are lower in fat like jelly beans, sherbets, hard candies, or fruits like grapes, bananas, or dates.

Meditation: A Single Thought Can Banish Urges

The average person has about 15,000 thoughts a day. If you're trying to quit, it can seem like every one of those thoughts is the same: Smoke!

But meditation can help you dampen that mental noise and help you become a nonsmoker, says Dr. Gersten.

Meditation is a form of concentration that allows you to focus your mind internally and step back from your thoughts and feelings, Dr. Gersten says. In its simpler forms, meditation uses pictures, words (mantras), objects (such as a candle flame), or sensations (such as breathing) to focus the mind. If your mind begins to drift, you refocus your attention on your chosen image or word.

Studies have shown that meditation can help reduce the severity of many medical conditions, including anxiety, asthma, migraines, high blood pressure, and chronic pain. And it can help you quit smoking, Dr. Gersten says. Every time you feel an urge to smoke, try this meditation. Each time you inhale, say the word "peace," and as you exhale, say "love." If your mind begins to wander, refocus it on the words. Do that for five minutes, and by then the urge to smoke may have passed or subsided to the point that you can resist it, Dr. Gersten says.

"This meditation will help you deal with the craving. You're not saying that the urge to smoke isn't there," Dr. Gersten says. "You're acknowledging that the urge exists, but you don't have to do anything about it. You just turn your mind back to your mantra."

Nicotine Fading: Letting Go Slowly

Although going cold turkey is your best bet, there is a gradual alternative that works for some people, says Dr. Orleans.

The process is known as nicotine fading, and Dr. Orleans calls it a form of "cool turkey" because it prepares you both physically and psychologically for the day when you finally quit altogether.

"Quitting abruptly on a target date is the best way to go," Dr. Orleans says. "But nothing says that you shouldn't prepare yourself for your quit date. Nicotine fading is one of the ways you can do that."

By making small weekly drops in nicotine, you avoid strong withdrawal symptoms when you quit, particularly if you smoke a high- or medium-nicotine brand.

High-nicotine brands include unfiltered cigarettes and any filtered brand that isn't labeled with the words "mild," "light," or "ultra-light." Medium-nicotine brands are labeled "mild" or "light." Low-nicotine cigarettes bear words like "extra mild," "ultra," and "ultra-light."

The program allows two weeks to complete the nicotine fading process if you smoke a high-nicotine brand, and one week for medium- or low-nicotine brands.

Let it fade. Fading is fairly simple, Dr. Orleans says. If you smoke a high-nicotine brand, switch to a medium for one week and then to a low brand for another week before you quit. That way you will cut your dose of nicotine by one-third each week. If you smoke mediums, switch to lows for a week, and if you smoke lows, try an ultra-low brand for a week.

Don't jump off too fast. Avoid going directly from a high-nicotine brand to a low one, Dr. Orleans says. If the nicotine in your body drops too rapidly, it can cause cravings and withdrawal symptoms, which will defeat the purpose of fading.

Be cautious. The way you smoke affects how much nicotine you take in, so keep your cigarette use on an even keel. Dr. Orleans warns that if you switch to lower-nicotine cigarettes but smoke more of them, you risk getting the same dose of nicotine that you were getting before. Also, avoid inhaling more often or deeply than you have in the past and try not to cover the tiny airholes near the bottom of the filter with your fingers or lips.

Keep that date. Having an absolute quit date is a must with nicotine fading, Dr. Orleans says. Without it, you may be tempted to think that cutting back on nicotine is good enough. It isn't. For the sake of your health, you need to shake the habit completely.

For more information on the Clear Horizons program write to: Fox Chase Cancer Center, 510 Township Line Road, Cheltenham, PA 19012.

Prescription for Prevention

Quitting smoking is the most important thing that a person can do to slash the risk of stroke, cancer, and heart disease. Even if you have smoked for years, quitting at 60, 70, or 80 can reverse many of the worst effects of smoking and improve the quality of your life.

Do:

- *Set a quit date and stick to it.*

- *Throw out all of your tobacco products on your quit date.*

- *Quit cold turkey.*

- *Plan out your day so that you'll be less tempted to smoke. Browse in a smoke-free shopping mall, for example.*

- *Eat like a nonsmoker. A balanced diet that includes at least five servings of fruits and vegetables like apples and carrots can help reduce your urge to smoke.*

- *Drink at least two 8-ounce glasses of orange juice daily. It will help flush nicotine out of your body. Orange juice, however, is not recommend if you are using the nicotine patch or gum.*

- *Persevere. Nicotine, a prime ingredient in tobacco, is one of the most addictive substances in the world. It may take several attempts to quit. But if you keep trying, you will become a nonsmoker.*

Don't:

- *Drink alcohol for at least 30 days after you quit smoking.*

- *Drink caffeinated beverages like coffee, tea, or colas. Caffeine can increase your urge to smoke.*

- *Let stress defeat your effort to quit. Practice relaxation techniques like meditation.*

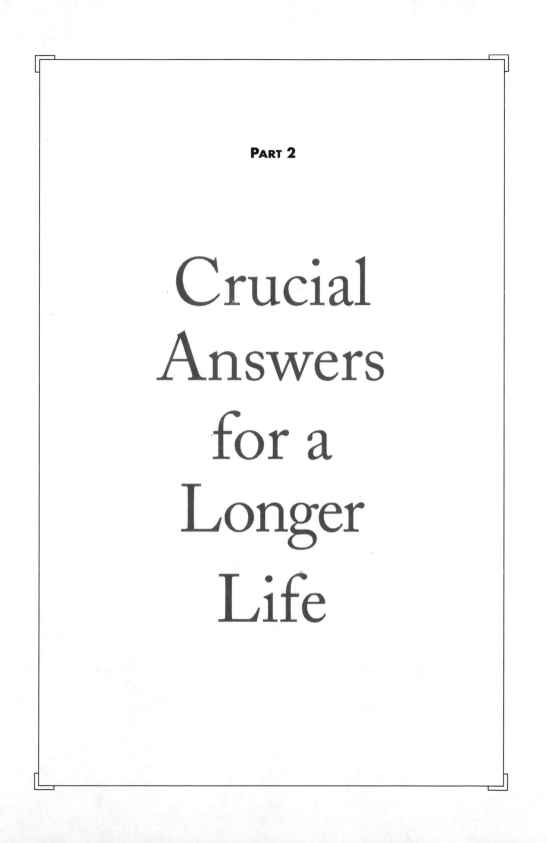

PART 2

Crucial Answers for a Longer Life

Chapter 10

Is Drinking Good or Bad for Me?

Think Mediterranean: blue sky, white beaches, sumptuous foods covered with sauces, and that bottle of red wine with every meal. Add to the idyllic picture an unexpected bonus—that the to-die-for Mediterranean diet may lower your risk of heart disease and stroke. It may even help fight cancer.

Part of the reason for the French paradox—the fact that rich French cuisine accompanies an unexpectedly low risk of heart disease—may lie in the vine, researchers believe. Or, more precisely, in the ethanol, the main ingredient in alcoholic beverages—the stuff that can make you light-headed.

Scientists also have found that some of the plant chemicals in wine provide protection from disease. While you're getting happy and relaxed, they go to work blocking the formation of harmful oxidized low-density lipoprotein (LDL) cholesterol and warding off cancers.

Bending the elbow at the dinner table may be part of the reason that people in Mediterranean countries can eat rich foods and still have low rates of heart disease.

Light to moderate drinking—a drink or two per day—may help you live longer, says J. Michael Gaziano, M.D., director of cardiovascular epidemiology at Brigham and Women's Hospital in Boston. "People who drink light to moderate amounts of alcohol have the lowest mortality—even lower than nondrinkers."

"In some instances the risk of heart attack is 20 percent to 30 percent lower in light drinkers than in people who don't drink," says Arthur Klatsky, M.D., senior consultant in cardiology for the Kaiser-Permanente Medical Center in Oakland, California.

When researchers at the Harvard School of Public Health studied

85,709 women over a 12-year period, they found that light to moderate drinkers had the lowest risk of fatal heart disease—even if they already had other heart disease risk factors.

Raise a Toast to the Health of Your Heart

"The cardiovascular benefits of alcohol come from the alcohol itself, no matter what drink it's in," says Dr. Gaziano. Ethanol raises the levels of high-density lipoprotein cholesterol, which helps to keep your arteries from filling up with plaque and, therefore, reduces your risk of heart disease. Dr. Gaziano's research shows that you get the same protective effects from wine, beer, and liquor.

Alcohol may help your circulatory system in other ways, too. Some data suggest that it reduces the blood's tendency to clot. And it may help keep the blood vessels more flexible. Furthermore, it's possible that a drink a day relieves stress. All of this could lead to lower risks of heart attack and possibly stroke.

"We know that the phytochemicals in wine are potent antioxidants that may help keep blood from clotting," says Andrew Waterhouse, Ph.D., a researcher in the Department of Viticulture and Enology at the University of California, Davis. Wine is rich in a group of phytochemicals called flavonoids, which also protect against cancer and prevent LDL cholesterol from oxidizing.

In one of his studies, Dr. Waterhouse tested the effect of California wines on the oxidation of the harmful form of human cholesterol, LDL. Both red and white wines blocked LDL formation by 46 percent to 100 percent, but three times as much white wine was needed for the effect.

Another "protective" factor: Researchers say that wine may attract a crowd that is more fit to begin with. "People who drink wine seem to have a healthier lifestyle in general," says Dr. Klatsky.

Some research suggests that you get the same antioxidant protection from nonalcoholic foods such as grape juice, fruits, and vegetables. That route will steer you clear of the risks of alcohol, including addiction, traffic accidents, and driving-under-the-influence citations.

294

Who Can Benefit from Alcohol?

Drinking alcohol may sound like a merry way to protect your health, but it's actually a serious, complex issue. No two people share identical risk for developing health problems or alcohol addiction, says Arthur Klatsky, M.D., senior consultant in cardiology for the Kaiser-Permanente Medical Center in Oakland, California. But according to Dr. Klatsky, these sample scenarios will help you make an informed choice about whether drinking is for you.

• You have had a cardiac episode. You don't have a history of alcohol abuse. You have given up smoking and followed your doctor's instructions to the letter. You even gave up wine, although you enjoy it. In this scenario, you're probably not at risk for alcohol addiction. Alcohol may help lower your risk of further heart problems. Your doctor will probably give you the go-ahead for a glass a day.

• You have no history of alcohol abuse. You drink occasionally, maybe once every few weeks. Ask your doctor whether you should drink more often to protect your heart. You'll probably get an okay.

• You've never abused alcohol. Your parents died of heart attacks, and you have high cholesterol. In this case, your doctor may advise a maximum of one drink a day to reduce your risk of cardiovascular problems.

• You have never had a drinking problem. You don't have heart disease, you don't smoke, you have low cholesterol, and your parents lived into their nineties. In this scenario your heart disease risk is probably not high. You probably don't need the protection of alcohol.

Just a Little Protects Your Heart

Alcohol is a bit like jalapeño pepper. A pinch adds spicy flavor. But more than that seems to set your system on fire.

"Luckily, light drinking doesn't affect blood pressure. But more than two drinks a day may make your blood pressure go up," says Dr. Gaziano.

It's not completely understood why a little alcohol is good for you while a lot can do big-time damage. But the fact is, heavy drinkers—people who

---

When You Can't Leave Alcohol Alone

Alcohol is a two-edged sword. Small amounts protect you. Too much will do you damage, increasing your risk of heart disease, cancer, and stroke as well as an assortment of other problems. If you can not stop after just one drink, here is what you can do, according to Arthur Klatsky, M.D., senior consultant in cardiology for the Kaiser-Permanente Medical Center in Oakland, California.

Get help. Ask your doctor for help or get in touch with an alcohol treatment program. For confidential information, write to Alcoholics Anonymous, P. O. Box 459, Grand Central Station, New York, NY 10163. To contact a local chapter of the organization, check your phone book.

Go public. Some experts think that it is easier to quit if you tell your friends and family that you have a problem and want to solve it. While you're at it, ask loved ones to help you avoid temptation by staying alcohol-free in your presence.

Tell it like it is. If someone offers you alcohol at a social gathering, just say, "I don't drink," and ask for something nonalcoholic.

---

put away three or more drinks a day—increase their risk of a variety of problems, including heart disease, stroke, esophageal cancer, and liver disease.

That's not all. In a study of more than 15,000 women up to age 74, researchers found that moderate drinking significantly increases the risk of breast cancer. And a lifetime average of even one drink a day increases the risk.

"For most people, light drinking is associated with a lower chance of prematurely dying because the benefits in terms of lower rates of heart disease outweigh any small risk of cancer," says Dr. Gaziano.

Get Maximum Protection

For some folks the best approach to alcohol is not approaching it at all. Drinking is off-limits to anyone who might abuse it, for instance. The advantages of alcohol are not so huge that a nondrinker should take up the habit, given the risks of addiction. But for many other people, a little can do a lot of good. So if you do drink, here is how to get the most protection from alcohol.

A little goes a long way. Alcohol concentrates in lean body tissue such as muscle, not fat. As you age, lean body mass decreases and fat increases. Not only are you more likely to feel the effects of alcohol when you're older, but also it is more likely to do damage to your system if you overindulge. "There's absolutely no reason for anyone, especially older people, to have more than a drink or two a day," says Dr. Gaziano.

Because women tend to have less body mass than men, along with a slightly different liver metabolism, they should have no more than a half to one drink per day.

Spread it out. "One reason that French and Italians have lower heart attack rates might be because they drink wine a little each day with meals, while northern Europeans drink large amounts on weekend nights," says Dr. Gaziano. "You wouldn't take all your cholesterol medicine on Saturday—you take it in very small doses every day."

Wine and dine. Having your drink with a meal is a doubly good idea. For one thing, large meals promote blood clotting, which increases your risk of stroke, says Dr. Klatsky. Drinking wine—either red or white—may help prevent that. "But wine's biggest benefit may be that it encourages people to eat more slowly, which also reduces risk," he says.

Imbibe in the evening. Have your drink (or part of it) with your evening meal. Beyond the digestive benefits, you cut down on other types of risk as well. "You're less likely to climb ladders, drive cars, and do other activities that increase risk," says Dr. Klatsky.

Call it a food. In some cultures people consume alcohol primarily in small amounts with meals. That keeps consumption within safe limits and may explain why there is less alcoholism in those countries. "In Mediterranean countries such as Greece and Italy, people think of alcohol as a food rather than something that you consume on the weekends for its mind-numbing effect," says Dr. Gaziano.

Switch to red? Because red wine is richer in flavonoids, some people

297

are choosing red over white for protection. So should you switch?

It's true that the more intense the color of the wine, the greater the antioxidant content. Red wine contains skins, seeds, and stems. All of this ferments, giving red wine color and flavor. Dr. Klatsky notes that the darker the wine, the greater the concentration of flavonoids.

White wine also contains flavonoids and other antioxidants, although in far lesser amounts than red. If you can't stand chianti but you would still like to add wine to your diet, chardonnay or another white variety should give you some of the same health benefits.

Prescription for Prevention

Just a little alcohol protects against heart disease and heart attacks. But just a bit too much can do major damage to your heart and other vital organs. It can also increase your risk of cancer.

As you get older, your body stores alcohol a little differently, making it especially important to keep consumption low.

Do:

- *Discuss your drinking habits with your doctor. If he feels it is safe for you to drink, limit yourself to one or two drinks per day.*

- *If your drinking is okayed by your doctor: Drink a little every day for maximum protection. Drink with a meal to lower risk of blood clots.*

Don't:

- *Drink more than two drinks a day because it will increase your risk of cancer, heart disease, and stroke.*

- *Drink if you have ever had a problem with alcohol addiction.*

Chapter 11

Will Aspirin Really Protect Me from Disease?

Once it was just a ho-hum over-the-counter ache-and-pain remedy. But in less than a decade, aspirin has been transformed into a superstar drug, touted for its tantalizing promise of preventing heart attacks, fending off recurrent strokes, and possibly deterring digestive cancers. But before you rush to your medicine cabinet, you should realize that researchers still have a lot of questions about this powerful and potentially toxic "wonder" drug.

Can it help some people prevent the three big killers? Probably. Is it for everyone? Nobody knows yet. Most researchers are cautious, but some advocates say that the existing evidence is compelling enough for broad recommendations.

"The real controversy with aspirin has been whether someone who isn't at high risk for these diseases should take it. In my estimation the medical establishment has been a bit too conservative about aspirin," says Tim Byers, M.D., professor of preventive medicine at the University of Colorado School of Medicine in Denver. "The risks of low doses of aspirin are fairly minimal, and the benefits may be high. I know I'm going to start taking aspirin regularly when I reach age 50. I think it's a reasonable choice to make for most people who are 50 and above."

It's Not Just for Headaches Anymore

Ironically, when it was first developed 100 years ago, aspirin was rarely used because doctors feared that it would weaken the heart. Now many physicians and scientists consider it to be a simple, cheap deterrent to cardiovascular disease.

In the landmark Physicians' Health Study, for instance, 22,000 healthy male doctors up to age 84 took either a standard 325-milligram aspirin or a placebo every other day. (A placebo is a look-alike tablet that has no medical effects.) After five years, those who had been taking the aspirin instead of the placebo had a 44 percent lower risk of suffering a first heart attack.

When the results of 25 similar studies of people who had previous heart attacks and strokes were pooled together, researchers found that those who took aspirin regularly had a 32 percent lower rate of subsequent nonfatal heart attacks. They also had 27 percent fewer nonfatal strokes and had a 15 percent reduction in death from cardiovascular diseases.

"I think what we know for sure right now is that in healthy people aspirin will prevent a first heart attack," says Charles Hennekens, M.D., Dr.P.H., professor of medicine at Harvard Medical School. "If you've had a prior heart attack, stroke, or unstable angina—the kind that occurs even when you're not exerting yourself—we know conclusively that aspirin will prevent a recurrence of all of those events and lower the death rate."

But whether aspirin reduces the probability of a first stroke is still questionable because researchers simply don't have enough information yet, Dr. Hennekens says.

Researchers do know that aspirin protects the heart in a couple ways, says W. Steven Pray, R.Ph., Ph.D., professor of nonprescription products at Southwestern Oklahoma State University in Weatherford and a columnist for *U.S. Pharmacist* magazine. First, the drug prevents blood platelets from sticking together and forming blood clots. Second, it may suppress the secretion of chemicals in the blood that contribute to the formation of atherosclerosis, hardening of the arteries, Dr. Pray says.

If you are having a heart attack, taking a 325-milligram aspirin while you're waiting for the paramedics to arrive may reduce the severity of the attack and save your life, Dr. Hennekens says.

"The benefits of aspirin are enormous in that situation," Dr. Hennekens says. "If it's a heart attack, aspirin will reduce the death rate by 23 percent if it is taken within 24 hours of onset and continued daily for 30 days. That alone could save 10,000 lives in the United States a year."

Can an Aspirin a Day Keep Cancer Away?

Researchers also are excited about aspirin's potential to squelch digestive tumors.

In an analysis of 662,000 white men and women, American Cancer Society researchers found that those people who took aspirin 16 or more times a month for a year had 40 percent lower rates of esophageal, stomach, colon, and rectal cancer than those who didn't use the drug.

Harvard University researchers found a 37 percent reduction of colon cancer risk after 10 years of regular aspirin use among 90,000 nurses up to age 72. The most effective dose appeared to be four to six aspirin tablets a week. A similar Harvard study of 48,000 male health professionals up to age 75 found that men taking two or more aspirin a week had a lower risk of colon cancer by 32 percent.

Other studies have shown that at least in animals and in people with a rare genetic predisposition to polyps, aspirin helps block the formation of precancerous polyps in the colon, says Michael Thun, M.D., director of analytic epidemiology at the American Cancer Society in Atlanta.

How aspirin protects the digestive tract isn't clear. The drug may inhibit the production of prostaglandins, hormonelike substances that may cause cancer cells to grow more rapidly. Another possibility is that aspirin boosts the body's immune system so that the body is better able to fight off tumors.

More studies are needed, however, before researchers can endorse aspirin as a preventive measure for digestive cancers, Dr. Thun says.

"Basically, there are good reasons to think that aspirin may have some role in the prevention of colorectal cancer," Dr. Thun says. "The catch is that we haven't proven it." Because aspirin will help some people and harm others, it's difficult to recommend its broad, regular use in the general population, he says. In some people even one adult aspirin (325 mil-

Stick with the Right Dose

Aspirin isn't kind if you overdo it.

"Some medications you can get away with taking too much of, but aspirin isn't one of those," says W. Steven Pray, R.Ph., Ph.D., professor of nonprescription products at Southwestern Oklahoma State University in Weatherford and a columnist for *U.S. Pharmacist* magazine.

Adverse reactions include kidney failure, hearing loss, ringing in the ears, vision difficulties, stomach irritation, gastrointestinal bleeding, confusion, dizziness, and headaches.

Never exceed the dosage recommended by the manufacturer or your physician, Dr. Pray says.

If you're taking the aspirin, avoid using other over-the-counter medications that contain the drug. These products can increase your risk of overdosing. Read the list of ingredients carefully. Look for words like aspirin, acetylsalicylic acid (aspirin's chemical name), or other salicylic acids like bismuth subsalicylate, which can interact with aspirin and cause many of same side effects, he says.

Some common brand-name products to avoid if you're taking aspirin include Alka-Seltzer, Aspergum, BC Powder, Cope, Ecotrin, Goody's Headache Powders, Halfprin, Momentum, Stanback Powders, Vanquish, and Pepto-Bismol, Dr. Pray adds.

Taking one of the pink antidiarrheal products can be particularly tricky, Dr. Pray says, because it's often not obvious from the label that they contain a salicylate. "So people who have upset stomachs, hangovers, or diarrhea may take one of them without realizing that it contains a salicylate. Then they'll take a couple of aspirin for their headaches. So they're actually doubling their dosage of salicylates. That sort of thing can be very troublesome," he says.

ligrams) daily can cause stomach bleeding or strokes from bleeding. There is still no certainty that these risks are outweighed by the potential benefit, except in people at high risk of heart attacks or strokes from clotting.

But Dr. Byers believes that it is only a matter of time before aspirin becomes generally advised to stave off cancer and cardiovascular diseases.

"The only questions that really remain are what is the proper dose and how often should you take it," Dr. Byers says.

Making It Work for You

Because researchers do suggest such a wide range of doses varying from 81 milligrams every other day (one chewable tablet) to 325 milligrams daily (one regular aspirin), consult your doctor before you begin taking aspirin routinely, Dr. Hennekens says. Your doctor will help you determine if taking the drug is a worthwhile step for you, and he can recommend a proper dosage.

Here are some other suggestions from medical experts.

Scope out your medicine cabinet. Check with your doctor or pharmacist before taking aspirin with any prescription or over-the-counter drugs, Dr. Pray says. Ibuprofen and other anti-inflammatory drugs, for instance, add to the adverse effects of aspirin.

Sit up. After age 60, it often becomes harder to swallow aspirin and other tablets. Stand or sit up when swallowing your aspirin. Take the drug with an 8-ounce glass of water at least an hour before bedtime or lying down, says Jacob Karsh, M.D., a rheumatologist and professor of medicine at the University of Ottawa in Ontario, Canada.

Munch on something. Aspirin is less likely to cause stomach pain, nausea, or other digestive upsets if you take it with food, Dr. Byers says. So have the drug with meals or during a snack.

Protect your stomach. Some aspirins are easier on your digestive tract because they have special coatings that allow them to pass through the stomach and digest in your small intestine, Dr. Byers says. Look for brands that are buffered or enteric-coated.

Go beyond aspirin. As promising as aspirin appears to be in preventing these diseases, it still needs your help, Dr. Hennekens says. Lifestyle changes such as low-fat eating, getting regular exercise, and not smoking can have more impact than any drug on your risk of disease.

Aspirin Allergy: Rare, but Potentially Lethal

Like all drugs, aspirin isn't for everyone. About 3 of every 1,000 people develop allergic reactions to aspirin. By age 60 most people who are allergic to aspirin know it because they have had at least one adverse reaction. But the allergy can develop at any age.

"It's like a bee sting. At any time, your body can develop an allergic reaction to aspirin even if you have never had a problem in the past," says W. Steven Pray, R.Ph., Ph.D., professor of nonprescription products at Southwestern Oklahoma State University in Weatherford and a columnist for *U.S. Pharmacist* magazine. "Many people develop hives or rashes, but it can be life-threatening. If you're allergic to aspirin, your airways can shut down so that you can't breathe."

People over 60 who have asthma should be particularly cautious about aspirin use, since they are 10 times more prone to serious allergic reactions than those who don't have asthma, Dr. Pray says. If you have hay fever, you are 5 times more likely to be aspirin-sensitive.

If you take aspirin and develop hives or a rash, stop using the drug and see an allergist or your family doctor as soon as possible. Seek emergency medical attention immediately if someone has difficulty breathing after taking aspirin, Dr. Pray says.

Prescription for Prevention

While doctors remain reluctant to recommend that all of us use aspirin on a daily basis, a growing stack of evidence suggests that this reliable drug may be more than just a remedy for muscle soreness and headaches. When used in combination with other healthy habits such as exercise and low-fat eating, aspirin may be a powerful preventive action against stroke, heart disease, and cancer for people over age 60.

Do:

- *Check with your doctor before taking aspirin on a regular basis.*

- *Take coated aspirin with food to protect your stomach.*

- *Take your aspirin with 8 ounces of water at least an hour before bedtime or before you lie down for a nap.*

Don't:

- *Take aspirin without checking about your other medications. Some prescription medications like Percodan and over-the-counter drugs like Alka-Seltzer contain aspirin (also called acetylsalicylic acid) or other salicylic acids like bismuth subsalicylate. If you're already taking aspirin, the additional aspirin in these products can cause adverse reactions like kidney failure or stomach upset. So read product labels carefully and check with your doctor.*

Chapter 12

How Important Are Screenings and Self-Exams?

L et's rephrase that question. What is the most important thing in your life? Your spouse? Your grandchildren? That little sports car you just bought? (Just because you are over 60 doesn't mean that you have to slow down.) Screenings and self-exams are just as important. They protect you from cancer, heart disease, and stroke—and make it possible for you to enjoy the good things in your life.

But you don't want to walk into your doctor's office and ask for every test in the book. Some tests just aren't worth taking. Here is a rundown of what you do and don't need.

Blood Pressure Screening

"Testing for high blood pressure is at the top of the list of needed tests," says Timothy A. McAfee, M.D., associate director of preventive care at the Group Health Cooperative of Puget Sound in Seattle, the nation's oldest and largest consumer-governed health maintenance or ganization (HMO). High blood pressure damages artery walls and dramatically increases your risk of heart disease and stroke.

It is easy enough to get a reading on the machine at the drugstore or take your own reading at home, but this test also is part of just about any visit to your doctor's office. Your doctor will place an inflatable cuff on your upper arm. When the cuff tightens, the doctor will get a reading of how forcefully your blood is being pumped by your heart. According to the American Heart Association, acceptable blood pressure falls within a range rather than a set number. For most adults, a reading that is less than 140/90 millimeters of mercury (mmHg) is good news. Talk to your doctor about what is a good blood pressure for you to aim for.

Blood pressure goes up and down over the course of the day, so a random reading may not be accurate. Here is how to get the best reading, says Lawrence LaPalio, M.D., medical director of geriatrics at Columbia La Grange Memorial Hospital in La Grange, Illinois.

Control consumption. Avoid stimulants that speed your heart rate, such as coffee or alcohol. A drink the night before can interfere.

Get comfortable. Five minutes before the test, sit in a comfortable, relaxed position with your arm at heart-height. Rest quietly.

Take the average. Ask your doctor to take several readings and average them. Get a reading before you head for home—you may be more relaxed. Or average the readings taken over several office visits.

Beware of the white coat. For some people, just being in the doctor's office causes nerves to surge and blood pressure to rise. "Unfortunately," says Dr. LaPalio, "if your blood pressure rises due to stress in the doctor's office, it may also rise in response to everyday events. If it goes up every time you drive in traffic or go to a new place, it should be treated."

Get the full picture. For high blood pressure, go for treatment immediately, says Dr. LaPalio. If you have mild to moderate blood pressure readings, get the true picture by monitoring your own blood pressure for a month or so. Follow this routine recommended by Dr. LaPalio.

Check it morning, noon, and night. Measure your blood pressure at different times of the day.

Use your moods. Measure when you are stressed, relaxed, happy, depressed, and active.

Keep a diary. Write down the readings, the time, and other relevant factors—what you ate and drank, if you exercised, if you took medications, and what you were doing when you took the measurement.

Breast Examination and Mammography

"A yearly mammogram and professional breast examination plus a monthly self-examination can reduce your risk of breast cancer death by

Get Yourself Covered

Many health insurance programs cover preventive care such as health screenings. So check your policy or call your agent. If you are age 65 or older or have a disability, you probably use Medicare. Although regulations may change in the future, this program routinely covers only a few screening tests. It doesn't cover checkups.

"But if you visit the doctor because something's wrong—if you have a symptom—Medicare will cover the visit," states an official of the Health Care Administration in Baltimore. "It covers tests your doctor decides that you need."

Here are the screening tests covered by Medicare.

Mammograms. If you are at low risk, the program picks up the tab for one mammogram every three years. High-risk women can get one every 11 months if they are age 64 or younger and once every 23 months at age 65 or over.

Cervical screening. Medicare covers one pap smear every three years, unless your doctor considers you to be at risk. In that case, there are no restrictions on how often you can have this test performed.

a third," says Joseph Aisner, M.D., director of clinical sciences at the Cancer Institute of New Jersey in New Brunswick. "Every woman age 50 and over should have an annual screening."

You need all the parts to get the whole picture: Tumors that distort the breast's structure or have absorbed calcium often show up on a mammogram. Physical examinations, by you and your doctor, can pick up what the mammogram misses. While this trio may not find all cancers, their use provides earlier diagnosis and saves lives.

For a mammogram the breast is compressed between two plates, which may be a little uncomfortable. A low-dose x-ray records two or three images of the tissues. Your doctor will also feel for any lumps in the breast as part of your annual physical examination.

Your risk of breast cancer increases as you get older. There is some controversy over whether screenings are needed, because few studies have been done of the over-60 population, but "from an individual's point of view, it makes sense to continue to get mammograms," Dr. McAfee explains.

Breast cancer is the most common cancer among American women. What can screening do? A 20-year study of breast cancer published by the American Cancer Society showed that screening results in a survival rate of 86 percent in women diagnosed with breast cancer.

Dr. Aisner suggests these methods for getting the best results from your examination.

Check for quality. Make sure that the facility you go to for a mammogram is accredited by the American College of Radiology. That tells you the machinery is adequate and the staff is trained.

Make one trip. Use a facility that develops the pictures on the spot. That way, if there is a problem with the film, the technician can reshoot. You don't have to return for a second test.

Tune your technique. Ask your doctor or nurse to show you exactly how to perform a self-exam. Or ask for a referral to a class, especially one where you can learn by using a "phantom," a silicone model in which several tumorlike BBs have been implanted. You can learn what to feel for in your own breasts.

Cervical Screening

"Pap smears have reduced death from cervical cancer by more than 95 percent in the past 35 to 40 years," notes Dr. Aisner. Yet, a lot of women stop getting this important test as they get older—not a good idea.

In this relatively painless test your doctor inserts a speculum into the vagina, opens it to reveal the cervix, and takes a small sample of cells from the vagina and the cervix. The cells are examined for cancer.

Here's what you need for protection.

Test further. Unless you have had a full or partial hysterectomy, your doctor should get samples both from the vagina and from the endocervix, which is the cervix at its opening, says Dr. Aisner. In premenopausal and menopausal women an endocervical sample is necessary. In postmenopausal women it may not be possible to obtain an

---

Get Free Protection

Think of it as the best bargain around. Some states get grants from the Centers for Disease Control and Prevention to provide screenings for breast and cervical cancer. That means free mammograms and Pap smears, says Joseph Aisner, M.D., director of clinical sciences at the Cancer Institute of New Jersey in New Brunswick.

Ask your doctor or call the American Cancer Society or an area hospital to check on the availability of low-cost or free mammograms and Pap smears. While you have them on the phone, ask about any other low-cost or free-of-charge screenings, too.

---

endocervical sample, he says. A vaginal Pap smear isn't always enough because the most common site for cancer is at the opening to the cervix.

Do a background check. Ask your doctor what tests were done and what the results were in your previous three exams. If they were interpreted as adequate and normal, you may need exams only once every three years. Otherwise, continue with yearly screenings, suggests Dr. Aisner.

Cholesterol Testing

Think of cholesterol as fat that comes in two forms. LDL (low-density lipoprotein) cholesterol latches onto artery walls and over time narrows them, thus increasing risk of heart attack and stroke. HDL (high-density lipoprotein) cholesterol is the good stuff that keeps the LDL in check. Protect yourself with low levels of total cholesterol and LDL, plus high levels of HDL. You'll need to donate just a very small sample of blood for a lab test to determine your levels of each.

A long-term study completed in 1992 indicated that people with HDL levels below 35 milligrams per deciliter (mg/dl) had a risk of dying from heart disease that was three times as high as for those with levels greater than 60 milligrams per deciliter. Low levels of total cholesterol, with a ratio of total cholesterol to HDL below 4.5, also protects you. In women, total cholesterol levels above 240 milligrams per deciliter increase risk of dying from heart disease by 80 percent.

Inexpensive home test kits give you the total cholesterol but not the level of important HDL cholesterol. Still, these tests may provide a starting point for you and your doctor to determine your risk, says Dr. La-Palio. If your doctor thinks that you are at risk for heart disease, more expensive cholesterol testing for HDL and total cholesterol will probably be covered by Medicare or other insurance.

Your cholesterol level varies. Ask your doctor to give you a second test one week to two months after the first. Average the results. If the difference between the two is over 30, take a third test and pool the three. Here's

---

Get Your Levels in Line

Here's a scorecard to help track your progress in controlling your cholesterol levels. To lower your risk of heart disease, you generally want higher levels of the beneficial HDL cholesterol and lower readings for total cholesterol and the harmful LDL cholesterol. (Your LDL level greatly affects your risk of heart attack. The key point to remember is: the lower your LDL level, the lower the risk.)

Here is a rundown of what the cholesterol readings indicate when you get a blood test, according to the American Heart Association.

Total Cholesterol (mg/dl)	Evaluation
Less than 200	Desirable
200 to 239	Borderline high
240 and over	High

LDL Cholesterol (mg/dl)	Evaluation
Less than 130	Desirable
130 to 159	Borderline high
160 or more	High

HDL Cholesterol (mg/dl)	Evaluation
50 to 60	Desirable for an average woman
40 to 50	Desirable for an average man
Less than 35	Low

how you can make your readings more accurate, suggests Dr. LaPalio.

Take a seat. Sit down for between 5 and 15 minutes before your test. Standing up or lying down can affect the readings.

Keep it low-key. Don't do strenuous exercise the day before your test—it will temporarily elevate HDL levels.

Stay alcohol-free. Stay away from alcohol for 48 hours before your test—it artificially raises HDL levels.

Colon and Rectal Screening

"Screening decreases colon cancer mortality. It can have the same life-extending benefits as breast cancer screening," says James E. Allison, M.D., clinical professor of medicine and assistant director of the internal medicine program at the University of California, San Francisco.

Colon cancer is the third leading cause of cancer death in the United States for men and women, despite the fact that this cancer often starts out as a benign polyp. Screening can make the difference. Here's advice for getting reliable results.

Take a sample. There are several ways to get a fecal occult-blood test. One involves the doctor taking a smear sample as part of your physical examination. Another test can be done at home using a kit from your doctor. You just wipe a stool sample on pieces of cardboard that are then analyzed by a laboratory.

Watch what you eat. Chemicals in the test kit react to some foods, says Dr. Allison. To get an accurate reading, change your diet a few days before the test. Stay away from red meat, turnips, horseradish, broccoli, radishes, cauliflower, cantaloupes, and other melons. But do eat lots of other fresh vegetables and fruits—it will help stimulate bleeding from lesions, which helps ensure that they will show up on the test.

Avoid conflicts. Test results may be skewed by vitamin C supplements (which will give false negatives), and aspirin and other nonsteroidal anti-inflammatory drugs (which will give false positives). Avoid medication that can cause gastrointestinal bleeding. If your hemorrhoids are flaring up, wait until they quiet down, suggests Dr. Allison.

There is a newer home test available at drugstores without a prescription that uses a specially treated pad that you drop into the toilet after a bowel movement. The manufacturer of one such test, EZ-Detect, says that there are no diet constraints and that the test results are not affected by vitamin C.

Many tests—both the off-the-shelf type and those available from your doctor—give a lot of false positives. They just look for blood in the feces, which could be caused by hemorrhoids, diverticulosis, or a host of other conditions. And no fecal occult-blood test picks up nonbleeding cancerous lesions.

Still, this is a test worth taking because it is very inexpensive—under $20 for the lab work. Even if you have to pay for the test, a positive reading means that the more expensive tests that give you maximum protection will probably be covered by Medicare and other insurance.

Take a look. Okay, now we are into the stuff that you don't want to read about: flexible sigmoidoscopy. And both men and women need to go through this about every three to five years, says Dr. Allison. In this procedure a thin, hollow lighted tube is inserted into the rectum and lower colon. There, it picks up precancerous polyps and removes them before they turn dangerous. (That development usually takes several years.) The device also spots cancerous lesions.

The downside is that it views only one-third of the length of the large intestine's left side, although that is where many cancers develop, notes Dr. McAfee. But this test is much less expensive and less uncomfortable than the more thorough colonoscopy.

Be thorough. "I think colonoscopy is probably the best screening examination," says Dr. McAfee. That is because the thin tube travels the length of your entire large intestine, allowing your doctor to snip off any polyps and identify any cancerous formations. So what if it is more uncomfortable than the other tests? Since colon cancer takes so long to develop, "you're home free for 5 to 10 years, maybe longer," he says.

Diabetes Screening

"Forty percent of people over age 65 have diabetes. It is a significant risk factor for heart disease," says Dr. LaPalio. When you have diabetes, the extra sugar in your blood tears up artery walls and leaves them more vulnerable to fatty deposits and blockages. How serious is one more risk factor? When you have three or four risk factors—like high blood pressure, high cholesterol levels, being overweight, lack of exercise, being a smoker, or having a family history of heart disease—you are 15 to 20 times more likely to develop heart disease than someone with just one risk factor.

Talk about easy—testing only requires one drop of blood. Ask your doctor to test levels of sugar in your blood if you show symptoms of diabetes: if you're overweight, get thirsty often, urinate more frequently than you used to, or just don't feel well, advises Dr. McAfee.

Electrocardiogram

An electrocardiogram gives a printout of your heart's activity. It lets you know whether your heart is working efficiently. But you need it only if you already have heart disease or risk factors for heart disease.

"It's reasonable to have this test if you have a family history of heart disease, if you smoke, if you have diabetes or are hypertensive," says Dr. McAfee. Medicare usually covers it.

Lung Cancer Screening

"We don't recommend chest x-rays or any screening for lung cancer anymore," says Dr. McAfee. Studies show that by the time you can see a lesion on an x-ray, it has already spread too far. Also, doctors worry that clean x-rays lull smokers into a false sense of security.

Oral Cancer Screening

You're at risk for oral cancer if you have been a tobacco user or if you have a history of alcohol consumption. "I've never seen oral cancer in a patient who didn't smoke or drink," says Dr. McAfee. All the same, he notes, there is no reason not to make this part of your visit. Your doctor will simply perform a visual check of the inner workings of your mouth to look for suspicious-looking growths or lesions.

Ovarian Cancer Screening

Your doctor may recommend an ultrasound examination if you have a close relative who was diagnosed with ovarian cancer at a young age, says Dr. McAfee. Since your family history puts you at extra risk, your insurance will probably foot the bill. In this test a probe is inserted into the vagina, transmitting images of the uterus and ovaries to a monitor. Your doctor will look for changes in the cells lining the ovaries.

Prostate Cancer Screening

Eighty percent of prostate cancer cases are diagnosed after age 65, and 40,000 men die from it every year. Testing is a simple two-part affair: Your doctor will perform a rectal exam to check the prostate. And a blood test, called the PSA (prostate-specific antigen) test, will measure levels of a protein produced by the prostate.

Many doctors do not actively recommend screening for prostate cancer, however. Screening is controversial because the disease develops slowly. Most men never experience any symptoms, and only 1 in 8 men diagnosed with prostate cancer dies of it. "Right now, we don't know that prostate surgery increases your chances of staying alive," says Dr. McAfee. "I'd avoid this test like the plague."

Further complicating matters, biopsied tumors that look dangerous under the microscope sometimes turn out to be slow-growing. And tumors that look easy going can suddenly shift into high gear, says Gerald W. Chodak, M.D., director of the Prostate and Urology Center at the University of Chicago Hospitals.

Even health organizations end up on opposite sides of the fence: The American Cancer Society recommends testing. The National Cancer Institute doesn't but has the question under study.

Dr. Chodak suggests considering these factors when deciding whether to test for prostate cancer. Get tested if:

- You want to minimize your risk of cancer and increase your chances of living as long as possible, regardless of side effects from prostate surgery or radiation, which can include impotence and incontinence.

- You expect to live for another 10 to 15 years.

- You and loved ones can handle the psychological burden of watching and waiting—one option for some slow-growing tumors.

Just say no if:

- You're more interested in the quality than the length of your life.

- You want to minimize your risk of complications from treatment to eradicate the tumor.

- You only want to take tests that have been proven effective. Prostate screenings miss 20 to 30 percent of cancers.

Skin Cancer Screening

"The difference between life and death is one-eighth of an inch," says Perry Robins, M.D., president of the Skin Cancer Foundation in New York City. We're talking not about that time you almost walked in front of the fast-moving truck but about minute changes in the moles and freckles that dot your body. Freckling occurs when the skin gets suddenly baked by the sun. Moles are malformed skin tissue. Little changes in these spots can signal the onset of malignant melanoma, a skin cancer that can be cured easily in its early stages but that quickly spreads.

Examine your body—from the top of your scalp to the bottom of your feet—twice a year. If anything looks suspicious, consult your doctor.

You're at extra risk if you spend a lot of time indoors and then go out and get "burned and blasted" by the sun, says Dr. Robins. "It's the sudden shock or intense exposure to sun that increases your risk." Also at risk are those who had bad sunburns as children or who sunburn easily or who have a family history of the disease. If you are in the high-risk group, ask your doctor to do a yearly skin check for you, says Dr. Robins. He will be able to get a better look at hard-to-see places.

For starters, you'll want to know the ABCs—and Ds—for skin cancer detection. The Skin Cancer Foundation has developed a self-exam guide called "The ABCDs of Moles and Melanomas."

A is for asymmetry. An irregular shape is a sign of trouble.

B is for border. Beware of irregular, scalloped, or notched borders.

C is for color. Different shades of brown or black signal a problem.

D is for diameter. Anything larger than the size of a pencil eraser may indicate a melanoma.

Here are other ways to detect trouble brewing.

Keep count. Count your moles. You're at risk if your total exceeds 100.

Check for changes. Keep a record. Use two line drawings of the human body, one of the back view and one of the front to make a chart (or ask your doctor for illustrations you can use). On the drawings make marks that correspond to the location of moles on your body. Draw a line from the mark to the margin and write down the size, color, and shape of each mole, along with the date of the examination. Use the chart to keep track of changes when you do your next self-examination.

Stroke Screening

A stroke fells someone in the United States every minute. Thirty-one percent of stroke survivors need long-term help to care for themselves. Fortunately, many people experience symptoms before a stroke. Here is what you and your doctor should look for.

Heed the mini-stroke. Your body does the screening for you. About 10 percent of strokes are preceded by transient ischemic attacks, or mini-strokes. Symptoms, which may last just a few minutes, include blurred vision, numbness or weakness on one side of the body, slurred speech, inability to talk, or difficulty in thinking. All these symptoms shout out that your brain isn't getting the blood supply it needs, says Dr. McAfee.

Beware the bruit. Your doctor can also use a stethoscope to listen to the carotid arteries on either side of the neck that carry blood to the brain. A soft, whooshing sound (called a bruit and pronounced *BRU-ee*) may indicate blockage in the arteries, says Dr. LaPalio.

If your doctor hears the sound, he will probably do an ultrasound test, using sound waves to provide a picture of the inside of the arteries.

Okay so far. But here's the problem: The surgery that is used to clear the blockage can also cause a stroke. And the jury is out on just how effective such surgery is. "So far, one good study has shown that screening in certain select populations and then operating on the carotid artery does lower the stroke rate, but we need to know more," says Dr. McAfee.

If surgery isn't your cup of tea, now is the time to make changes in your lifestyle to lower your risk of the big one.

Prescription for Prevention

Having the right screening tests can dramatically cut your risk of heart disease, cancer, and stroke. They can let you know if you need to make protective changes in your lifestyle and identify small problems before they mushroom out of control.

Do:

- *Get your blood pressure checked yearly.*
- *Have yearly breast examinations and mammography screenings.*
- *Check your HDL and LDL cholesterol levels every year.*
- *Get a Pap smear every year.*
- *Use an inexpensive fecal occult–blood test to check for colon cancer.*
- *Have a sigmoidoscopy done every 3 to 5 years or a colonoscopy done every 10 years.*
- *Get a simple blood test to check for diabetes.*
- *Check your skin for changes.*

Don't:

- *Automatically get every test in the book. Discuss the positive and negative aspects of some tests, such as those for prostate cancer.*

Chapter 13

Do Environmental Hazards Really Cause Disease?

Pollution is civilization's oldest companion. The ancient Greeks and Romans spewed massive amounts of toxins into the air as they extracted silver from lead ore. During the Civil War an abandoned canal in Washington, D.C., was so clogged with animal carcasses and household waste that the stench permeated the White House.

In the past 45 years alone, more than 70,000 new chemical compounds—including many that cause cancer in laboratory animals—have been invented and spread throughout the environment. So how does this affect your risk of cancer, heart disease, and stroke as you creep beyond age 60? A lot more than you might think.

While estimates vary, some researchers believe that up to 25 percent of all cancers might be prevented if Americans reduced their exposure to smog, pesticides, secondhand smoke, and other hazards that we breathe, drink, eat, and absorb into our bodies, says Devra Lee Davis, Ph.D., senior fellow and program director at the World Resources Institute, an environmental research center in Washington, D.C. Reducing exposure to toxins also might prevent thousands of heart attacks and strokes each year, she says.

"Unlike some things that have been identified as causes of cancer, stroke, and heart disease that you can't control—like family history—environmental factors are often things you can do something about," Dr. Davis says. "Even after age 60, it represents an opportunity for prevention that, in many ways, is easy to achieve."

What We're Doing to Ourselves

All of us carry residues of a few toxins in our cells. DDT, for example, an insecticide suspected of promoting breast cancer, has been banned in the United States since 1972. Yet because traces of it can linger in food and water for more than 50 years, virtually all people in this country still have some DDT in their bodies, Dr. Davis says.

In most cases these minute amounts of toxins probably won't harm you. Only 30 chemicals, for instance, have been proven to cause cancer in humans. But at least another 400 have been shown to cause cancer in laboratory animals and are suspected of promoting tumors in us.

Here's a sampling of intriguing findings.

Pollution increases heart attack risk. Automotive air pollutants, such as carbon monoxide, can reduce the ability of the blood to carry oxygen and trigger heart attacks and angina in people over age 60, says Robert Morris, M.D., Ph.D., director of the Center for Environmental Epidemiology at the Medical College of Wisconsin in Milwaukee. Long-term exposure to carbon monoxide also may promote more blood clots in the arteries and possibly lead to stroke.

In his three-year study of 204,000 Medicare patients, 65 and older, in seven American cities, Dr. Morris found up to a 30 percent increase in hospital admissions for congestive heart failure as carbon monoxide levels rose.

"There's a steady increase in hospital admissions as carbon monoxide goes up," Dr. Morris says. "There's no question that if you're exposed to excessive amounts of carbon monoxide, your heart is going to have to work harder to deliver oxygen to the cells. So if an older person has an underlying heart condition, carbon monoxide can push the heart to a dangerous extent."

Breast cancer rates may be higher in industrial areas. Postmenopausal women in Nassau County, New York, who live within a mile of a chemical, petroleum, rubber, or plastics facility are 60 percent more likely to develop breast cancer than postmenopausal women who lived in other parts of Long Island, according to a study by New York State Department of Health researchers.

"This study adds credibility to the suggestion that environmental exposure may be important in the development of breast cancer," says Elizabeth Lewis-Michl, Ph.D., lead author of the study and a research scientist at the Center for Environmental Health at the New York State Department of Health in Albany.

Some cancers are more common among farmers who use pesticides. In a 16-year study of 70,000 Canadian farmers, those who routinely sprayed more than 250 acres with herbicide were 2.2 times more prone to develop prostate cancer than farmers who didn't use pesticides, says Howard Morrison, Ph.D., chief of behavioral risk assessment, Cancer Bureau, at Health Canada, the equivalent of the U.S. Department of Health, in Ottawa. In another 16-year study, 143,000 herbicide-using farmers, most of whom were at least in their sixties by the end of the study, were twice as likely to develop a life-threatening cancer of the lymphatic system known as non-Hodgkin's lymphoma than their colleagues who did not spray with herbicides.

Other studies have found that farmers who work with insecticides have higher rates of leukemia, bone marrow cancer, and brain cancer. Some of these same chemicals are used in lower doses by household gardeners, Dr. Davis says.

"It's absolutely established that many herbicides are carcinogens," says Philip Landrigan, M.D., director of environmental and occupational medicine at the Mount Sinai School of Medicine of the City University of New York in New York City. "It just doesn't make any sense to expose yourself to these compounds at any age."

Radon is linked to lung cancer. Swedish researchers found that people up to age 74 who lived in homes with high levels of radon were 80 percent more susceptible to lung cancer than those who lived in houses containing little or no radon. Radon is an invisible, odorless radioactive gas that seeps into homes from the decay of underground uranium deposits.

"Radon is clearly a carcinogen. There's no doubt about it, but the degree of risk of lung cancer from residential exposure is not clear," says Aaron Blair, Ph.D., chief of the occupational studies section at the National Cancer Institute in Bethesda, Maryland.

321

Many Questions Remain Unanswered

Although these studies strongly suggest the powerful impact of environmental hazards, scientists are still struggling to determine the thresholds at which many of these toxins cause trouble.

"That's the $64,000 question," says Jane Koenig, Ph.D., professor of environmental health at the University of Washington in Seattle. "In a lot of cases we don't have the answers yet."

A few, like carbon monoxide and asbestos, a potent carcinogen that causes a rare form of lung cancer, have no known safe exposure levels. For others, like radon, the Environmental Protection Agency (EPA) has set exposure limits. But in general, the magnitude of your risk depends on what you have been exposed to, how much and how often you are exposed to it, and your age.

Certain occupations, for example, can come back to haunt you, even if you have long been retired. Workers who installed asbestos insulation in the 1940s and 1950s have tremendously high rates of lung cancer. Textile workers who are exposed to benzidine-related dyes have unusually high rates of bladder cancer, according to Max Costa, Ph.D., chairman of the Norton Nelson Institute of Environmental Medicine at New York University Medical Center. Furniture workers who are exposed to wood dust may be susceptible to nasal and sinus cancers for up to 40 years after their first exposure. Some hobbyists who frequently use paints, solvents, and solders also are more prone to cancers than the general population, he says.

Toxins Carry More Clout As You Age

The damage that these hazards inflict on the body often increases as you get older. That's because as you age, your lungs, liver, kidneys, and other organs gradually lose much of their ability to rid the body of cell-damaging toxins, says Jonathan Samet, M.D., chairman of the Department of Epidemiology at Johns Hopkins University School of Medicine in Baltimore.

Although doctors still aren't sure how these toxins trigger cancer, heart disease, or stroke, they suspect that hazardous substances may cause gradual changes in DNA, the genetic building blocks that cells use to reproduce. Over decades, these changes might cause mutations in cells that may spark cancer and might accelerate atherosclerosis, hardening of the arteries, says Chris Schonwalder, Ph.D., assistant to the director of the National Institute of Environmental Health Sciences of the National Institutes of Health in Research Triangle Park, North Carolina.

These pollutants also may weaken the immune system so that it is less capable of destroying abnormal cells that eventually could become cancerous, says Mary Wolff, Ph.D., a toxicologist and professor of community medicine at the Mount Sinai School of Medicine of the City University of New York.

Keep Your Guard Up

Even if you have been exposed to massive amounts of environmental hazards in your lifetime, it's not too late, Dr. Landrigan says. If you eliminate an environmental hazard like pesticides from your life now, you may be able to prevent that one final exposure that would set you on a collision course with one of the three killers.

"Older people need to engage in prudent avoidance and try to minimize their exposure to environmental hazards," Dr. Davis says. "That doesn't mean you have to live in a bubble. But if you pay attention to your environment—as well as exercise regularly, eat well, and don't smoke—you will be healthier."

Here's a closer look at several environmental hazards that are known or suspected of causing the big three killers and what you can do about them.

Smoking Is Never Passive

Tobacco smoke is one of the most dangerous and most pervasive environmental hazards.

Fifty-three thousand people die of passive-smoking-related causes each year, according to Stanton Glantz, Ph.D., professor of medicine at the University of California, San Francisco, School of Medicine. That's

10 Toxic Jobs That Can Damage Your Health

Here's a look at a few occupations that expose workers to substances that may increase the risk of cancer and heart disease. Even if you're retired, consult your doctor if you suspect that you have worked in an industry that may have exposed you to hazardous materials, says Max Costa, Ph.D., chairman of the Norton Nelson Institute of Environmental Medicine at New York University Medical Center.

Occupation	Hazardous Substances	Risks
Agriculture worker	Arsenic, pesticides, carbon monoxide, carbon disulfide	Lung, liver, skin cancers; increased atherosclerosis
Assembly line worker	Halogenated hydrocarbon solvents	Heart arrhythmias
Automotive mechanic	Cadmium, carbon monoxide, halogenated hydrocarbon solvents, chromium, polycyclic aromatic hydrocarbons	High blood pressure; increased atherosclerosis; arrhythmias; lung, bladder, skin cancers
Ceramics worker	Arsenic, cadmium, nickel	High blood pressure; nasal, skin, lung cancers

because sidestream or secondhand smoke from burning tobacco emits virtually all of the same toxic chemicals and carcinogenic substances into the air that you get from taking a puff. A nonsmoker who regularly inhales these secondhand fumes has a 30 percent greater risk of developing lung cancer and heart disease and may be more likely to develop breast cancer

Occupation	Hazardous Substances	Risks
Construction worker	Asbestos, polycyclic aromatic hydrocarbons, halogenated hydrocarbon solvents	Lung, bladder, skin cancers; arrhythmias
Dry cleaner	Benzene, carbon disulfide, halogenated hydrocarbon solvents	Leukemia, increased atherosclerosis, high blood pressure
Dye or ink maker	Benzene, chromium, nickel, carbon disulfide	Leukemia, lung and bladder cancers, arrhythmias
Leather worker (tanner)	Benzene, chromium, arsenic, halogenated hydrocarbon solvents	Leukemia, lung cancer, high blood pressure
Textile mill worker	Arsenic, cadmium, nickel, halogenated hydrocarbon solvents, carbon disulfide	Lung, nasal, and bladder cancers, arrhythmias, increased atherosclerosis
Welder	Arsenic, benzene, nickel, chromium	Leukemia, lung and nasal cancers

than nonsmokers who live in smoke-free homes, he says.

"Passive smoking increases the need of the heart for oxygen and decreases the body's ability to use it effectively," Dr. Glantz says. "So if you already have some heart disease or atherosclerosis and then you throw in secondhand smoke, this could easily push you over the edge."

Enjoy Crafts the Safe Way

Hobbies are fun, relaxing, and rewarding. But unless you are wary, pastimes involving ceramics, jewelry, paint remover, solders, metals, or clays also can be hazardous to your health.

"Certain hobbies can expose you to solvents and dust that may contain cancer-promoting compounds," says Michael Thun, M.D., director of analytic epidemiology for the American Cancer Society in Atlanta. "So you need to use some common sense when you're working at a hobby to minimize your risk of inhaling or coming in contact with these compounds."

Here are a few safety precautions to reduce your risks.

Read the label and follow directions. Before you buy, make sure that the most dangerous toxic chemicals aren't in the product. Avoid using art materials that contain known or suspected carcinogens such as benzene, carbon tetrachloride, trichloroethylene, or dioxane, Dr. Thun says. Choose nontoxic art materials whenever possible. Read and understand the package directions fully before you begin using the product.

Keep air circulating. Good ventilation is a must when working with toxic or cancer-promoting substances like lead, cadmium, or nickel found in clays and metals. Work in a space that can be easily ventilated like a garage or large hobby area. Before you begin, open adjacent doors and windows. Use a large floor fan to disperse the toxins, Dr. Thun says.

Wear protective clothing. Don a ventilation mask, heavy-duty overalls, and latex gloves, available at most hardware stores. These items will help prevent you from accidentally inhaling or coming in contact with many carcinogen-containing dusts and fumes while doing your hobby, Dr. Thun says. Wash your clothing separately in hot water after you finish.

Mop up. Sweeping stirs up harmful dusts and toxins, Dr. Thun says. Wet mopping is a safer way to clean up.

According to Dr. Glantz, studies have found:

- Exposure to secondhand smoke thickens artery walls and promotes the formation of artery-clogging plaque. It also lowers blood levels of HDL, the "good" cholesterol that normally would prevent plaque buildup in the arteries.

- If a heart attack occurs, previous exposure to sidestream smoke magnifies heart damage and complicates recovery.

In addition, at least 3,000 lung-related deaths among nonsmokers each year are attributable to secondhand smoke, according to the Environmental Protection Agency.

Persuading household smokers to quit is the best way to protect nonsmokers like young grandchildren. But until that happens, here are a few things you and your nonsmoking loved ones can do to reduce these risks.

Take it outside. Allow smokers to puff away outdoors only, says C. Barr Taylor, M.D., professor of psychiatry at Stanford University School of Medicine and author of *The Facts about Smoking*. As an alternative, designate a well-ventilated room in your home not normally used by others where they can light up. Ask your guests who smoke to use the room, too.

Create a breeze. If possible, open windows or install strong exhaust fans to quickly clear smoke out of your home, Dr. Taylor suggests.

Eat in self-defense. Eating at least seven servings a day of fruits and vegetables, such as apples, pears, carrots, and broccoli, that are rich in antioxidants may help a nonsmoker counteract some of the risks of breathing secondhand smoke, says James Scala, Ph.D., a nutritional biochemist and author of *If You Can't/Won't Stop Smoking*. Antioxidants fight off the effects of the free radicals found in tobacco smoke that rob cells of oxygen.

Air Pollution Steals Your Heart

Inhale. Exhale. You do that about 17,000 times in an average day. And what are you breathing? Carbon monoxide, sulfates, and other dangerous pollutants that can strain your heart and lungs to the breaking point.

"Studies have consistently shown that there are increased numbers of

Get the Chlorine Out of Your Water

In 1969, Neil Armstrong walked on the moon. But back on Earth, he couldn't swim in horribly polluted Lake Erie, just a few miles from his home.

We have cleaned up our act since then, and the bulk of America's water supply is safe, says James M. Symons, Sc.D., author of *Drinking Water: Refreshing Answers to All Your Questions*, and former director of the drinking water treatment program for the U.S. Environmental Protection Agency in Cincinnati.

But at least one chemical used to purify tap water may provoke cancer, heart disease, and stroke, says Michael Klaper, M.D., director of the Institute of Nutrition Education and Research in Manhattan Beach, California.

Yes, chlorine kills bacteria and other germs in the water. But it might cause cholesterol to cling to artery walls and accelerate atherosclerosis. Chlorine also can combine with other chemicals in drinking water to form cancer-promoting substances, Dr. Klaper says.

"If an older person has cells on the verge of becoming cancerous, how do you know that one more glass of water containing these cancer-promoting substances won't push him over the edge?" he says. "If I were an older person, I wouldn't drink chlorinated water, especially if I had a history of these three diseases."

Use bottled water instead of tap, he suggests. Bottled water is purified by a process called reverse osmosis and usually contains little or no chlorine. As an alternative, consider getting a reverse osmosis water filter, available at many department stores. It's an inexpensive way of ridding chlorine from tap water, Dr. Klaper says.

deaths associated with increasing levels of particulate material in the air. One to 3 percent of the deaths that occur on days with high levels of particulate material are due to cardiac problems in people over age 65," Dr. Koenig says.

Researchers have also found that people who live in cities with high air-pollution levels die an average of 2½ years earlier than those who live in the least-polluted areas, Dr. Koenig says.

"Air pollution is similar to secondhand smoke. The more you breathe it, the more toxic effects it is going to have on your body," Dr. Koenig says. "So you should do everything you can to reduce the amount of air pollution that you breathe, particularly if you're 60 or 70 and already have an underlying heart or lung condition that could be exacerbated by breathing dirty air," Dr. Koenig says. Here's how to lower your intake of air pollutants.

Stick to side streets. Regular exercise such as walking strengthens the heart. But avoid strolling along busy streets where carbon monoxide levels are higher. Head for a secluded park or neighborhood, Dr. Morris says.

Dodge rush hour. The more cars on the road, the more air pollution you are likely encounter. Try doing outdoor activities such as walking and gardening at off-peak times like the middle of the day so that you avoid being exposed to fumes from the morning and evening rush hours, Dr. Morris says.

Stay smoke-free. Tobacco smoke contains large amounts of heart-damaging carbon monoxide. "Certainly one of the biggest sources of carbon monoxide you can be exposed to is the end of a lit cigarette," says Dr. Morris. So avoid secondhand smoke, and if you smoke, quit, he says.

Snatch pollutants out of the air. Even indoors you can be exposed to air pollutants that seep into your home, Dr. Koenig says. Consider getting a high-efficiency particulate (HEPA) filter. About the size of a footstool, HEPA filters collect many of the worst pollutants. They are available at most hardware or building supply stores and cost less than $200.

Relax. Scan the newspaper or watch television weather reports for pollution alerts in your area. When a pollution alert is declared, stay indoors, cut back on your regular activities, and take more frequent rest breaks so that you reduce the amount of air you breathe and don't overexert your heart and lungs, Dr. Koenig says.

Pesticides: Look to Natural Alternatives

A foggy mist of DDT engulfing beaches, campgrounds, and parks once was a sure sign that summer had arrived.

329

Some trucks belching out this potent concoction actually displayed signs proclaiming, "DDT: powerful insecticide, harmless to humans."

But far from being harmless, DDT, now banned in the United States, and many other pesticides that are still in use like dimethoate can provoke cancers, Dr. Landrigan says.

"You're never so old that you're immune from the effects of pesticides," Dr. Landrigan says. "My advice to people is reduce their use as much as possible. If you must, use the minimal amount necessary and integrate other, more natural approaches into your effort to control pests."

In a study by Dr. Wolff, women who had elevated blood levels of DDE, a residual component of DDT, were four times more likely to develop breast cancer than women who had lower blood concentrations of the residue.

"The older you are, the more DDT you have," Dr. Wolff says. "We're still uncertain whether DDT actually causes breast cancer. But it's something that we need to understand better because there is still plenty of it around. Although it is banned in the United States, it is still widely used in Mexico and other Third World countries. So it can still get into this country."

Some researchers speculate that substances called xenoestrogens in DDT and other pesticides may promote breast, prostate, and other hormonally linked cancers, Dr. Wolff says.

These xenoestrogens may mimic sexual hormones in the body and fuel cancer development by damaging DNA or helping cancer cells form new blood vessels that are needed for tumor growth, Dr. Davis says.

Here's how you can battle back.

Load up on vegetables and soy. Broccoli, cauliflower, cabbage, and soy products like tofu have compounds that may enhance the body's ability to repair damaged DNA and fend off the worst effects of xenoestrogens, Dr. Scala says. Eat at least five servings of these foods a day, he suggests.

Lay off meat. Pesticides tend to accumulate in animal fats like in beef, pork, and chicken. Try to eat no more than one 3-ounce serving of meat a day, Dr. Scala says.

Do a striptease. Carefully wash and peel all fruits and vegetables be-

Steer Clear of the Dirty Dozen

Here, in order from most to least toxic, are the 12 fruits and vegetables loaded with the highest amounts known of suspected cancer-causing pesticide residues, according to the Environmental Working Group, a nonprofit environmental research organization in Washington, D.C. Since many of these foods are American favorites, the Working Group recommends limiting, rather than eliminating, consumption of these fruits and vegetables. You also may consider trying some of the nutritionally equivalent, less toxic alternatives listed. In some cases the Working Group recommends avoiding certain fruits from a specific country (listed in parentheses).

Food	Alternatives
1. Strawberries	Blueberries, blackberries, oranges, kiwifruit, grapefruit
2. and 3. (tie) Bell peppers	Green peas, broccoli, romaine lettuce
Spinach	Broccoli, brussels sprouts, asparagus
4. Cherries (U.S.)	Oranges, blueberries, raspberries, grapefruit, kiwifruit
5. Peaches	Nectarines, U.S. cantaloupe, tangerines, watermelon
6. Cantaloupe (Mexico)	U.S. cantaloupe in season (May to December) or watermelon
7. Celery	Carrots, romaine lettuce, broccoli, radishes
8. Apples	Pears, oranges, nectarines, bananas, virtually any fruit that isn't one of the dirty dozen
9. Apricots	Nectarines, U.S. cantaloupe, tangerines, oranges
10. Green beans	Green peas, broccoli, cauliflower, asparagus, potatoes, brussels sprouts
11. Grapes (Chile)	U.S. grapes in season (May to December)
12. Cucumbers	Virtually any vegetable

Keep Your Hands Off Asbestos

Once considered safe and efficient, asbestos insulation now tops almost every list of environmental hazards in this country.

That's because asbestos fibers can cause a rare form of cancer that is both painful and deadly.

"Asbestos has been an absolute disaster. Ultimately, there will be 300,000 to 400,000 deaths in this country due to asbestos before this epidemic burns itself out in the twenty-first century," says Philip Landrigan, M.D., director of environmental and occupational medicine at the Mount Sinai School of Medicine of the City University of New York in New York City.

Mesothelioma, a cancer that arises from the linings of the chest, heart, and abdomen, affects about 2,000 people annually in the United States, says Joseph Testa, Ph.D., senior member of the Department of Medical Oncology at Fox Chase Cancer Center in Philadelphia. Construction workers and shipbuilders who have had years of exposure to asbestos are more prone to get the disease. But people who live in homes built prior to 1972, when asbestos was phased out of use in household construction, also may be at risk.

Homeowners probably won't be able to distinguish asbestos from other types of insulation, says Pat Eiding, business manager of the Insulators and Asbestos Workers Union in Philadelphia. But if your

fore eating, says Dr. Schonwalder says. That should eliminate most of pesticide residues on the food.

Keep your kitchen pesticide-free. You may be unwittingly contaminating your meals if you use pesticides on kitchen counters and other food preparation areas, Dr. Davis says. Instead, keep your kitchen clean at all times and use less-toxic pest-control methods like boric acid dust, available at most hardware stores, which will slowly kill ants and cockroaches without harming you. Boric acid dust should be used carefully and not in-home was built before the early 1970s, there is a 50 percent chance that it is insulated with asbestos. As long as the insulation remains sealed and intact, asbestos can't harm you.

If you live in an older home and notice a piece of tattered or worn insulation, carefully cover it with duct tape. Then seek the advice of an asbestos removal contractor listed in the yellow pages of the telephone book, Dr. Landrigan says

Trying to remove asbestos yourself can create more of a hazard than leaving it alone, Dr. Landrigan says. If removal is done improperly, asbestos fibers can flake off the insulation, lodge in your lungs, and possibly spark a cancer.

"Asbestos removal is a complex job that requires specialized skills and equipment. It's not for amateurs," Eiding says.

Professional asbestos removal is expensive, sometimes costing more than $8,000, Eiding says. Get several bids, ask the contractor for references, and avoid letting price dictate your selection. An unusually low bid might be a sign that the contractor is more concerned about profit than your safety, he says.

Insist on an air-quality test after the job is finished to make sure that no asbestos fibers are in your household air, he says.

haled, says Jay Feldman, executive director of the National Coalition against the Misuse of Pesticides (NCAMP). For more information on other natural pest-control techniques, write NCAMP, 701 E Street SE, Suite 200, Washington, DC 20003.

Create a barrier. Skin barriers, a thin nonpenetrable solution similar to petroleum jelly, can prevent pesticides from soaking into your skin, Dr. Schonwalder says. Used by petrochemical workers, skin barriers are available in most drugstores.

Remove Indoor Carcinogens Naturally

You don't have to install high-tech gadgetry, rip up walls, or spend a fortune to banish cancer-promoting substances from your home. All that you may need is a green thumb.

"Plants can have a vital role in clearing carcinogens and other unstable organic chemicals from household air," says B. C. "Bill" Wolverton, Ph.D., a former NASA senior scientist who has studied plants and pollution treatment for more than 20 years. "They can make a significant difference in the pollution levels in your home."

Here are few suggestions from Dr. Wolverton to help these plants work most effectively for you.

Pick the right plant. Lady palm, peace lily, *Ficus alii*, golden pothos, and areca palm are easy to grow, insect-resistant, and can absorb many of the cancer-causing chemicals like benzene, arsenic, and formaldehyde found in secondhand smoke and other household pollutants, says Dr. Wolverton, author of *How to Grow Fresh Air*. Azalea, Boston fern, spider plant, chrysanthemum, philodendron, and mother-in-law's tongue also clean the air but may require more diligent care, he says.

Keep it in your breathing zone. A typical houseplant can filter about 6 cubic feet of air—about the area of a lounge chair. Make sure that you place the plant on a table or on the floor beside your bed or favorite chair to maximize the amount of clean air around you, he suggests.

"If you want a healthier indoor environment, place those plants in your breathing zones, where you spend most of your time. Then you will have significant air-quality improvement with just one or two plants."

Keep a fan nearby, too. Plants can remove the invisible chemicals like benzene from the air but will do little to dissipate smoke and other visible particles, Dr. Wolverton says. For that, consider getting a high-efficiency particulate (HEPA) filter. These filters, available at many hardware stores, quickly remove all particulates from the air.

"Ideally, you would have cleaner indoor air if you used a HEPA filter in conjunction with two or three indoor plants in each room," he says.

Don't track in trouble. "Most houses are so airtight these days that once a pesticide gets into your home, it's there to stay," says Dr. Schonwalder. After applying pesticides, take off your shoes before entering your house. Remove all your clothing in an entryway and wash them in hot water as soon as possible. Then take a shower to remove any remaining residues from your body, he suggests.

Radon: Close the Door on This Cancer Culprit

After a construction engineer set off radiation detectors as he walked *into* a nuclear power plant in Limerick, Pennsylvania, in 1984, investigators narrowed their search for the contamination down to a startling culprit.

It was radon seeping into the man's home, exposing his family to 50 times the annual radiation levels allowed for uranium miners. Although the family quickly fixed the problem, they may have an elevated risk of developing lung cancer for years or decades, Dr. Landrigan says.

"Radon isn't a small problem," says Charles T. Hess, Ph.D., professor of physics at the University of Maine at Orono, who has studied the health effects of radon for more than 20 years. "It's in the air. It's in the water. It's one of the biggest sources of radiation exposure in the United States."

Radon is a naturally occurring gas produced by radioactive decay of uranium in soil and water throughout the country. It is the second most common cause of lung cancer after smoking, contributing to 10,000 deaths a year. Smoking and radon exposure more than doubles your risk of developing lung cancer, Dr. Landrigan says.

Because it is a gas, it can easily slip into a home through cracks in floors and walls, construction joints, and gaps around pipes. It also is commonly found in wells or municipal water systems that use groundwater, Dr. Hess says. Up to six million homes in the United States may exceed EPA standards for radon exposure.

"If you have excessive radon in your home, it is prudent to take corrective measures to get it out, no matter what your age. It's just a gas, and you can get rid of it very easily," says Dr. Landrigan, who is also co-author of *Raising Children Toxic Free.*

335

Be snoopy. Call the county or city health department and ask if they have received any reports of high radon levels in your neighborhood, says Richard Sextro, Ph.D., a staff scientist at the Lawrence Berkeley Laboratory at the University of California, Berkeley. Ask neighbors if they have taken recent radon measurements. Since radon levels can fluctuate dramatically from house to house, this isn't a foolproof method. But at least it will give you a better idea of whether you should test.

Check it out. Get a radon detector, available at many hardware stores, and place in the basement or lowest living areas of your home, Dr. Landrigan says. Detectors that accumulate radon for 2 to 90 days will give you a general idea of your risk. If that reading is high, get a detector that will measure radon levels for 6 to 12 months. Since radon levels can vary day to day, a long-term test will give you a better idea of your year-round radon exposure. When the detector is ready, you mail the device off to a lab that analyzes the contents and then sends you a report.

Radon is measured in units called picocuries per liter. If your test results are greater than 4 picocuries per liter, the highest exposure recommended by the EPA, you should consider ways to fix the problem. In most cases it can be done for $500 to $2,500, according to the EPA.

Stop those leaks. Seal large cracks in your basement with caulk to prevent radon from pouring in, Dr. Hess suggests. In basements with porous or cracked concrete, apply several layers of epoxy paint or masonry sealer to the floor or walls.

Get some fresh air. Open all the windows, particularly in the basement, and use a window fan to flush the radon out, Dr. Landrigan suggests.

Take it out before it gets in. Installing a 4-inch plastic pipe through the foundation and venting it to a small fan in the roof will suck the gas away before it gets in the house, Dr. Sextro suggests. You may want to consider having this done professionally, since pipe and fan size can be dependent on house size and local codes.

Bathe wisely. If you get your household water from a well, a long, hot shower can make radon levels in the your bathroom soar more than 28 times higher than normal, Dr. Hess says. That's because some wells and other groundwater sources are loaded with the radioactive gas.

When you bathe or shower, turn on the fan and water, then leave the room while the water warms or the tub fills, Dr. Hess suggests. Shower for no more than 5 minutes, grab a towel, and dry off in another room. That should reduce your radon exposure in the shower to about 20 percent. Be sure to close the bathroom door while you are showering or whenever you leave the room so that the gas won't seep into the rest of the house. Take warm rather than hot showers. Hot water releases more radon.

Prescription for Prevention

Radon, secondhand smoke, asbestos, and other environmental toxins can increase the risk of stroke, heart disease, and certain forms of cancer, especially after age 60. But even if you have lived or worked around hazardous materials for years, you can still make lifestyle changes to dampen your chances of getting ill.

Do:

- *Make your home a smoke-free zone.*

- *Exercise in secluded parks or neighborhoods away from congested or busy streets that have high concentrations of carbon monoxide.*

- *Get a HEPA filter. It will eradicate many of the worst pollutants.*

- *Carefully wash and peel all fruits and vegetables before eating them. This should prevent you from inadvertently digesting pesticides.*

- *Get a radon detector. If levels of the gas in your home are high, open windows and seal all cracks in the foundation and basement flooring.*

Don't:

- *Exercise in morning or evening rush hours. Pollution is highest at those times.*

- *Use pesticides on kitchen counters. That can contaminate foods.*

- *Abuse pesticides. In large amounts, they can poison you. Follow label.*

Chapter 14

How Do Genes Affect My Risk of Cancer, Heart Disease, and Stroke?

The shape of your nose, the color of your eyes, and other traits of your family are passed on from generation to generation like newspapers rolling off a printing press.

It seems so simple but actually is so complex that scientists are still mystified by some aspects of the process. What they do know is that genes, composed of millions of encoded nitrogen molecules, carry your reproductive blueprints. And they are busy. Every day, your body's 100 trillion cells rely on genes to tell them what they are supposed to do. What could possibly go wrong?

Plenty.

"The genetic code is a set of instructions that tells cells how to function properly. A cell follows those instructions rigorously. But if one of the instructions is wrong, it then messes up how the cell functions. These mistakes can cause disease—if they prevent the cell from carrying out important tasks—or cause the cell to die," says Richard H. Myers, Ph.D., professor of neurology at Boston University School of Medicine.

Mistakes in genes are called mutations. They develop over a lifetime due to aging or exposure to harmful substances like tobacco smoke. But these spontaneous mutations are seldom passed from one generation to the next, Dr. Myers says.

A very small percentage of the time, however, the mutation is caused by a mangled gene passed on to you from one or both of your parents. People who inherit these defects, which can remain dormant for decades, are more prone to certain diseases after age 60, including some types of cancer, heart disease, and stroke, researchers say. But even if you have a family history of one of these three diseases, you are not doomed.

"Having a mutation doesn't mean that you're absolutely going to get the disease. It should just make you more cautious about monitoring your health. If you're truly concerned about your family history, there is genetic testing and counseling available that in some cases may help ease your mind," says Glenn A. Miller, Ph.D., head of the clinical studies laboratory at Genzyme Genetics, a genetic research and testing company in Framingham, Massachusetts.

Unraveling the Mystery

Researchers know less than you might think about your genes. Just sorting out what every one does is an enormous task. Each one of your cells has up to 100,000 genes. Scientists who are trying to locate and identify all of these genes believe that they won't be finished until at least 2005. For now, researchers have found and developed detection tests for only a handful.

"This effort is a marathon, and the starting gun has just gone off," Dr. Miller says. "We're still only a couple of hundred yards down the track."

But here is a look at some of this pioneering research that may help some of us forestall or combat these diseases, Dr. Miller says.

Heart disease and stroke can be all in the family. In ongoing research at the Framingham Heart Study, which has been tracking the lives of 5,209 Massachusetts adults, many now in their eighties and nineties, for almost 50 years, investigators found that strokes were three times more common among men and women whose parents had had heart disease.

In a second Framingham report, researchers concluded that people were 29 percent more likely to develop heart disease if a parent also had had cardiovascular ailments, says Dr. Myers, lead author of the study.

"I don't think we're going to find a single gene that causes these two diseases. But there are a number of genes that increase blood pressure and

339

How to Snuff Out a Genetic Malady

Although we can't turn off genes that contribute to stroke, heart disease, and cancer, we can at least slow one down, according to French researchers.

A gene that causes excessive production of fibrinogen, a blood protein that contributes to heart disease and stroke, may be more active if you smoke, says François Cambien, M.D., director of research at the Institut National de la Santé et de la Recherche Medicale in Paris. This may help explain why people who smoke have more heart attacks than nonsmokers.

One in five people carried a mutation of the beta fibrinogen gene in Dr. Cambien's study of 565 men who had heart attacks and 668 healthy men up to age 64. Fibrinogen, which is present in all of our bodies, thickens blood by making blood platelets stickier. The more fibrinogen in your blood, the more likely you are to develop atherosclerosis and form blood clots that can lead to heart attack and stroke, Dr. Cambien says.

Among those who don't smoke, the gene seems to have only a small influence on cardiovascular diseases. But if you smoke, its impact is greater and may be just enough to trigger cardiovascular problems.

A test for this gene isn't on the horizon. But quitting smoking would significantly reduce your fibrinogen levels even if you don't carry the gene, he explains.

"People who smoke have elevated levels of fibrinogen anyway. So if you can quit smoking, you'll positively affect your risk of coronary disease and stroke," Dr. Cambien says.

others that affect cholesterol. So the presence of the same genes may result in heart disease in some people and stroke in others," Dr. Myers says.

Researchers find a pair of breast cancer genes. Only 5 percent of breast cancers are hereditary. But among women who have families with a history of breast cancer and carry either the BRCA1 or BRCA2 gene (*BRCA* stands for "breast cancer"), the lifetime risk of breast cancer is about 80 percent, says Raymond L. White, Ph.D., director of the Huntsman Cancer Institute at the University of Utah Medical Center in Salt Lake City.

"Women who have an inherited breast cancer gene do tend to get the disease 10 to 15 years earlier than other women. But it's also true that close to half of the women who inherit the BRCA1 gene won't get their breast cancer until after age 60," Dr. White says. "Overall, the great majority of these breast cancers will develop between the ages of 50 and 70."

Other researchers have isolated genes linked to melanoma and colon and ovarian cancer, Dr. White says.

It's All Relative

But for most of us, the odds of developing an inherited form of cancer or heart disease is about as likely as winning the lottery and being struck by lightning on the same day.

To grasp how unlikely it is that you will inherit one of these diseases, think of your genetic risk in terms of a fire hazard, Dr. Miller says. If the house down the street is in flames, you probably wouldn't abandon your home. But if the fire is next door and flames are leaping onto your roof, it's time to take emergency measures.

"For the great majority of us, genetically predisposed cancers and heart disease are fires that are burning well down the block," Dr. Miller says. "Only a small number of individuals are at risk."

But if it appears that your family is prone to a particular disease, it may be worth taking some precautions, Dr. Myers says.

"If my mother or father had died of a heart attack, or my brother died of a stroke at a young age, I'd certainly tell my doctor about it. I'd also try to make some modifications in my lifestyle such as regular exercise, eating well, and not smoking," Dr. Myers says.

So before you decide to seek genetic counseling and testing, it's important to take an up-close-and-personal look at your family history. Here is how to do it.

Ask for volunteers. The more information you have, the better. Compiling all the family history that you would want can be a big job.

341

"If you're looking at a breast, ovarian, or other female cancer, for example, you really need to have a broad reach. So you wouldn't look only at mothers, sisters, and aunts but at first cousins, second cousins, and great-aunts," says Katherine Schneider, a genetic counselor at Dana Farber Cancer Institute in Boston.

Information about fathers, uncles, and grandparents can provide vital clues, too. Ask family members to help, she suggests. Elect a family historian to pull together all the pieces of information that others gather.

Glance forward as well as back. Most of the health information that you will need is buried deep in your family's past. But don't forget to record the health of your children and grandchildren. If they have a history of heart disease, cancer, or stroke, it may be time to seek genetic counseling, says Mary Daly, M.D., director of the Family Risk Assessment Program at Fox Chase Cancer Center in Philadelphia.

"We have some families where the daughter gets breast cancer before the mother, and then the mother goes on to get it, too," Dr. Daly says. Discovering that you carry the same mutated gene as your ill children may help you consider your options, she says.

Check everything out. If you know only that your aunt died of "female" cancer or that your grandfather had "cancer all through his body when he died," that won't help you very much, Schneider says.

"A lot of family myths about death are passed on from generation to generation," Schneider says. "It could turn out that the relative had a completely different cancer than family legend claims. It could be that he didn't have cancer or heart disease at all."

Get as many official documents as you can, including the death certificates, suggests Schneider. Your best bets are local hospitals, coroners, or the state department of vital statistics.

Dig deeper. Check out diaries, letters, old photographs, anything that will give you clues about how your relatives lived. Did they smoke? Where did they live? What were their occupations? What did they eat? Were they overweight? Did they have high blood pressure? Did they have high cholesterol levels? These questions will help you figure out if lifestyle or genetics played a bigger role in their pattern of disease, Dr. Hopkins says.

342

"If they all developed lung cancer, but they also smoked for 20 to 30 years, you can probably bet it wasn't inherited," Schneider says.

Is Genetic Testing Worthwhile for You?

Once you compile your family history, you might notice some patterns of heart disease, stroke, and cancer that can't be accounted for by poor diet, smoking, and other risk factors. If this is the case, you may want to consider taking the next step—genetic counseling and testing. But for most of us it is probably unnecessary, Dr. Miller says. For the most part, these diseases are caused by lifestyle factors like smoking.

Genetic counselors are available at most major medical and cancer centers, says Schneider. A counselor can help you evaluate your family history of disease and determine if genetic testing is appropriate.

If genetic testing seems apt, a laboratory technician will either draw some of your blood or use a small brush to swab a few cells from the inside of your mouth. Both methods will disclose the same genetic information, Dr. Miller says. A lab could then evaluate a sample of your cells for known genetic markers of cancer and heart disease.

It takes anywhere from three weeks to six months to get your initial results, depending on what type of testing you have. Cancer, for example, is very complex, says Dr. Myers. Researchers have to analyze thousands of genetic patterns to find the mutation that they are looking for. But once a defective gene has been detected in one family member, it usually takes only one to four weeks to check for that mutation in other relatives. Here are a couple of things to keep in mind before you seek counseling and testing.

Ask yourself why you are doing this. Before seeking genetic testing, it's important to think about all of the possible emotional and economic consequences for you and your family, says Dr. Daly.

Consider how genetic testing might affect you or your children's ability to get insurance or find employment, Dr. Daly says. Imagine how it might affect your relationship with your sister, daughter, or spouse.

Think about what you will really do with this information. Some people do nothing. Some begin getting more frequent checkups to detect these diseases early. Others opt for preventive surgery to remove cancer-prone organs, Dr. Daly says.

Imagine how you might react to positive test results. Take time to seriously contemplate these issues before making a decision to undergo testing. A certified genetic counselor will help you to understand the risks and benefits of genetic testing for you.

Get a referral. This process isn't cheap—up to $200 for counseling and more than $1,500 for testing. Ask your doctor to refer you to a genetic research project that will help pick up the tab for you, Schneider suggests.

Prescription for Prevention

Genetic defects that cause inherited forms of cancer and cardiovascular diseases are rare. Genetic testing can detect some of these mutant genes that are passed on from one generation to the next. But even if you carry a mutated gene, it doesn't mean you are doomed to develop one of these diseases. A healthy lifestyle that includes not smoking may help keep these genes dormant.

Do:

- *Think carefully about the economic and social consequences of genetic testing on you and your family.*

- *Get a referral to a genetic testing study at a major medical center.*

- *Gather specific information about your ancestors and how they lived and died.*

Don't:

- *Panic. The vast majority of cancers, heart attacks, and strokes are not caused by inherited genetic defects. Focus on living as healthy a life as you can.*

Chapter 15

What Other Maladies Contribute to These Killer Diseases?

You know your enemies—cancer, heart attack, and stroke. But in reality, these diseases are more like the four-star generals of the opposing forces. In any army the big brass may get all the attention, but foot soldiers lead the assault. Cancer, heart disease, and stroke couldn't wage their battles without lots of help from other medical conditions that get on the front line for these killer diseases.

Here is a rundown of the other culprits that help pave the way for these high-profile diseases. The good news is that if you control them, you can outflank the big three.

Atherosclerosis

Atherosclerosis is just the fancy name for hardening of the arteries. And that's what happens—they get stiff and narrow. But that's not all. "Bad" low-density lipoprotein (LDL) cholesterol starts the process, attaching to artery walls and even attracting other cells to the site. The walls thicken and stiffen. Tiny shards of bone actually form within the walls, which become inflamed. The body tries to repair the damage but ends up making plaque, the stuff that can break loose and form a clot—and increase your risk of a heart attack or stroke.

The destructive process picks up speed if you already have high blood pressure, diabetes, or high cholesterol levels. But you can fight the effects, says John Cantwell, M.D., director of preventive medicine and cardiac rehabilitation at Georgia Baptist Hospital in Atlanta.

Get hormonal protection. Until menopause, estrogen provides women with protection from hardening of the arteries. Hormone replacement therapy will help restore the benefits.

Slow it down with exercise. Exercise slows the progress of atherosclerosis. It doesn't matter whether you go to an exercise class, take walks, or just work in the house or garden. Strive for 30 minutes or more of vigorous exercise just about every day, says Dr. Cantwell.

Get control. If you can control your high blood pressure and cholesterol, you will help put the brakes on this condition, says Dr. Cantwell, who notes that just being 20 percent overweight can trigger insulin resistance or diabetes, key contributors to hardening of the arteries.

Adjust your diet. If you cut cholesterol and animal fats, you will also cut your risk, advises Frank Barry, M.D., a family practice physician in Colorado Springs and author of *Make the Change for a Healthy Heart.* You increase the effects of insulin resistance and diabetes (both of which speed up hardening of the arteries) if you consume a lot of polyunsaturated oils, such as corn, safflower, and sunflower oils. Monounsaturated fats, such as olive and canola oils, provide a healthy alternative.

Take vitamin E. Vitamin E spurs insulin activity and can prevent LDL cholesterol from being oxidized in the body, notes Dr. Barry. One study designed to find out how much vitamin E is necessary for this protection found that 400 international units of vitamin E is the minimum needed to prevent damage. It also found that 800 to 1,200 international units of vitamin E provided more protection. But talk with your doctor first, especially if you are already taking anticoagulant drugs, says Dr. Barry.

Think small. Large meals send insulin and blood sugar up steeply, giving your system more problems to deal with, especially if your cells aren't taking in insulin and sugar as effectively as they used to. Smaller, more frequent meals will take off some of the pressure, says Dr. Barry.

Atrial Fibrillation

With atrial fibrillation, your heart loses its sense of rhythm—and your risk of stroke shoots up. According to the American Heart Association, this disorder is responsible for 75,000 strokes a year.

Symptoms of atrial fibrillation are subtle, including palpitations and shortness of breath. Oftentimes, you don't know that you have it until a routine physical picks up the irregular beat or an electrocardiogram maps it out.

This condition increases your risk of a stroke because blood tends to pool and be more likely to congeal.

Atrial fibrillation usually goes along with other heart problems. You're at risk if you have had a stroke, heart attack, high blood pressure, congestive heart failure, hyperthyroidism, heart valve or rheumatic heart disease, or if you have abused alcohol.

Your doctor will probably prescribe an anticoagulant, followed by a regimen of drugs to help your heart keep its steady beat.

Barrett's Esophagus

It seems pretty innocent at first—little benign tumors on your esophagus, the pipe that moves food from mouth to stomach. The growths frequently start out as irritations caused by digestive juices that spurt upward from the stomach. Symptoms include heartburn and difficulty in swallowing.

But, as in the case of many cancers, harmless little lumps can turn malignant. Doctors once thought that this condition also increased your risk for colon cancer. But the good news is that a study performed in five French hospitals suggests that is not the case.

Chronic Infections

When your body's cells are damaged, repaired, then damaged again on a frequent basis, you're setting the stage for cancer, says Dr. Cantwell. Pay attention to skin sores, especially if they are exposed to the sun. Scar tissue, too, is more at risk.

"We know that chronic ulcerative colitis, an inflammatory disease of the colon, seems to be associated with increased risk of cancer. It is very likely that all of the body's tissues react the same way to chronic irritation," says Dr. Cantwell.

Colds and Respiratory Infections

In an English study of 96 older men and women, researchers found that the increased risk of winter colds may make the blood more likely to clot in the arteries that supply the heart. That may be caused by increased levels of fibrinogen and factor VIIc, substances in the blood that lead to increased clotting.

Fibrinogen actually provides the scaffolding around which clots form, and it is linked to higher rates of heart disease. An Israeli study, for instance, followed more than 3,000 male heart patients for three years. The 111 men who died during the study all had higher levels of fibrinogen than did the survivors.

One theory is that respiratory infections trigger the body's infection-fighting mechanisms, which also increase blood clotting. But the increase in winter strokes and heart attacks could also be due to seasonal variations in high blood pressure, weight gain, and lack of activity when the temperature drops.

One common bacterium, *Chlamydia pneumoniae,* may be tied to higher rates of heart disease. This bacterium causes upper and lower respiratory tract infections. It increases the concentration of fibrinogen and sialic acid in the blood, which is also associated with higher rates of heart disease. Furthermore, research shows that people with the high levels of fibrinogen may have twice the amount of the harmful LDL cholesterol. Their levels of protective high-density lipoprotein (HDL) cholesterol are lower than normal, too.

Still, experts aren't willing to put too much emphasis on colds and bacterial infections as risk factors for heart disease, cancer, and stroke. "It's much less significant than other factors, such as high blood pressure, cholesterol, and diabetes," says Dr. Cantwell.

All the same, you can make changes in your lifestyle to keep fibrinogen levels down: Lose weight and eat a diet low in saturated fat and high in unsaturated fat. Include vegetables, fruit, and fish in your diet, says Dr. Cantwell.

Depression

You may already know that the go-go-go type A personality weighs heavy on the heart. But depression is actually worse on the heart, says Robert Carney, Ph.D., professor of medical psychology at Washington University School of Medicine in St. Louis. "Depression appears to be a risk factor for heart disease," he says. "It's more important than a type A personality, but probably not as significant as high blood pressure and cholesterol." Still, he notes that depression is often treated long before patients show signs of heart disease. All the same, depressed people may have higher risk for heart trouble not because of their emotional states alone but because they're more likely to smoke and ignore doctors' recommendations.

Depression takes more than a mental toll. If you're depressed, the nervous system becomes more active and the heart beats faster—and it's more likely to beat irregularly. "Any kind of chronic illness or problem affects the nervous system and adds to risk," says Dr. Carney. Depression differs from normal mood changes. You may be depressed if you experience some of these symptoms for two weeks or more, says Dr. Carney.

- Loss of interest in things you normally enjoy
- Inability to concentrate
- Trouble sleeping
- Lack of appetite—you may lose 5 pounds or more
- A hopeless and helpless feeling, crying for no apparent reason

Even though you will need to see your doctor, you can help reverse depression. Here's how.

Do what's good for you. Even though it's hard to stick to it when you are depressed, exercise and a healthy diet will help bring you out of the depths, advises Dr. Carney.

Get emotional support. People who are depressed feel isolated, as if they don't have anyone who cares for them. Ask for support from family and friends. "You need someone to put an arm around you and help you get through this," says Dr. Carney. "It's a lot easier if you ask for help and know that someone hears you, understands you, and is with you."

Admit it to yourself. Often, just acknowledging to yourself that you are depressed helps, particularly if your depression stems from a specific event, such as an illness. "This kind of depression can be treated quickly and effectively," says Dr. Carney. It may require short-term psychotherapy or antidepressants.

Keep it simple. If you are depressed, you may feel out of control or overwhelmed. "Focus on simple tasks and goals, things you can accomplish," says Dr. Carney. "If you tell yourself that you have to stop smoking right now, you may not feel that you're in control enough to do so. You'll set yourself up for a failure and add to your depression."

Instead, try to cut down. If you smoke 30 cigarettes a day, try to smoke only 25 a day. "That way you can feel that you're making progress and setting goals that you can accomplish," he says.

Make a list. Depression robs you of your concentration and makes it hard to remember things, says Dr. Carney. Keep a list of just a few tasks that you want to accomplish each day. Mark them off when you finish them. Don't overdo it—keep your list short and easy to accomplish. Tell yourself, "I may not be coping very well with this right now, but here are some things I can do to help myself. If I accomplish them, I'll feel more in control and less depressed."

Make your own meaning. When you're depressed, you may feel that life has no meaning. Make a list of your personal reasons for living—the positive things you look forward to, says Dr. Carney. "For instance, that you can still enjoy your grandkids and you still play cards with friends," he suggests. When you feel down, pull out your list and read it to yourself.

Diabetes and Insulin Resistance

Insulin resistance often leads to diabetes—and that's not all. "Insulin resistance and the abnormalities associated with it accelerate atherosclerosis, which leads to heart disease and stroke," says Gerald Reaven, M.D., a researcher at Stanford University. He estimates that insulin resistance affects 25 percent of all Americans.

Both insulin resistance and diabetes wage guerilla warfare on your circulatory system and significantly increase your risk of heart disease or stroke. They also produce a domino effect in your body as other systems go haywire.

Here's what happens in your body. If you have insulin resistance, your system doesn't respond to the insulin you make. That's a problem because insulin is the substance that makes it possible for sugar to get into your cells and provide important nourishment. Think of insulin as the key that unlocks the door to your body's cells and allows nutrients to get in, says Dr. Reaven.

Your system is no slacker, so your pancreas gets the signal to work overtime to produce extra supplies of insulin because the insulin it makes is insufficient to do the job. Over time, it may not be able to sustain the extra insulin production, and you end up with not enough insulin. That's when insulin resistance turns into diabetes.

Though both insulin resistance and diabetes involve insulin, they are two different diseases affecting the body differently. First, let's look at the problems created by diabetes.

The lack of insulin means that blood sugar can't get into the cells where it is needed for energy, and it builds up in the blood. In type II diabetes, the most prevalent kind, some of this sugar gets into the cells by sheer force.

The blood sugar outside the cells exerts pressure—kicking the door down, so to speak, when the insulin key doesn't work. Having blood sugar levels that are either too high (hyperglycemia) or too low (hypoglycemia) is not good for your body.

As if that weren't enough, diabetes seriously increases your risk of developing cardiovascular disease. According to the American Heart Association, approximately 80 percent of people with diabetes die of some type of heart or blood vessel disease. This is because diabetes increases triglyceride levels and lowers helpful HDL cholesterol levels.

Diabetes is also the leading cause of blindness, kidney failure, and nerve damage.

Insulin resistance leads to its own share of problems. Several studies show that insulin resistance and high blood levels of insulin appear in as many as half of the patients with high blood pressure.

You'll want to alleviate insulin resistance because it changes the size of your LDL cholesterol, which is a risk factor in coronary heart disease. In this instance the LDL cholesterol particles become smaller and denser and more easily oxidized, allowing them to grab on to artery walls and narrow them.

If you are insulin-resistant, you have more insulin floating around in your system trying to get that blood sugar into the cells. This is not good because insulin raises levels of triglycerides, fats in the bloodstream that help clog up the works. High levels of triglycerides are normally associated with low levels of HDL cholesterol.

High insulin levels and insulin resistance interfere with your body's system for breaking up clots in the bloodstream.

But there is much you can do to help your body use sugar and insulin more efficiently, reversing insulin resistance and preventing or minimizing diabetes.

Get active. People who exercise can enhance how their bodies use insulin, decreasing their insulin resistance, says Dr. Reaven. In addition, physical activity can lower triglyceride and insulin levels, help lower blood pressure, and increase levels of "good" HDL cholesterol in the blood. The American Heart Association recommends that people get 30 to 60 minutes of aerobic exercise three or four times a week.

Lose weight. Being overweight is not the only factor that can lead to insulin resistance, but it is an important one. If you are overweight and subsequently lose weight, your body will improve its sensitivity to insulin, and you will become less insulin-resistant, says Dr. Reaven.

Where your body stores fat may be more important than how much your body stores. People who store fat in their upper body usually have more features of insulin resistance than those who store fat on their hips and thighs.

Check your inheritance. There is a genetic component to insulin resistance and diabetes. Your risk of developing insulin resistance or diabetes is higher if you are of non-European ancestry. If that fits your family's description, be particularly careful to lower your risk, advises Dr. Reaven.

Put out the cigarettes. Another good reason to quit now: Smoking increases insulin resistance, makes triglyceride levels go up, and makes HDL cholesterol levels go down, says Dr. Reaven.

Hepatitis

This highly infectious disease comes in several forms. Two kinds, hepatitis B and C, are linked to liver cancer. You get type C through blood transfusion or sharing contaminated needles. Type B can get into your system through blood transfusion, sexual contact, or sharing contaminated needles or instruments.

High Blood Pressure

Many people think that high blood pressure is a natural part of getting older. But it doesn't have to be that way. When you lower high blood pressure, you can cut your risk of heart disease and stroke in half or more, says Dr. Barry. That may seem hard to believe. After all, you can have high blood pressure and still feel great. But doctors don't call it "the silent killer" for nothing.

"When you blow up a balloon too much, you put too much pressure on a structure that's not built to take it. It pops," says Dr. Barry. "That's what high blood pressure does to your arteries."

The pressure rises when the muscles in your blood vessels constrict. Blood vessels narrow, and your heart works overtime, pumping more vigorously just to get enough oxygen and nutrients to your body's cells.

Because the blood is under more pressure, it travels more turbulently through your arteries. Imagine a wide river that suddenly narrows through a slender gorge. That wild river ride is close to what happens in your ar-

Don't Get X'd Out

Your grandchildren might be Generation X. But the X you really want to keep your eye on is *Syndrome X,* a cluster of medical conditions that dramatically increase your risk of heart disease and stroke.

Syndrome X is composed of several conditions, including high blood pressure, high triglyceride levels, low high-density lipoprotein (HDL) cholesterol levels, and premature coronary heart disease. Researchers see indications of this syndrome even in children, but it usually doesn't become a major problem until much later in life.

"All the components of Syndrome X are related to insulin resistance," says Gerald Reaven, M.D., the researcher at Stanford University who coined the term and has pioneered the research into Syndrome X. When insulin can't get into the cells, the body gets the message and mistakenly thinks it needs to make more.

High blood levels of insulin lead to high levels of triglycerides, fats in the blood. This high triglyceride level is related to a low HDL cholesterol level—that is, the level of good cholesterol in the blood.

"You can make a big improvement with lifestyle changes, such as eating a healthy, low-fat diet and doing some aerobic exercise," says Dr. Reaven.

teries. And other things start to go wrong. The smooth walls of your blood vessels get torn up and become more accessible to debris, or plaque, that builds up on artery walls—which narrows them still more.

Under extra pressure, the plaque may rupture. As it breaks lose, it turns into the stuff clots are made of, and your risk of heart attacks and strokes rises.

Sometimes high blood pressure doesn't start in your arteries. If your kidneys don't work right, they can produce hormones that tell the muscles in your blood vessels to tighten, constricting the arteries, and putting on the pressure. Stress can be another common cause of increased constriction of the blood vessels.

Your blood pressure also rises in response to things in your life that you can change. Here's how to take off the pressure.

Lower stress. Studies show that stress gets your heart pumping and your pressure rising, says Dr. Barry. As stress raises your heart rate and blood pressure, hormones may make the coronary arteries constrict, especially if they have been damaged by atherosclerosis (hardening of the arteries). The combination of reduced blood supply and greater demand for blood can lead to a heart attack.

Cut the salt. As you get older, your system becomes more sensitive to salt and hangs on to it longer. The average American diet contains 3,500 to 5,000 milligrams of salt a day. Consuming 1,000 to 1,500 milligrams a day puts you in the low-salt and high-health range. So check those nutrition labels when you shop and look for no-salt or low-salt products, suggests Dr. Barry.

Add the potassium. Low potassium intake can also increase blood pressure, says Dr. Barry. Get it from your diet: fresh fruit and vegetables, particularly bananas and potatoes.

Drop some pounds. Being overweight can contribute to high blood pressure, says Dr. Cantwell, and a weight loss of just 5 to 10 pounds can actually make blood pressure medication unnecessary in some cases.

Get active. Physical activity lowers high blood pressure. "If you're not doing anything, start to do something physical," says Dr. Barry. "Just accumulate 30 minutes of activity a day. This needn't be marathon running. You can walk, ride an exercise bicycle, work in the garden, or mow the lawn."

Reduce the fat. If you have been wondering why you've put on weight over the years, ponder this tidbit: 37 percent of most people's daily calories comes from fat.

To lower high blood pressure (and get your cholesterol down), Dr. Barry suggests that you try to get your fat consumption down to 10 percent of calories, the amount recommended by Dean Ornish, M.D., to reverse heart disease. Get into the habit of checking the labels on processed food—they will fill you in on the fat content.

Up the antioxidants. Some researchers suspect that high blood pressure is caused, in part, by a shortage of disease-fighting antioxidants in your system. Free radicals, compounds that antioxidants disarm, block your body's production of nitric oxide and prostacyclin, both of which relax blood vessels to help keep blood pressure down. You can get antioxidants through your diet by eating foods rich in beta-carotene and vitamins C and E, such as carrots, cantaloupe, broccoli, red bell peppers, and sweet potatoes. A multivitamin and a vitamin E supplement at 400 international units will also increase your intake, says Dr. Barry.

High Cholesterol

"High cholesterol is the number one risk factor for heart disease," says Dr. Barry. While HDL cholesterol protects you, LDL cholesterol and other fats do big-time damage to your arteries. Here's what happens.

The insides of your arteries start out with a smooth, elastic lining. Over time, it loses the elasticity and gets roughed up. The barrier between the cells in the lining breaks down. Fat cells get trapped within the lining and thicken artery walls. Microscopic fatty deposits even form on the artery surface. The result: narrowed, plaque-filled arteries.

If these deposits break free, they can lodge in the blood's passageway, causing a heart attack or stroke. The good news is that one form of cholesterol, HDL, actually helps the body get rid of the harmful stuff before it can do damage.

Here is what you can do to keep cholesterol levels where they belong.

Eat less fat. Eat the standard American diet, and you take in gobs of fat, typically accounting for 37 percent of your calories. Your body makes a valiant effort to deal with the problem, but there is just too much. So it ends up as cholesterol.

Taking fat out of your diet is the most important change that you can make because it helps lower cholesterol (especially LDL) levels.

Cut the fat. Not all fats affect the body equally. Saturated fat, which you get in red meat and dairy products, is the real culprit. Eat less of these foods, and you lower your total and LDL cholesterol levels, says

Dr. Barry. Unfortunately, polyunsaturated fats (corn oil, for instance) are also problematic because they lower the beneficial HDL. If you need or crave fat, then lean toward monounsaturated fat instead (olive and canola oils), and you will get LDL levels down and also raise HDL levels. Keep in mind that you should eat as little fat as possible, even if it is monounsaturated.

The American Heart Association (AHA) recommends that you keep fat consumption to 30 percent of calories or less each day. But you will do your system even more favors if you get total fat intake below the AHA guidelines, down to 10 percent of calories, says Dr. Barry.

Stop smoking. No surprises here. Snuffing this habit tops doctors' lists, says Dr. Barry. Nonsmokers have higher levels of the beneficial HDL cholesterol, 5 to 9 milligrams per deciliter (or mg/dl, how doctors measure cholesterol) above that of most smokers.

Lose weight. HDL—the "good" cholesterol—protects your heart, so you need as much of it as you can get. The problem is that if you gain weight, your HDL levels actually drop. A study showed that men's HDL cholesterol levels drop by 4 percent for every 5 pounds they gain. Women lose 2 percent. Lose the weight, and the HDL levels go back up.

Raise a glass. Studies show that very light drinking raises beneficial HDL cholesterol by up to 15 percent and lowers risk of heart attack. But more than a couple drinks a day may do more harm than good, says J. Michael Gaziano, M.D., director of cardiovascular epidemiology at Brigham and Women's Hospital in Boston.

Add fiber. Fiber in your diet can lower cholesterol levels, says Dr. Cantwell. Go for oats, oat bran, barley, legumes, prunes, apples, carrots, and grapefruit. If you like, add products rich in psyllium seeds, which are often sold as laxatives.

Get an E. In a small study, researchers found that vitamin E supplements combined with a diet high in monounsaturated fat blocked LDL cholesterol and kept it from oxidizing. Some doctors recommend 400 international units of vitamin E a day for their patients that have coronary heart disease.

(continued on page 360)

357

Protect Yourself with a Low-Stress Life

How do you lower stress? It depends on what motivates you, says Frank Barry, M.D., a family practice physician in Colorado Springs and author of *Make the Change for a Healthy Heart.* "Some people, in their heart of hearts, decide that it's easier to take a pill to reduce high blood pressure. Others prefer to make lifestyle changes."

Whatever your approach, you will feel less stress if you feel in control of your life, notes Dr. Barry. Get that control by establishing goals, writing them down, and working toward them, giving less attention to little things that aren't really important to you. Ask yourself, "What do I want to accomplish in life?" Here are techniques that many people find effective in relieveing stress, says Dr. Barry.

Relax and enjoy. Believe it or not, relaxation and enjoyment take some effort—or at least some calculation. "A lot of people realize that if they sit in a chair all day, they will make their health worse. But in the years of work, they have forgotten how to enjoy themselves," says Dr. Barry. "If you enjoy life and develop a sense of playfulness and humor, you'll be less prone to stress, anxiety disorders, and depression."

Make a study of what really relaxes you and what you really enjoy—the types of places (say, museums or parks) or activities (like cards, golf, or quilting). Then deliberately build those things into your day. Remind yourself that it is okay to have fun—you deserve it.

Lend a helping hand. You may get your greatest satisfaction from helping your children or grandchildren. But if you are considering providing financial assistance, think carefully: Will you find that satisfying or just stressful? "But I've seen patients who have never had such joy as when they gave their grandchild a new car. In that case, money can be a stress reducer," says Dr. Barry.

Pay attention to changes. Stress goes up with major life changes, such as the first few months after retirement. "Your routine changes immediately, but your mind and body are still tuned to the habits that may have taken 65 years to form," says Dr. Barry. Often, just acknowledging the stress helps to bring it down.

Remember, less is more. Many older people feel the stress of a fixed income. "Take advantage of the burgeoning simplicity movement," says Dr. Barry. When you sit down and think about what makes you happy and what makes you worry, you may find that you don't need the second car, the cabin in the mountains, or the new furniture. You may find that what makes you happy are family and friends, and fewer material things. Letting go of what's not important helps cut costs and stop stress.

Get on with life. Especially when you retire, you may be tempted to live vicariously through your children and grandchildren. That always produces stress because it doesn't work. Instead, live your own life. Do volunteer work to establish a larger circle of friends and responsibilities. Take courses at your local college.

Change your inner environment. Biofeedback or meditation will relax you mentally and lower stress, says Dr. Barry. Try reducing the psychological stress that raises your blood pressure by repeating a sound, word, phrase, or muscle activity while you passively disregard other thoughts.

Say good-bye to beepers. A lot of people feel as though they are always on call, says Dr. Barry, thanks to pagers, cellular phones, and the like. Take a break from technology, perhaps spending a restful day with the phone unplugged. Get unbusy. Allow yourself time to do nothing.

Make like a B. People with type A personalities suffer stress more often. Type A's are impatient, competitive, hostile, easily angered, and constantly struggling against the demands of real or imagined deadlines. (If you ever had to work for one, they gave you stress.) Type Bs, on the other hand, are more relaxed, accepting, and less impatient.

If you're a type A, practice being assertive but not hostile, advises John Cantwell, M.D., director of preventive medicine and cardiac rehabilitation at Georgia Baptist Hospital in Atlanta. You'll be more pleasant to be around—and you'll reduce stress, giving your heart a break.

Are You Hot?

The standard tests that doctors use to tell whether you are an easily stressed "hot reactor" (and at greater risk for disease) are pretty simple, so take your pick, says Frank Barry, M.D., a family practice physician in Colorado Springs and author of *Make the Change for a Healthy Heart*. For the first two tests, you'll want to take a blood pressure reading twice—once before the test and once during the test for comparison.

Test 1: Chill out. In Test 1, put your hand into a cold bucket of water for 1 minute and have someone measure your blood pressure right after you have done it. If it goes up into the high range in response to physical stress, you are a hot reactor.

Test 2: Do some math. Test 2 is a little more cerebral. Start with the number 100 and mentally subtract 7, then continue to subtract 7s until you get to 2. In the midst of your figuring, have your blood pressure taken. "There's no exercise, no threat to your life, but a lot of people still feel mental stress and their blood pressures shoot up," says Dr. Barry.

Test 3: Talk to yourself. You can also test yourself without the shock of cold water or the mental anguish of math. Ask yourself: Are you working toward your own true goals or someone else's? If you are busy trying to keep up with the Joneses, "you're still in the rat race, even if you have retired. You're much more likely to feel the effects of stress regardless of whether you're a hot reactor," says Dr. Barry.

Soy to the world. Rather than a hamburger, reach for a soy or tofu burger. Soy protein is low in fat and rich in genistein. While this substance has received a lot of attention because it may lower the risk of breast cancer, researchers believe that it also decreases total cholesterol.

Stomach Ailments

Results from one study suggest that stomach cancer may be tied to a type of common bacteria, *Helicobacter pylori*. The little organisms produce chronic upset that may eventually allow cancerous cells to take over. In an American study, doctors found that half of the people who visited their family doctors for stomach complaints had these bacteria to blame. Antibodies that your body produces to fight the bacterial infection may actually stimulate cancer cells in the stomach. Good news: The infection can be treated with antibiotics.

Stress

In the film *West Side Story,* members of the Jets, a New York street gang, urge each other to "stay cool." Researchers who study stress say the same thing: Stress can make you vulnerable to heart disease, cancer, and stroke.

Feeling stressed or overwhelmed raises your blood pressure and can even trigger heart arrhythmias. "We know that stress can contribute to increased cholesterol and hypertension," says Dr. Carney.

People who react strongly to stress are called hot reactors by cardiologists and psychologists. Their stress triggers an extra release in the flight-or-fight hormones that gave your Stone Age ancestors an edge over saber-toothed tigers. The hormones tell your heart to pump faster, which increases your blood pressure.

Stress also releases free fatty acids into your system, giving your body the energy boost it needs. But unless you're really going to wrestle a prehistoric feline, your body doesn't have a use for these compounds. They turn into dangerous, artery-clogging cholesterol.

Chronic stress may also decrease your body's immune response, leaving you more vulnerable to a cancer. Researchers at the National Institute of Mental Health in Bethesda, Maryland, found that stress activates hormones that allow viruses and cancerous cells to get to work.

Thyroid Imbalance

In a study of 2,000 men and women age 60 and over, researchers found that thyroid imbalance can interfere with the rhythm of your heart's beat. Those with slightly overactive thyroids were most at risk, a condition called subclinical hyperthyroidism. If you have it, your thyroid releases a low level of thyrotropin, a pituitary hormone that controls the production of the thyroid hormone. Your doctor can prescribe medication to regulate hormone production.

Prescription for Prevention

Cancer, heart disease, and stroke don't arrive out of the blue. Lots of little problems pave the way for these major maladies. All the little things you can do to assure your general health play important protective roles.

Do:

- *Keep cholesterol, blood sugar, blood pressure, and body weight within normal limits.*

- *Exercise regularly to prevent the circulatory slowdowns that lead to heart disease and stroke.*

- *Take vitamin E at 400 international units daily to activate your insulin reserves and protect your cells from damage.*

- *Eat small meals to help your system take in insulin and sugar more efficiently.*

Don't:

- *Smoke.*

- *Let winter weather make you inactive.*

- *Be a hot reactor.*

- *Get low on potassium. You risk getting high blood pressure.*

Chapter 16

How Dangerous Is Sun Exposure at My Age?

I t's easy to get burned. Just stick an uncovered hand into a 550°F oven for a second or two. That's why we use pot holders.

The sun is 20 times hotter than a broiling oven. Sure, it's 93 million miles away, but in just 10 minutes it can toast you more thoroughly than a marshmallow over a campfire. And even after age 60, a rich brown tan or charring burn can ignite cancer-causing skin damage.

That's why doctors urge you to use sunscreen and take other precautions.

"At this age, people want to live an active lifestyle. And I don't blame them. You don't have to live in a cave, but there are certain measures that you can take to protect yourself while you are enjoying the outdoors that will drastically reduce your risk of skin cancer," says Craig Eichler, M.D., a dermatologist at Cleveland Clinic Florida in Fort Lauderdale.

The Bronze Age Is Over

For years, our heroes were bronze: Burt Lancaster, Cary Grant, Mickey Mantle, Natalie Wood, and Racquel Welch. Tans were in. Pale was out. But all that sun worshiping has sparked an epidemic of skin cancer, Dr. Eichler says. Skin cancer is the most common type of cancer in the United States. Americans over age 65 were expected to account for about half of the 838,000 new cases of skin cancer in 1996. In the same year about 9,400 Americans—more than one an hour—were expected to die of some form of skin cancer, according to the American Cancer Society.

Almost all of this is unnecessary because without sun damage, skin cancer, wrinkles, and liver spots would be virtually nonexistent, Dr. Eichler says.

Indoor Tanning Isn't a Bright Idea

The Bahamas beckon. Surf, sand, and lots of sun. You certainly don't want a nasty sunburn to spoil your fun. So before you leave, you visit the neighborhood tanning parlor a few times to brown your skin.

A smart move?

"It may seem like a perfectly reasonable thought. The problem is that it doesn't work," says James Spencer, M.D., a dermatologist and director of Mohs Micrographic Surgery at the University of Miami School of Medicine. "The tan you get at a tanning parlor only provides an SPF (sun protection factor) of about four. So it won't protect you from burning, and tanning itself is a sign that the skin has already been damaged."

Most tanning parlors are unregulated and use UVA light in the mistaken belief that these rays are less harmful than other forms of radiation, Dr. Spencer says. In reality, UVA penetrates deep into the skin and can significantly increase the risk of melanoma and other skin cancers.

If you live for a tan, however, try bronzers, chemical dyes that brown the skin without sun. They are available over the counter at most drugstores.

"Some people tell me that they absolutely don't feel healthy unless they have a tan. For them, bronzers containing dihydroxyacetone (DHA) are worth trying. They are much better than they were years ago when they tended to give an orange-carrot-type look to the skin. Nowadays, these dyes are much more natural looking and are a nice alternative for some people," says Craig Eichler, M.D., a dermatologist at Cleveland Clinic Florida in Fort Lauderdale. But remember that you still need the protection of sunscreen.

To get an idea of how this damage accumulates, imagine sun exposure on a 100-point scale. When you're born, you have 0 points. When you reach 100 points, you get skin cancer, says Michael Kaminer, M.D., assistant professor of dermatology at Tufts University School of Medicine in Boston.

Every time you expose your unprotected skin to sun, it damages the skin a bit, and you add on points. One bad sunburn in your teens, for instance, might add 50 points to your lifetime total. Even tanning, which is really the skin's reaction to sun exposure, is a sign that harm has been done and more points are piling up, Dr. Kaminer says.

So if you are age 60 and your sun exposure score is 90, wearing sunscreen and taking other precautions may stop you from getting those last 10 points that would push you irreversibly toward skin cancer, Dr. Kaminer says.

The problem is that you never really know where you are on that imaginary scale. You can look perfectly fine but could be getting close to topping 100 points and developing a skin cancer. That's why it is important to start or continue taking sun precautions after age 60, Dr. Kaminer says.

"A lot of my patients in this age range say, 'Well, I'm old and it doesn't matter how much sun I get anymore.' The point is that it does matter very much at that age," says Nancy Silvis, M.D., assistant professor of dermatology at the Arizona Cancer Center in Tucson.

How the Sun Does Its Damage

Sunlight contains two types of harmful ultraviolet rays: UVA, a long-wavelength ray that penetrates deep into the skin; and UVB, a medium-wavelength ray that is absorbed by the upper skin layers. Both scramble DNA, the genetic code that cells use to reproduce, and increase the likelihood that your skin will form abnormal cells. At the same time, these rays suppress the immune system so that your body will be less able to defend itself, says Kevin Cooper, M.D., chairman of the Department of Dermatology at Case Western Reserve University and University Hospitals of Cleveland.

Over years or decades, these skin changes can develop into one of three types of cancer. Basal cell carcinoma, the most common type, is also the least serious form of skin cancer and rarely spreads to other organs. Squamous cell carcinoma is a bit more aggressive than basal cell and is more likely to spread to the lymph nodes and other parts of the body. Both of these types of skin cancer are usually easily cured but can leave disfiguring scars when removed. Melanoma is tougher. The most tenacious of all skin cancers,

Keep Your Eyelids under Cover

Sunscreens, hats, long pants, and shirts can protect 99.9 percent of your skin. But unless you don a pair of strong sunglasses, your eyelids will be vulnerable to the ravages of skin cancer.

"The eye is an easy pathway into the brain. That's why a tumor on the eyelid can be particularly dangerous," says René Rodriguez-Sains, M.D., chief of the Ocular Tumor and Orbital Clinic at Manhattan Eye, Ear and Throat Hospital in New York City.

For optimal eye and eyelid protection, sunglasses should wrap around the face, fit snugly and comfortably as close to the forehead as possible, and absorb at least 99 percent of the sun's ultraviolet rays, she says.

When you are doing your monthly skin self-exam, don't forget to inspect the eyelids. See an ophthalmologist or dermatologist if you notice any lumps, growths, and discolorations, Dr. Rodriguez-Sains says.

"Nine times out of 10, it will be nothing to worry about. It will probably just be the barnacles of life that go along with aging skin. But sometimes it will be a lesion that will need prompt attention," Dr. Rodriguez-Sains says.

melanoma can quickly spread to the lungs, brain, and other vital organs if it isn't corralled early. It was expected to kill more than 7,300 in 1996.

"Once melanoma spreads to a vital organ, it is resistant to radiation and chemotherapy. At that point, there is really nothing you can do. But if it is caught at the start, there is virtually a 100 percent cure rate," says James Spencer, M.D., a dermatologist and director of Mohs Micrographic Surgery at the University of Miami School of Medicine.

Lighten Your Risks

Most of the skin damage that leads to skin cancer occurs before age 20. But even if you have never taken one precaution in the sun, there are still plenty of reasons to start doing it now, Dr. Kaminer says.

Sun exposure, for instance, can increase your risk of certain skin cancers after age 60, according to researchers at the British Columbia Cancer Agency in Vancouver. In a study of 586 men up to age 79, the researchers found that those who reported spending 24 hours or more a week outdoors during the summer months were twice as likely to develop squamous cell carcinoma in the next 10 years than men who got less sun exposure.

But taking preventive measures even at a late stage may help repair seriously damaged skin before it turns cancerous, Dr. Silvis says. For six months, Australian researchers tracked 588 people up to age 93 who had precancerous skin lesions called actinic keratosis. Those who began using sunscreen developed fewer new precancerous lesions and were 53 percent more likely to have existing actinic keratosis disappear.

"Studies like this have shown that patients over age 60 who use sunscreen are actually helping their skin recover," Dr. Silvis says. "But among patients who don't use any protection, the skin isn't doing the needed repair work because it is continually being damaged."

Here are a few ways to lower your risk of skin cancer yet still enjoy the warmth of the sun.

Make 15 your lucky number. Use a sunscreen with an SPF (sun protection factor) of at least 15, Dr. Kaminer says. That means it will protect your skin in the sun for about 150 minutes, or 15 times longer than if you didn't wear it. Although sunscreens with SPFs up to 50 are available, a 15 should do the job. It will block out 93 percent of the sun's harmful rays. In comparison, an SPF of 35 only gives the skin about 4 percent more protection. If you really want 100 percent protection, choose a sunblock that contains either zinc oxide or titanium dioxide.

Make it a daily routine. Sunscreen is easy to forget unless you make it a part of your morning ritual. After you bathe and dry off, apply sunscreen to every part of your skin that will be exposed to the sun before you dress for the day, Dr. Cooper suggests. Allow at least 20 minutes for the lotion to soak into your skin before going out in the sun so that the sunscreen will stay on better once you swim or start sweating.

Don't let the clouds fool you. Wear sunscreen even on overcast days, since the sun's rays penetrate clouds and can still damage your skin, Dr. Eichler says.

Don't Get Burned by Your Drugs

Medicines can do wonders for arthritis, high blood pressure, heart disease, and other ailments that are common after age 60. But when some drugs collide with the sun, your skin may pay a big price.

Certain oral drugs like antibiotics and diuretics can increase your sun sensitivity. That magnifies your chances of getting a cancer-promoting sunburn, says Nancy Silvis, M.D., assistant professor of dermatology at the Arizona Cancer Center in Tucson.

Ask your doctor or pharmacist if you should avoid the sun while taking any drug. Here is a sample list of common medications that can increase sun sensitivity.

Drug Class	Generic Name	Brand Name
Diuretics	Furosemide	Lasix
	Hydrochlorothiazide	HydroDIURIL
Sulfonylureas	Chlorpropamide	Diabinese
(for diabetes)	Tolbutamide	Tolbutamide
Antibiotics	Tetracycline	Achromycin V
	Doxycycline	Vibramycin
	Sulfamethoxazole	AZO Gantanol
	Nalidixic acid	NegGram
	Griseofulvin	Fulvicin
Nonsteroidal anti-	Naproxen	Aleve
inflammatory drugs	Piroxicam	Feldene
Antidepressants	Doxepin	Sinequan
	Imipramine	Tofranil
Anti-arrhythmic drugs	Amiodarone	Cordarone
(for irregular heartbeat)	Quinidine	Quinaglute

Smear it on. Many people, particularly in this age group, spread sunscreen on much too thinly, Dr. Kaminer says. Put at least one heaping teaspoon on your face and neck together, another heaping teaspoon on your chest, and yet another heaping teaspoon on your back. Then use a half-teaspoon to cover both hands, another half-teaspoon to cover both feet, a half- to a full teaspoon for each leg, and a half-teaspoon for each arm and shoulder, he suggests. For men with lots of body hair, more might be needed on the arms, chest, and legs because the sunscreen is absorbed by the hair before reaching the skin.

Do the hands, neck, and ears first. "Three places where older people often forget to put sunscreen on are the neck, ears, and the back of their hands," Dr. Kaminer says. "So I tell my older patients to apply sunscreen to those areas first. It's important, especially on the back of the hands, because a lot of skin cancers develop there."

Start all over again. Reapply sunscreens at least every 2 hours to maintain maximum protection, Dr. Kaminer suggests. If you are swimming or perspiring heavily, you may need to do it every hour that you are in the sun. Some sunscreens are water-resistant or waterproof, but even these should be rubbed into your skin every couple of hours, he says.

No matter your color, beware. People who have naturally dark skin pigment develop fewer skin cancers than fair-skinned individuals, Dr. Spencer says, but it isn't perfect protection.

"African-Americans rarely develop skin cancers because their dark skin provides natural sun protection," he says. "Hispanics can and do develop skin cancers, so they should use sunscreen if they're going to be out in the sun for extensive periods, like fishing on a boat all day."

If you are African-American, keep an eye on lighter portions of your skin such as scars and the palms of your hands, which are often less resistant to sun damage, Dr. Spencer suggests. No matter your skin coloration, see your doctor if you develop any unusual spots or growths on your body.

Check the weather. Look for the UV Index in your local weather report, Dr. Silvis suggests. It is a forecast from the National Weather Service of how much ultraviolet light will reach the ground in your area at midday. It will help you decide when and for how long you may want to go out that day. The index ranges from 0 to 15. Zero to 2 is minimal risk, meaning 1 hour of unprotected sun exposure may cause skin damage in sun-sensitive people.

At high noon, take cover. When the sun is directly overhead, its rays are traveling through less atmosphere than when it is on the horizon. That is why sunlight is considered more intense and damaging at midday than at sunrise or sunset, Dr. Eichler says.

"I suggest that my patients only go out in the sun when they cast a shadow that is longer than they are tall. It is an easy rule of thumb to remember, and it will protect you from the most damaging ultraviolet light," Dr. Eichler says.

Put a lid on it. Hats are essential in the sun to cover your scalp and shade your neck and ears, particularly if you are over age 60, Dr. Kaminer says. Wear one that has at least a 3-inch brim all the way around the base.

Reapply sunscreen regularly. Certainly, long-sleeve shirts and pants offer more protection from the sun than bare skin, Dr. Silvis says. But not much more—a dry T-shirt provides an SPF of 6 to 8, and only 2 to 3 when wet.

"Most people think that their clothing is enough to protect them from the sun," Dr. Spencer says. "But if you hold a white T-shirt up to the sun, you can see right through it. And if you can see through it, that means light is going through it."

So be sure to regularly apply sunscreen every couple of hours underneath your clothes. Some mail-order clothing manufacturers such as Sun Precautions, however, do make tightly woven clothing with an SPF of 30 even when wet. For a free catalog, write Sun Precautions, 2815 Wetmore Avenue, Everett, WA 98201.

"Sun-protective clothing is an excellent option," Dr. Silvis says. "The clothing provides a broad range of protection from both UVA and UVB light."

Soothe the sizzle. If you do get a sunburn, only time will really relieve your symptoms, Dr. Spencer says. Your best bet? Take a 325-milligram aspirin every 4 to 6 hours and apply cool-water compresses to the burn as needed. You also might try over-the-counter moisturizers such as aloe vera to mollify the burn.

Pore over your skin. Conduct a self-exam of your skin once a month and see a dermatologist at least once a year for a professional evaluation, Dr. Spencer recommends.

"It's so simple to do a head-to-toe. It doesn't take long, it doesn't hurt, and you can save yourself a lot of trouble," he says. "Remember that most skin cancers are very easy to cure if they're detected early."

Look for any new growths and changes in size, shape, color, texture, or thickness of existing moles, freckles, and birthmarks on any part of your skin. If you do find a suspicious spot, have it checked out by a dermatologist promptly, Dr. Spencer says.

Prescription for Prevention

Americans over age 65 account for more than half of all new cases of skin cancer. Skin damage accumulates as you age. The more unprotected sun exposure you have, the greater your risk of skin cancer. But even after age 60, you can stop this process and reverse some skin damage if you begin taking precautions in the sun.

Do:

- *Use a sunscreen with an SPF of at least 15. Apply it to your skin 20 minutes before sun exposure. Reapply every 2 hours when outdoors.*

- *Look for the UV Index in your local newspaper. It will help you decide when and for how long you may want to go out that day.*

- *Wear a broad-brim hat in the sun.*

- *Conduct a self-examination of your skin once a month. Look for any new growths or changes in moles, freckles, and birthmarks. See a dermatologist if you have any suspicious growths.*

Don't:

- *Let clouds fool you. Sunlight penetrates clouds, so wear sunscreen even on overcast days.*

- *Forget to apply sunscreen to your ears, neck, and back of the hands. These spots are just as vulnerable to sun damage as other parts of your body.*

Chapter 17

Should I Take Hormone Replacement Therapy?

History is full of great teams. There's Burns and Allen, Lewis and Clark, Barnum and Bailey—and estrogen and progesterone, two hormones that, until menopause, coordinate the activities of a woman's reproductive system.

During your reproductive years, these two hormones formed a tag team to trigger your monthly menstrual cycle. During the first part of the month, estrogen levels rose. Your uterus walls thickened to provide nourishment for an anticipated embryo. At ovulation your estrogen levels dropped then rose two days later, and production of progesterone (the synthetic version is called progestin) shifted into high gear to maintain a pregnancy. If you weren't pregnant, toward the end of the cycle, levels of estrogen and progesterone both went down. Your uterus shed the extra lining—and you got your period.

Hormone replacement therapy (HRT) mimics this process. Earlier forms of the therapy were thought to present risks: Going on the therapy would increase your risk of uterine and, perhaps, breast cancer. But there was a trade-off, because the extra hormones also cut your risk of heart disease, strengthened your bones, and possibly gave you more energy—which is why doctors typically recommended it. A hard choice? You bet it was.

Today, the bite has been taken out of the cancer risk that used to go along with estrogen replacement therapy.

Part of that is because doctors used to think that only estrogen by itself helped protect women against heart disease and other risks. But researchers have found that when estrogen and progestin team up, they do just about as well. Together, they form one of the all-time great teams for protection: Estrogen protects your heart and bones, while progestin keeps your uterus safe from cancer.

In terms of cost alone, this dollar-a-day lifelong preventive therapy is clearly preferable to treating such diseases. And the cost of hormone replacement therapy is often picked up by insurance, particularly if you have medical reasons such as risk factors for heart disease.

But even in the old days when women had to weigh one risk against the other, one clear-cut winner emerged.

Keep Your Heart Healthy with Hormones

Doctors agree—hormone replacement therapy protects your heart, providing up to a 50 percent reduction in heart disease risk.

In one study doctors focused on women who began using estrogen as early as 1969 and followed them for more than 17 years. "The women on HRT had a lower mortality rate," says Gary D. Friedman, M.D., a researcher at Kaiser-Permanente Medical Care Program in Oakland, California, who worked on the study.

Dr. Friedman adds that these women did show a higher rate of uterine cancer. "We expected to see that because most women had started taking estrogen so long ago, before the combination of estrogen and progestin virtually eliminated the added risk. But most of those cancers were cured. It is a lot easier to cure uterine cancer, if caught early, than coronary heart disease. The death rate from heart disease is much higher, and heart disease is much more common."

"Every woman should consider hormone replacement therapy. The benefits far outweigh the risk," says Trudy Bush, Ph.D., professor of epidemiology and preventive medicine at the University of Maryland School of Medicine in Baltimore. She is the principal investigator for the Heart and Estrogen/Progestin Replacement Study at the Johns Hopkins Women's Research Core in Lutherville, Maryland.

Here is what hormone replacement therapy does to cut your risk of heart disease and stroke.

> ## Keep Cellular Division on Target
>
> It sounds like a bad riddle: Why does estrogen increase risk of one cancer and decrease the risk of others?
>
> Estrogen is like the lawman of old TV westerns—it keeps the citizens, or cells, in line. Researchers note that cells are most vulnerable to cancer when they are dividing. Estrogen helps control cell division and prevent uncontrolled growth, the body's equivalent of riots in the streets.
>
> The exception? Estrogen's other job is to build up the lining of the uterus. As part of that process, it encourages cell division. As cells divide and replicate rapidly, there is more opportunity for a mutation that can lead to cancer. That is why progestin is commonly included in the therapy. It causes the body to shed the lining of the uterus, protecting you from cancer.

HRT controls cholesterol. "Estrogen tends to reduce the levels of the 'bad' low-density lipoprotein (LDL) cholesterol and raise the 'good' high-density lipoprotein (HDL) levels. That is one way that estrogen may help to prevent coronary heart disease," says Dr. Friedman. Scientists note that low HDL and high LDL are key culprits in increased heart disease risk. You get nearly as much benefit if you were on estrogen-plus-progestin therapy as you would from estrogen alone.

It is blood pressure–friendly. Good news: Hormone replacement therapy has very little effect on blood pressure. In fact, it may actually lower it. Researchers note that it actually seems to relax the blood vessels, opening them up so that the blood is under less pressure.

HRT reduces clot risk. One study suggests that hormone replacement therapy reduces the blood's tendency to clot, which might lower heart attack and stroke risk. Researchers think that is because the therapy causes a change in blood flow and other factors that affect clot formation.

It protects your arteries. In a tantalizing study, researchers found that hormone replacement therapy may actually keep the important carotid arteries from thickening and narrowing, reducing your risk of a stroke. Researchers used ultrasound to examine the thickness of artery walls. "As atherosclerosis develops, you see a lot of bumps and thickenings along the artery walls. In women who were using the therapy, that didn't happen. But it progressed in women who were not using it," says Mark Espeland, Ph.D., professor of biostatistics at the Bowman Gray School of Medicine of Wake Forest University in Winston-Salem, North Carolina, who conducted the study.

In general, women who take hormone replacement therapy have more flexible arteries than those who don't.

"It's not clear whether that translates into a reduced risk of stroke," says Dr. Espeland.

Beat the Cancer Risk

Nothing is perfect, and hormone replacement therapy has long been linked with the risk of cancer. Here is a breakdown on how cancer links up with HRT and what you can do to avoid the risks.

Endometrial cancer. "This is really a nonrisk," says Alvin F. Goldfarb, M.D., professor in the Department of Obstetrics and Gynecology at the Jefferson Medical College of Thomas Jefferson University in Philadelphia. If you have a uterus, he says, your doctor will prescribe an estrogen/progestin hormone replacement therapy.

Estrogen taken without progestin (often referred to as unopposed estrogen) causes the lining of the uterus to become too thick, which may increase the risk of cancer. Progestin helps the uterus to shed the extra lining every month. (It's exactly what used to happen during your menstrual cycle.)

Of course, a woman who has had her uterus removed doesn't have to worry about this form of cancer. She can take estrogen by itself for maximum heart protection.

Colon cancer. Hormone replacement therapy may lower your risk of colon cancer. "We think there is a strong connection between estrogen and reduced risk," says Dr. Bush. In a study of 41,070 Iowa women ages 55 through 69, researchers found lower levels of colon cancer among HRT users. In the lab estrogen prevents the "wild cell growth of cancer cells,"

Live Better with Hormones

While protection from heart disease and stroke are important reasons to think about hormone replacement therapy, these hormones are more complex and beneficial than you might think.

Remember when you held down a job and balanced taking care of the house and kids? Estrogen is about that busy doing good deeds. Here is what else it can do for you and why experts recommend hormone replacement therapy for most women.

Keeps your brainpower strong. Researchers think estrogen may keep your brain at its best. It may help ward off Alzheimer's disease and dementia. It also protects short-term memory. "We don't know if the protection comes from estrogen receptors in the brain and how much comes from the fact that hormone replacement therapy improves the blood flow to the brain," says Trudy Bush, Ph.D., professor of epidemiology and preventive medicine at the University of Maryland School of Medicine in Baltimore.

Adding to the excitement, researchers at the University of Maryland note that a small section in rats' brains shuts down when it doesn't get estrogen.

Strengthens your bones. Hormone replacement therapy protects your bones. Doctors note that it can reduce your risk of fractures caused by osteoporosis by 30 to 50 percent.

Provides more zest. Some women say that they have much more pep and energy than they did before they started hormone replacement

---

she says. Because colon cancer cells interact with estrogen, it may help keep them from getting out of control—and stop cancers before they start to grow.

Lung cancer. "In our study we found a slightly lower than normal risk of lung cancer in women who took hormone replacement therapy," says Dr. Friedman. He emphasizes that the evidence is slight and inconclusive.

Breast cancer. "We're finding that many cancers, including breast

therapy, says Dr. Bush. But it's hard to know if there is a universal effect, she adds.

Keeps the weight off. Researchers note that women on hormone replacement therapy tend to gain less weight as they age and retain more of their lean body mass, which is important to reduce the risk of heart disease, cancer, stroke, and diabetes.

Ends incontinence. Estrogen improves bladder function because it strengthens the bladder's tissues. It also keeps the tissues in the urinary tract from atrophying. This appears to reduce urinary tract infections, says JoAnn Manson, M.D., associate professor of medicine at the Harvard Medical School.

Beats the heat. Because estrogen helps regulate the body's internal clock, it keeps you from experiencing hot flashes. Even though you are well into menopause, you may still be feeling the symptoms, notes Roger Duvivier, M.D., associate professor in obstetrics and gynecology at the Albert Einstein Medical Center in New York City and author of the book *Midlife, Madness, or Menopause.*

Fights insomnia. Hormone replacement therapy helps get rid of insomnia, a frequent side effect of menopause.

Makes sex enjoyable. Hormone replacement therapy helps eliminate vaginal dryness and reduce the thinning of the vaginal walls that can make sex painful.

cancer, have a strong genetic component. Estrogen may not be much of a factor," says Dr. Goldfarb. Still, if a woman is genetically at risk, it is possible that estrogen may activate the gene that gets breast cancers started, he adds. "If a patient's mother and sister had breast cancer, I would caution her that hormone replacement therapy may increase her risk," he says.

"We see a modest increase in breast cancer in women who have used hormone replacement therapy for more than five years. But the benefits appear to outweigh the risk for women who don't have close relatives who have had breast cancer," says JoAnn Manson, M.D., associate professor of medicine at the Harvard Medical School. She worked on a study that found that, after five years of hormone therapy, the average 65-year-old woman has a 3 percent chance of developing breast cancer. If she had never used hormones after menopause, the risk would have been 1.8 percent.

Researchers at Harvard University also concluded that the average woman's lifetime risk of breast cancer is 11.3 percent if she is not on hormone replacement therapy. If she is, the risk jumps to 16 percent. But her lifetime risk of developing coronary artery disease is 46 percent. HRT lowers it to about 30 percent.

Pick the Right Products

"Oral hormone replacement therapy products are the only ones that improve cholesterol levels, and they appear to give cardiovascular benefits," says Dr. Manson. "The estrogen skin patch does help protect you from osteoporosis, but we don't have evidence that it helps the heart." Neither do the vaginal ointments that help strengthen the vaginal walls to prevent dryness and discomfort during sex.

Still, if you go on hormone replacement therapy, you may get your period again, returning to your youth in the one way that you would rather not. You might also experience the side effects that used to accompany your period. Here is a breakdown of what products are available and how they will affect your system.

Unopposed estrogen therapy. If you don't have a uterus, the choice is clear: estrogen by itself. This way, you get the most heart protection and eliminate the possibility of side effects, which come from the progestin that protects the uterus from cancer.

Continuous hormone replacement therapy. If you have a uterus, you need the combination of estrogen and progestin to protect from uterine cancer. Continuous hormone replacement therapy gives you low daily doses of both estrogen and progestin.

You may get a little less heart protection than you would from estrogen alone, because progestin keeps HDL from rising as much as it would otherwise. "But the difference is modest," says Dr. Manson.

If you're lucky, you won't get a return of your period, either. "About one-third of women on continuous hormone replacement therapy don't get their periods, one-third get regular periods, and one-third experience irregular bleeding," says Dr. Bush.

It is usually worth putting up with the inconvenience, advises Dr. Manson. Irregular bleeding with continuous therapy almost always stops after six to nine months. After that, most women have no more bleeding—period.

You may also start to reexperience premenstrual symptoms such as bloating and mood changes. "There is no way of predicting whether your symptoms will be more or less than those that you had with your natural periods," says Dr. Manson.

Your body may let you know it is uneasy with the change through periodic twinges of nausea. "You probably won't throw up," says Dr. Bush. "You just may feel a little queasy at times." Some women also report tenderness and discomfort in their breasts. Most symptoms subside within three months.

If your symptoms really bother you, ask your doctor to prescribe the lowest possible dose of progestin. "You still need progestin to protect your uterus, but it is what causes most of the symptoms," says Dr. Manson. If you're on a continuous program, your doctor may be able to lower your symptoms by dropping your progestin dose to 2.5 milligrams.

Cyclic hormone therapy. If you can't tolerate the irregular bleeding that may accompany continuous hormone replacement therapy, try cyclic hormone therapy, advises Dr. Bush. On this form of therapy, you recycle your body's old reproductive routine and return to the days when you had a regular menstrual cycle. You take estrogen pills for most of the month and then switch to progestins for the remainder.

On cyclic therapy you may get the old side effects of your menstrual cycle, thanks to the progestin. If you're very uncomfortable, ask your doctor to lower your progestin dose to 5 milligrams, says Dr. Manson.

Prescription for Prevention

Hormone replacement therapy lowers bad cholesterol levels, increases good cholesterol, and appears to protect you from heart disease and stroke. It may also guard against colon cancer, although it may be linked to a slight increase in breast cancer risk. It also keeps your bones strong, helps prevent incontinence, may protect against Alzheimer's disease, and makes sex more enjoyable.

Do:

- *If you have a uterus, use a combined estrogen/progestin regimen to protect against uterine cancer.*

- *If your uterus has been removed, use an estrogen-only product for maximum heart protection.*

- *Use oral products, if possible, for heart protection, not products applied to the skin.*

Don't:

- *Use hormone replacement therapy if you are genetically at high risk for breast cancer (if your mother or sister had it).*

- *Use hormone replacement without progestin if you have a uterus. It will increase your risk of uterine cancer.*

Chapter 18

How Safe Is Snow Shoveling at My Age?

Down comes the snow, out comes the shovel, and then comes the heart attack. It's a pattern that Stephen Hargarten, M.D., sees all too often.

"After a heavy, wet snowfall, we'll get five to six times the number of heart attack cases that we would on any other typical winter day," says Dr. Hargarten, associate professor of emergency medicine at the Medical College of Wisconsin in Milwaukee.

At least 75,000 heart attacks occur each year during or shortly following strenuous physical exertion. About 1 in every 3 of those heart attacks are deadly, says Murray Mittleman, M.D., a researcher at the Institute for Prevention of Cardiovascular Disease at Beth Israel Deaconess Medical Center West in Boston. Many of these heart attacks and deaths occur among people over age 60 who have been shoveling snow.

"A lot of people think, 'Oh, it's just snow. I can take care of this.' They think of it as just another domestic chore like mowing the lawn," Dr. Hargarten says. "But snow shoveling is a lot more strenuous an activity than power mowing. Shoveling causes changes in blood circulation that are a lot more stressful on the heart."

Those changes in blood flow can be particularly risky for people over age 60 who are sedentary or who are unaware that they have heart disease.

"As you move along in years, you tend to get less exercise, and activities like snow shoveling become more dangerous," Dr. Hargarten says.

A study of 10 sedentary men in Michigan, for instance, found that just 2 minutes of shoveling snow raised heart rates above the limit commonly recommended for safe exercise.

And if you are out of shape, the chances that you will have a heart attack in the hour following a physically draining task like snow shoveling

Blowing That Snow Away Isn't Necessarily Better

Snowblowers may make your work easier and put less stress on your heart rate and blood pressure. But even with power assistance, the demands of snow removal can still be too high for inactive people who have heart disease, says Barry Franklin, Ph.D., director of the Cardiac Rehabilitation and Exercise Laboratories at the Beaumont Hospital Rehabilitation and Health Center in Birmingham, Michigan. Plus, these devices may have limited value with extremely deep snowfalls.

"In sedentary men manual shoveling increases heart rates up to 175 beats a minute. But using a snowblower can elevate your heart rate to 120 beats a minute, and if you have a heart condition that could still be a real problem," he says.

So remember: Before you decide to clear any snow, ask your doctor if it is safe for you to do, Dr. Franklin says.

are 53 times greater than that for a person who is physically active, Dr. Mittleman says.

"If you live in an area like Boston where snowfall is inevitable, it is important to get regular exercise throughout the year so that your cardiovascular system will be better prepared to handle the demands of shoveling in the winter," Dr. Mittleman says.

How Shoveling Strains Your Heart

When you shovel snow, you tend to hold your breath as you lift, Dr. Hargarten says. That increases pressure in your chest and reduces blood flow to your heart. At the same time, cold air constricts your blood vessels. All of this pushes up your blood pressure and forces the heart to work even harder. If your heart arteries are damaged or partially blocked with plaque, these things can combine to set you up for a heart attack.

Doctors are uncertain if physical exertion like snow shoveling also contributes to the onset of a stroke, Dr. Mittleman says.

So is snow shoveling a good idea if you're older than 60? If you're exercising regularly, you're living a healthy lifestyle that includes low-fat eating, you're getting regular physical exams, and you do not have any signs of heart disease, high blood pressure, or diabetes, you can probably safely do it, Dr. Hargarten says. Otherwise, it is smarter to get someone else to do it for you.

If you choose to shovel, here are some things to consider.

Get an annual checkup. Before the first snow flurries begin to fall in your area, get a physical and ask your doctor if you can shovel snow during the upcoming winter, Dr. Hargarten recommends.

Let morning snow go. If at all possible, avoid shoveling snow immediately after you awaken, Dr. Hargarten says. Most heart attacks occur early in the morning because blood is more prone to clotting after you have been sleeping. Take your time getting around to shoveling. Stretch, take a warm shower. Allow yourself an hour or two before tackling this task.

Lay off the smokes and java. Avoid drinking caffeine or smoking tobacco for at least an hour before and after shoveling. Coffee and cigarettes can elevate your blood pressure and pulse rate and increase the risk of a heart attack, Dr. Hargarten says. In addition, smoking elevates your carbon monoxide level, which further compromises the delivery of oxygen to the heart muscle.

Eat lightly. Wolfing down a big meal may seem like a great way to rev yourself up for this exhausting chore, but you may be doing yourself more harm than good, says Barry Franklin, Ph.D., director of the Cardiac Rehabilitation and Exercise Laboratories at the Beaumont Hospital Rehabilitation and Health Center in Birmingham, Michigan. Eating draws blood into the stomach, which means that less blood is circulating to the rest of your body. So if you shovel after eating, you are more apt to strain the heart, he says.

Stretch out. Before you begin shoveling, take 5 minutes to stretch and warm up your muscles, says John Emmett, Ph.D., an exercise physiologist and associate professor of physical education at Eastern Illinois University in Charleston. Stretching will help open up blood vessels and improve circulation to the heart. Try doing 20 to 25 knee bends and other

383

stretching exercises before tackling the white stuff, he suggests. (To learn a warm-up routine, see "Warm Up for Comfort" on page 228.)

Dress in layers. Dress in easily removable layers so that you don't become overheated as you work, Dr. Mittleman suggests. As you shovel, your body will warm up. But you don't want to get too warm, because if you get overheated, your blood vessels will dilate, blood will pool in your legs, and your blood pressure will drop. All of that forces your heart to pump harder and increases your risk of a heart attack. If you start sweating or feeling warm, it's time to shed a layer of clothing, he says.

Find the right tool. The smaller and lighter the shovel blade, the lighter the load you will lift. And the lighter the load, the less strain you will have on your heart and back, says Dr. Emmett. Specially designed snow shovels that have a bend in the handle can lessen the strain on the body even more. These shovels are available at most hardware stores, he says.

Be sure that the shovel is the right height so that you don't have to stoop too much, Dr. Emmett says. Here is one rule of thumb: Grasp the handhold at the end of the shovel with one hand. Place your other hand about 18 inches from the point where the handle meets the blade. If your hands are a little more than a shoulder-width apart, you have the right shovel for you.

Work smart. Start slowly and work your way up to a faster pace, Dr. Emmett says. During the first 5 minutes of shoveling, take half as many scoops as you would when you are going full speed. When you lift the shovel, bend at the knees and lift with your legs. That will put less strain on your arms, back, and heart, Dr. Franklin says.

Try to keep the load as close to your body as possible. Avoid twisting and turning as you work. Instead, shovel in the direction that you want to toss the snow and throw it out straight from the shovel blade, Dr. Emmett suggests. Take a 5-minute break from shoveling every 15 to 20 minutes.

Watch for the warning signs. Immediately phone for an ambulance or go to an emergency room if you feel dizzy, light-headed, or short of breath or if you sense tightness or burning in your chest, arms, or back, Dr. Mittleman says.

"Don't worry about feeling embarrassed about coming into the emergency room for a suspected heart attack. It is better to be embarrassed and safe rather than be sick and dead," Dr. Hargarten says.

Prescription for Prevention

Heart attacks triggered by snow shoveling are quite common, particularly among people over age 60 who don't regularly exercise or who are unaware that they have heart disease. If you live a healthy lifestyle that includes regular physical activity, low-fat eating, and not smoking, you probably can safely shovel snow. If you don't, ask someone else to do it.

Do:

- *Get a physical and ask for your doctor's consent before shoveling.*
- *Dress in layers to prevent overheating.*
- *Stretch and warm up before shoveling.*
- *Work smart, not hard. Use the right equipment, start slowly, and take frequent breaks.*
- *Be on guard for the warning signs of a heart attack, including tightness or pressure in the chest.*

Don't:

- *Smoke. And don't drink caffeinated beverages such as coffee or overeat for at least 1 hour before or after shoveling.*
- *Shovel snow within 1 hour of waking in the morning.*

Don't Let It Happen Again

Chapter 19

Heart Attack

To Prevent a Recurrence, Tailor Your Lifestyle

Okay, you've had a heart attack. But that doesn't mean that you have to live the rest of your life in slow gear. After all, Lyndon Johnson served as vice president and president of the United States after surviving a heart attack. Other survivors have competed in marathon races.

"You can go on to a whole new, enjoyable life after a heart attack," says Andreas T. J. Wielgosz, M.D., Ph.D., head of the Division of Cardiology at Ottawa General Hospital in Canada.

Researchers are finding that lifestyle changes will speed your recovery and even shield you from another attack. And if you don't make these changes after a heart attack? Your risk of another attack skyrockets.

"If you've had a heart attack, your risk of a second one is three or four times greater than it is for someone who has never had an attack," says Daniel Levy, M.D., director of the Framingham Heart Study in Massachusetts, the nation's most important long-term study of heart disease. "You have to take aggressive steps to minimize your risk."

The idea that lifestyle changes can lower your risk of a second attack isn't all that new. Heart attack survivors were once urged to recuperate at health spas, with a regimen of relaxation, exercise, and special diets—not too different from what contemporary cardiologists prescribe. But patients also underwent some treatments that by today's standards seem just plain peculiar—long, hot baths in saltwater, for instance.

Even today, researchers note that spa time seems to speed recovery. That's not surprising when you consider that life at the spa includes many elements that cardiologists believe are crucial if you want to avoid another heart attack.

- The calm, ordered life that frees spa residents from daily stresses

- A ready-made social support system, critical to prevention in today's world

- Regular exercise, also an essential part of today's regimen for recovery

If you've had a heart attack, here is how to lower your risk of a recurrence.

Take Charge of Cholesterol

When you lower your low-density lipoprotein (LDL) cholesterol count to 100 milligrams per deciliter (mg/dl) or less, keep your protective high-density lipoprotein (HDL) cholesterol above 35 milligrams per deciliter, and add exercise to the mix, something magical happens—you could help to reduce your risk for a second heart attack by 89 percent, says Tom LaFontaine, Ph.D., manager of disease prevention and community wellness at Boone Hospital Center in Columbia, Missouri.

"Cholesterol is a major risk factor for heart attacks. We've become much more aware in recent years of how important it is to lower cholesterol," says Dr. Levy. A diet and exercise program can lower your cholesterol by 10 to 15 percent. If that's not enough, a combination of diet, exercise, and cholesterol-lowering drugs can do the trick.

"When you lower your cholesterol levels, you can stabilize or even reverse the atherosclerotic process," says Dr. LaFontaine.

That process is a big part of what got your heart into trouble in the first place. Here is how your system got started down the road to a heart attack: Over the years cholesterol, or fats, in the blood found a home in your artery walls. These squatters really gummed up the works. Their population swelled as they built up thick deposits on your artery walls. Along the way, they turned into the hardened plaque that made your arteries stiffer and less flexible. They started to take up space that your blood needs to flow to your organs and tissue. That raised your blood pressure, leading to extra wear and tear on the artery walls.

And here's the worst part of the scenario—if the built-up plaque ruptures and breaks free, it can make a clot all by itself. Chances are, that's what caused your first heart attack. When the blood flow gets blocked, the heart muscle is denied the oxygen its cells need to stay alive and healthy. Beyond 20 to 30 minutes, the longer the heart muscle goes without oxygen, the more cells die, the more damage to the muscle—and the slower your recovery.

Since you've had a heart attack, it's a safe bet that other arteries have filled with plaque and become vulnerable to blockages. You need to get rid of the squatters—or at least stop the population explosion.

"You have to do everything you can to slow down the process that allows fats to oxidize and attach to your artery walls," says Dr. LaFontaine. "And it can be done. We're seeing that not only can you stabilize the plaque, but also you can make changes in the way you live to make it less likely to rupture and cause clots." You should start to see lower levels of cholesterol in your blood just a few weeks after you begin a cholesterol-lowering diet.

Regardless of your age or how much cholesterol has been setting up shop in your artery walls, getting the cholesterol down still lowers your risk. "In one study the oldest adult in the project got the most benefit from lowering cholesterol," says Dr. LaFontaine.

Here's how to get your cholesterol down.

Make a list. After your heart attack, your dietitian probably prepared a list of menus and foods that you should eat to protect your heart. Make a list of what you are eating now and compare it with those recommendations. If you threw the list away when you started to feel better, ask your dietitian to review your current diet. As time passes, it is easy to fall into old habits, says Dr. Wielgosz.

Take your spouse. If you recently had a heart attack, you will meet with a dietitian or nutritionist to help plan a protective diet. Don't go alone—ask your spouse to go with you, suggests Dr. Levy. After all, both of you will probably end up eating the heart-protecting diet that you'll be given. It will be easier for both of you to stick to the diet if your spouse understands how important the new diet is to your future health.

Play the percentages. Read package labels and compare nutritional content. Choose low-fat, low-cholesterol, and low-calorie products over those that contain higher amounts, suggests Fredric J. Pashkow, M.D., medical director of the Cardiac Health Improvement and Rehabilitation Program at the Cleveland Clinic Foundation.

Buy low-fat dairy products made from either skim or 1% low-fat milk. Try nonfat or low-fat yogurts. Choose cheeses that feature 3 grams of fat or less per ounce—and plan on a 1-ounce serving, suggests Dr. LaFontaine.

Pay particular attention to artery-clogging saturated fat. Make that less than 7 percent of your day's total calories.

You can automatically lower the amount of fat in your diet just by substituting foods high in starch and fiber. Increase your consumption of breads, cereals, pasta, grains, fruits, and vegetables.

Divide and conquer. Shave off a third of your fat intake, and you may help beat high cholesterol, experts say. Here's how to do it.

Figure out the calorie and fat content of a day's worth of food. If you're eating 2,000 calories a day, your fat content should total no more than 400 calories, or 20 percent of your total food intake. Make that figure—or a lower one—your daily target, says Dr. LaFontaine. Look at product labels that show "calories from fat."

You'll get even greater results by switching to a diet with fat levels at a super-low 10 percent, the level recommended by Dean Ornish, M.D., who devised a widely known program for reversing heart disease. Dr. Ornish's programs are so successful that they're finding favor with insurance companies. Some reimburse subscribers for the cost of participating in the programs, which focus on making changes in lifestyle through diet, exercise, and meditation.

Count calories. Just reaching for the low-fat products on grocery store shelves isn't enough by itself. You can choose low-fat foods and still end up with too many calories. Researchers from the National Center for Health Statistics note that in the 1970s, Americans took in about 36 percent of calories from fat. In 1990 they took in only 34 percent of calories from fat. Sounds like an improvement, until you realize that calorie consumption jumped and fat intake actually increased. What's more, unburned calories get stored in the body as fat, perpetuating the problem.

Drop dietary cholesterol. When you read the label, you'll see that many foods contain cholesterol, in addition to fat. That's not as bad for your system as fat, but it still adds to the assortment of harmful fats in the bloodstream. Look for products with low cholesterol. Try to consume less than 200 milligrams a day, says Dr. Pashkow.

Eat more often. Eat smaller meals more often, suggests Dr. Wielgosz. Emphasize fruits and vegetables. Your overall food consumption will probably drop, and your body will have an easier time burning the calories you take in.

Stay low on oil. Choose products that are low in oils. Read the labels to make sure that oils appear far down on the ingredient list, a sign that they played a small part in the food's production. All fats aren't created equal either. "Substitute monounsaturated fats for unsaturated or polyunsaturated fats," says Dr. LaFontaine. "Monounsaturated fats, such as olive oil or canola oil, don't seem to contribute to fats in the bloodstream the way other fats do."

He cautions that most of the studies showing the benefits of monounsaturated fat have centered on the Mediterranean diet. While this eating approach is high in monounsaturated fats and low in other kinds, it is also loaded with protective fruits and vegetables, which lend protection against high cholesterol. So far, researchers haven't determined whether the heart-saving benefits come from the oil or the other foods it flavors.

Avoid products that don't specify the kind of oil they contain. They're probably high in the artery-clogging kind, says Dr. LaFontaine.

Stay liquid. Keep away from oils such as shortening that come in cans and are solid at room temperature. They're particularly high in the harmful kinds of fat.

Cut the fat. Buy "select" and "choice" cuts of meat because they are lower in fat than prime cuts, which are marbled with fat. Better yet, just generally cut down on the amount of meat you eat. Make portions smaller or, several days a week, prepare meatless entrées, suggests Dr. LaFontaine. Instead of relying on meat for your protein needs, look to beans and other vegetables. Not only will you take in less fat but also you'll consume more fiber, which also protects your heart.

Make substitutions. Small changes can make big differences in helping to get the cholesterol levels down. For instance, instead of eating whole eggs, use egg whites or egg substitutes. Switch to filtered coffee. The paper filters trap substances that are high in cholesterol. And buy fat-free salad dressing and fat-free margarine, says Dr. Pashkow.

Fortify with fiber. When you eat a high-fiber diet, you're also picking foods that are generally low in cholesterol. Try to take in 25 to 35 grams of fiber a day. "You can get that by eating a lot of vegetable protein, consuming soy and other bean products, for example," says Dr. LaFontaine. "You can also get fiber in fruits, vegetables, and cereals. Evidence suggests that the fiber you get from cereal may be particularly important for protecting your heart."

Step on the scales. Every time you stand on the bathroom scale, you get an instant readout of your cholesterol risks. "The best way to lower cholesterol is to burn off as many or more calories than you take in," says Dr. Wielgosz. What stays in the system can turn into fat and clog up your arteries.

Get reminders. Tell friends and family about the changes that you are making in your diet—and that they can help keep you alive and healthy with their support and encouragement. Ask them to remind you if you start to slip into your old eating patterns. Experts think that social support is one of the biggest motivators in keeping people on track.

Call for help. Your doctor or dietitian should be an important part of the support system that keeps you on the path to heart recovery. Choose a doctor who invites your calls, checks on your progress, and is interested in whether you are sticking to the lifestyle changes that you have made to protect your heart. You'll get encouragement and psychological support just from the fact that you know your doctor cares about how you are doing.

Take the Pressure Off

Not that long ago, doctors thought that high blood pressure was okay as you got older. The theory was that you needed the extra pressure to keep the blood flowing. But study after study shows just how important it is that you get your blood pressure down into the normal range to lower your risk of a second heart attack. "Even if you're 80, your blood pressure can be similar to what it would be for someone 40 years old," says Dr. Pashkow.

Here's how to bring high blood pressure down.

Tip the scales. If you're overweight, lose it. Not only will excess baggage make you more prone to high blood pressure, it will increase your risk of diabetes, which will raise your risk of a second heart attack even more, says Dr. LaFontaine.

Add the fiber. Fiber is one of those all-purpose substances. Not only does it lower your cholesterol but also it helps reduce your blood pressure.

Focus on fat. Make sure that you're getting no more than 20 percent of your calories from fat—an eating approach that will lower both your cholesterol levels and your blood pressure, says Dr. LaFontaine.

Cut the salt. For heart protection stay away from high-salt, high-fat foods, such as potato chips, anchovies, sauerkraut, pickles, and salami as well as other highly processed foods, says Dr. Wielgosz. Your total daily sodium intake should be under 2,400 milligrams, according to the National Academy of Sciences. Your system may also be salt-sensitive, something that often contributes to high blood pressure. Talk with your doctor or dietitian about cutting back on your salt consumption.

Check your supplement. High blood pressure is linked to low levels of potassium, calcium, magnesium, and vitamin C. Eat foods rich in these nutrients. Make sure that they are in your daily multivitamin, but discuss changes that you plan to make with your doctor. And don't consume more than these daily levels recommended by Jeffrey Blumberg, M.D., associate director and chief of the Antioxidants Research Laboratory at the U.S. Department of Agriculture Human Nutrition Research Center on Aging in Boston: 1,200 to 1,500 milligrams calcium, 400 milligrams magnesium, 3,500 milligrams potassium, and 250 to 1,000 milligrams vitamin C.

Stop the Stresses

Researchers have identified stress as an important risk factor for heart attacks. Researchers found that how someone responds to mental stress gives as clear a picture of heart attack risk as does the traditional exercise stress test, says Dr. Wielgosz. This finding under- scores just how important a stressful environment may be in heart at- tack risk.

"While you can't eliminate stress a lot of the time, you can change how you cope with it and manage it. That may be an important factor in reducing your risk for a second heart attack," he says.

Here's how you can cut your risk.

Take time out. During the day spend a few minutes for quiet reflec- tion, contemplation, or isolation from daily life. In your office, bedroom, or outdoors, tune out stress-provoking pressures and thoughts. Focus on pleasant thoughts. Many people relax by repeating a single thought or a prayer over and over again, says Dr. Wielgosz.

Walk the dog. Fido may not be up for a brisk, nonstop, 10- to 20- minute walk, the kind of workout that is intensive enough to benefit your heart. But even leisurely dog-walking has beneficial aspects: It will help you reduce stress. You'll benefit from the repetitive action of your muscles as you walk. You'll enjoy the scenery. But most important, you'll have so- cial interaction with another being, says Dr. Wielgosz.

Find a hobby. A hobby can refresh you and help clear out stress. Write down a list of things that you enjoy, suggests Dr. Wielgosz. Knitting? Reading? Volleyball? Dancing lessons? Pottery? Continuing education courses?

"An amazing number of cardiac patients can't name anything that they do to relax and unwind," he says. "They don't have a hobby or other ac- tivity that's unrelated to the demands of their daily life. Think about what you might get pleasure and satisfaction from."

Enjoy the moment. Practice getting enjoyment out of routine activi- ties, such as preparing dinner. "It's easy to see everything you do as one more thing to be checked off on the agenda," says Dr. Wielgosz. "But you end up not enjoying anything, whether it's watching your grandchild in a school recital or eating dinner."

Dr. Wielgosz speculates that enjoyment of eating may explain the French paradox—the fact that people in France and Italy eat a lot of fat but have fewer heart problems. "These people have more *joie de vivre* at the table," he says. "Their meals take longer. There is more socializing around the dinner table. People enjoy the moment and live in the moment."

Get Moving

You'll need a two-part program of strength training and aerobic exercise to help optimize your recovery from a heart attack, says Dr. LaFontaine. Strength training builds a larger musculature, which burns more calories and helps to keep weight down—which is important to reduce risk. Aerobic exercise strengthens your cardiovascular system and actually reduces the levels of atherosclerosis that contributed to your first attack.

"If you have had a heart attack or have coronary artery disease, you have to do more exercise, not less," says Dr. LaFontaine. "Of course, you have to work up to it gradually."

"If your cardiologist didn't automatically refer you to a cardiac rehabilitation exercise program after you left the hospital and didn't recommend exercise, call him or her for a referral," adds Dr. Pashkow. "Even if your heart is severely damaged and you don't think that you can tolerate exercise, you should get into a program."

Cardiologists sometimes assume that older patients are too frail or won't participate in an exercise program. But it can mean the difference between life and death for you. "Researchers in Finland did a 15-year follow-up study and found that people who participated in a cardiac rehabilitation exercise program and risk factor–reduction program had a significantly lower risk of death," says Dr. LaFontaine.

While exercise will help your heart get healthy, there is a catch. To get the job done, you'll have to put the pump to work for 2 to 5 hours a week. "Studies show that people with coronary artery disease show the most benefit from this amount of exercise," says Dr. LaFontaine. "That's the threshold at which their atherosclerosis stabilizes or even regresses. If you do less exercise, the atherosclerosis continues and more plaque builds up in the arteries."

As you are burning off calories, your levels of the beneficial HDL cho-

Get the Right Cardiologist

Having the right cardiologist in your corner will go a long way toward avoiding a second heart attack, says Fredric J. Pashkow, M.D., medical director of the Cardiac Health Improvement and Rehabilitation Program at the Cleveland Clinic Foundation.

Knowing that your doctor and recovery program are the best that you can get provides important reassurance. And, if you do experience additional heart problems, you'll know that you will get up-to-date quality care. Here are more pointers.

Check credentials. To check the credentials of a cardiologist, call the local medical society or hospital physician referral service to get a guide to the doctors in your area. You can find out about their education, training, and, sometimes, their specialities.

Look at the diplomas. Check to see if the cardiologist has degrees from quality institutions. Quality education and training can make a difference in a practitioner.

Research the hospitals. Ask whether the hospitals that the cardiologist is affiliated with—the ones where you will end up—are accredited by the Joint Commission on Accreditation of Healthcare Organizations. That indicates that the hospital meets criteria for staffing and safety requirements. If possible, choose a cardiologist associated with a hospital that features a cardiac care center.

Then visit the hospitals. Talk to friends who have been to the hospitals where your cardiologist works. If there is a regional or national heart health center in your area, discuss it with your doctor. This is especially important if you have complex problems or advanced coronary disease.

lesterol go up. That's the stuff that helps keep your arteries clean and helps stop plaque buildup. The effort that you expend through exercise also helps lower triglycerides, harmful fats in the blood.

While several short daily bursts of activity (10 to 15 minutes in length) seem to help prevent cardiac problems in the first place, it is not sufficient to reverse risk if you have already had a heart attack, says Dr. LaFontaine.

If you have been inactive for a long period of time, you won't have the capacity to exercise as strenuously as you need to. You won't burn calories at as high a rate as someone with more exercise tolerance. This means that you will have to exercise for longer periods at a moderate level to get similar results. So talk with your doctor about the exercise level appropriate for you. It's important to make sure that you are not overdoing it, advises Dr. LaFontaine.

Exercise also benefits your system in another way, by speeding up your metabolism, says Dr. Pashkow. As you get older, your metabolism shifts into lower gear. "That seems to accompany a drop in the beneficial HDL cholesterol," he says. Higher metabolic rates are tied to higher levels of the protective HDL cholesterol.

The changes in your metabolism also help fight off diabetes. As you get older, some of your systems don't work as well as they used to. You don't metabolize carbohydrates as efficiently, which can lead to insulin insufficiencies and diabetes, a major risk factor for heart problems, says Dr. Pashkow. "When you change your metabolism, you also make it easier for your body to use carbohydrates over the next 24 hours," he says.

Here's how to get the most out of your workout.

Get attention. When you start an exercise program, you may be going against a lifetime of habits. You'll have the most success in sticking with your efforts if your cardiologist provides extensive follow-up and support. If this kind of follow-up isn't a routine part of your cardiologist's program, ask for it.

"We get patients in four times a year just to monitor their progress because it helps them stay on track," says Dr. LaFontaine. "We ask them about their exercise and diets, check their symptoms, and look for improvement." This follow-up procedure is particularly important once you recover from the heart attack and start to feel fine. It will be tempting to go back to your old habits. "In the early months people have a lot of incentive to stay with the program. They see the heart attack as a wake-up call to make lifestyle changes. But it is easy to revert to former habits when

---

On Your Own? Work It Out

Sure, it helps to have workout pals egging you on and charting your physical progress. But what if that's not possible? Here are some strategies to increase your odds of sticking with the program, suggested by Tom LaFontaine, Ph.D., manager of disease prevention and community wellness at Boone Hospital Center in Columbia, Missouri.

Make a display. Keep exercise clothes and equipment where you can see them. They will provide constant reminders in case you start to lapse. Park your stuff by the front door, in the living room, in front of the TV, or in the den, at least until exercise becomes an ingrained habit.

Set a time. Exercise at the same time every day. You will be less likely to forget or become sidetracked. Exercise will become as much a part of your daily routine as brushing your teeth.

Most heart attacks happen in the morning, but you can help condition your heart by light exercise, such as walking during those early hours. Save the strenuous stuff until later in the day, says Andreas T. J. Wielgosz, M.D., Ph.D., head of the Division of Cardiology at Ottawa General Hospital in Canada.

Tour the mall. Try getting your exercise by walking in an enclosed mall, especially if the weather is particularly hot or cold. You may find local mall-walking programs that welcome cardiac patients. "These organized exercise programs are particularly important because they also get people out in a group, helping to reduce social isolation, which is itself a major risk factor," says Dr. Wielgosz.

Walk with energy. You'll probably include walking as a major component of your exercise program. The more energy you expend, the more benefit your cardiovascular system receives. Consult your doctor to find your optimal energy level, says Dr. Wielgosz.

---

everything seems back to normal," he says.

Get rhythm. You can get your aerobic workout through walking, bicycling, working out on ski machines, or using other exercise equipment.

"What makes exercise aerobic is that it's rhythmical, can be sustained for 30 minutes, and burns about 300 calories in a session," says Dr. La-Fontaine.

Build slowly. "At first, do what you can handle," says Dr. Pashkow. "You may not be able to work up to 45 minutes of aerobic activity five times a week—what I recommend for people who have had a heart attack. If you can just do 10 minutes, start there."

Regardless of how long your exercise, make it fairly intense, says Dr. Pashkow. "The exercise stress test that you had in the hospital and in follow-up visits will let you know what you can safely handle. The kind of exercise that helps prevent another heart attack is different from just strolling in the mall and window shopping."

Choose with care. Sticking with an exercise routine will be a lot easier if you get support from your rehabilitation group or exercise program as well as friends and family. "It's probably as hard to stay with exercise as it is to stop smoking," says Dr. Pashkow. After a year, you have a 1-in-3 chance of returning to inactivity. After four years, your chances of going sedentary are about 1 in 13.

So if you have a choice of rehabilitation centers, pick one that will help you stay with the program. "We know that can make a big difference. We put a lot of effort into getting to know the patients, having special events and dinners with them, and recognizing their birthdays," says Dr. La-Fontaine.

Take the time. If your local hospitals don't offer a rehabilitation exercise program beyond the standard 8- to 12-week regimen, discuss other programs with your doctor. The ideal program is a Phase 3 or Phase 4 cardiac rehabilitation program, also called a maintenance program. (Your in-hospital program is classified as a Phase 1 program, and the 8- to 12-week program conducted at the hospital or in another institution is the Phase 2 program.)

Phase 3 programs are usually supervised and may be geared specifically for people who have had heart attacks or coronary procedures. They are often offered through community centers and generally aren't covered by insurance, but the costs are usually very low, says Dr. Pashkow.

Heed the Warnings

If you experience a second heart attack or stroke, you need to get treatment as quickly as possible to minimize the impact. The longer your heart or brain goes without oxygen, the more tissue is damaged.

When you are over age 60, the symptoms of a heart attack are often different than they are in younger people.

"Instead of the classic crushing, heavy feeling in the middle of the chest, you may get a cluster of subtle symptoms. They may not seem serious when you consider them individually, but call your doctor if you experience several of these minor symptoms together. Equally important, don't put off making the call," says Andreas T. J. Wielgosz, M.D., Ph.D., head of the Division of Cardiology at Ottawa General Hospital in Canada. Every second counts.

Watch for these symptoms.

- A heavy fullness or pressure in the center of your chest that radiates to your left arm or shoulder
- Weakness or lethargy
- Nausea
- Clammy perspiration
- Shortness of breath
- Pain traveling down the left or right arm
- Back pain or deep aching in the left or right biceps or forearm
- A feeling of doom, as though something awful is about to happen
- Angina that continues for more than 15 to 20 minutes
- Dizziness
- Confusion
- Pain in the neck, jaw, or shoulder
- Some people, just the feeling of indigestion or difficulty breathing

In a Phase 4 program you exercise on your own, perhaps at home or in an unsupervised group.

Your only options may be the YMCA or community center programs designed for the general public, not heart patients. Ask your cardiologist to discuss your exercise treatment with the class leaders. They can work together to set up target goals and monitor your progress through periodic telephone calls, says Dr. Pashkow. It becomes a low-cost program tailored just for you. Follow-up involvement from your cardiologist and class leader provide an important psychological incentive for you to keep at it.

Find safety in numbers. Regardless of where you are in the recovery process, you're better off exercising with a group. "Group exercise sessions give you social interaction, as important for recovery from a heart attack as the exercise itself," says Dr. Pashkow. This can help you ward off the feelings of social isolation and depression that often come with a heart attack and dramatically increase your risk of another one, he says.

Go high-tech. If you live in a rural area or if it is hard for you to get to group exercise sessions, look for a cardiac center that has developed "transtelephonic" programs. In these programs patients exercise at home, in their physician's office, or in a medical clinic. Regardless of where they are, a telephone link allows their cardiologist to monitor their activities with an electrocardiogram readout. Four to six people can exercise together, even though they are in different settings. Participants can also communicate with each other during exercise, which is important to provide the social support that helps them stay with the exercise program and keeps them healthier in general, says Dr. LaFontaine.

Spread the word. Tell your loved ones and friends that you are starting an exercise program to help your heart. Ask them to remind you to exercise if you lapse, says Dr. LaFontaine. Ask them to ask you about your progress. Let them know that their support is important to your success. Not only will their support help you stay with exercise but also it will reinforce your sense of having friends and family, which will help you fight off the depression that often follows a heart attack.

Tell Tobacco Good-Bye

If you smoke, the habit played a big part in your first heart attack. If you have since continued to smoke, you just have to snuff out the habit.

What about Sex?

Six weeks after a heart attack, most people have most of their strength back. "If you can climb three or four flights of stairs without panting and puffing, you can have normal sex," says Tom LaFontaine, Ph.D., manager of disease prevention and community wellness at Boone Hospital Center in Columbia, Missouri.

Your heart rate and blood pressure do go up during sex, but only for about 30 seconds during orgasm. But there is an important caveat, and an even greater reason for staying with one partner. Researchers found that the heart rate escalates far more with new partners or extramarital encounters. "Those levels could, theoretically, be dangerous," says Dr. LaFontaine.

If your heart attack resulted in severe damage and your exercise tolerance is quite low, you may need to adjust your sexual activities, perhaps playing a passive role or taking nitroglycerin before you have sex.

"Studies show that even in people age 75 and over, quitting smoking reduces the chance of recurrent cardiac problems. That's the most important thing that you can do to prevent future attacks," explains Dr. LaFontaine.

"If you continue to smoke, you will have a sevenfold increase in risk for a second heart attack and a threefold increase in the risk of dying within the first year after the attack," explains Dr. Wielgosz.

Keep trying. "We know that smokers go through phases to quit. And often it takes many attempts. So, if you have tried and tried but haven't been able to quit, don't be discouraged—it's part of the normal process," says Dr. Wielgosz.

Take the three-pronged attack. You are most likely to stop smoking if you take the three-pronged approach, consisting of counseling, group therapy, and wearing the nicotine patch, recommends Dr. Wielgosz.

Look for a cardiac rehabilitation program that puts all the pieces in place to help you quit. Your health insurance may cover the costs, says Dr. LaFontaine.

Think long-term. Cardiologists agree that you can claim to have kicked the habit only if it has been a year or more since your last puff. Even then, there is a 50-50 chance that you will fall back into your old ways. Minimize the risk by joining a heart attack survivors' discussion group, says Dr. Wielgosz. You'll get important psychological support from other heart attack survivors.

If you start smoking again or feel the urge, call your cardiologist immediately. Ask for a referral to a smoking-cessation group (possibly covered by insurance) and jump-start the stopping process.

Take Mental Control

Researchers believe that your mental outlook can make a big difference in whether you experience a second heart attack. "Depression and social isolation put you at greater risk for a second heart attack than even smoking," says Dr. Wielgosz. "If you fall into that category, you have the highest mortality rate after a heart attack."

People with heart disease who become depressed are four to six times more likely to die than those who don't, regardless of other risk factors, says Robert Carney, Ph.D., professor of medical psychology at Washington University School of Medicine in St. Louis. He adds that when you're depressed, you'll be more likely to smoke and have a more difficult time following your doctor's instructions and staying on medication that you need. More important, researchers believe that depression affects the autonomic nervous system that regulates heartbeat and heart rhythm.

Most people who have a heart attack go through bouts of depression. But if your depression lasts one week or longer, contact your cardiologist— you may need help to break free. Let your cardiologist know if you experience some of these symptoms, says Dr. Carney.

- Depressed mood
- Loss of interest in things that you normally enjoy

(continued on page 408)

Be Prepared

You're going to do all you can to prevent a second heart attack. But just in case, prepare your own plan of attack to minimize damage and risk, say medical experts. Here is how to do it.

Choose a hospital. Look for a hospital with a strong cardiology department to deal with future heart problems or in case of an emergency, says Fredric J. Pashkow, M.D., medical director of the Cardiac Health Improvement and Rehabilitation Program at the Cleveland Clinic Foundation. Find out whether the physicians in the cardiology department are board certified, an indication that the doctor has completed a specified course of training in his field.

Compile the data. Prepare a list of instructions for the hospital staff and include the following information, advises Dr. Pashkow.

- Information about any clot busters administered to you during your first heart attack—if you received streptokinase, administering it again may produce an allergic reaction.
- Your doctor's telephone number and those of close friends and relatives—ask hospital personnel to call them as soon as you're admitted.
- Any history of bleeding.
- Name of the cardiac surgeon recommended by your doctor.
- A copy of your electrocardiogram (EKG), a readout of your heartbeat—if you've had one heart attack, your EKG may look abnormal. A copy will help the hospital staff determine if you've had another attack.

Get an assist. Have your spouse, family member, or close friend learn cardiopulmonary resuscitation (CPR), suggests Daniel Levy, M.D., director of the Framingham Heart Study in Massachusetts. "Many people who have a heart attack live in enormous fear that they'll have a recurrence, and so do their spouses," he says. Having friends or family members who know how to administer CPR often provides reassurance. CPR should be administered the minute someone collapses with an attack.

Contact your local office of the American Heart Association to find out how to get CPR training. You might also want to become certified in Basic Life Support, available through local community centers or adult education programs, adds Dr. Pashkow.

Make it obvious. Now, before you have a second heart attack, is the time to check the exterior of your house, says Dr. Pashkow. Make sure that your house number is clearly visible and that your outside lights work. If you have an episode at night, turn on the outside lights to help the ambulance driver locate the right house.

Make it fast. The time between the attack and your arrival at the hospital determines the amount of damage to your heart. That's because the longer your heart goes without oxygen, the more cells die, explains Dr. Pashkow. Some medications that actually stop a heart attack, such as clot busters, are best given within a few hours of the attack.

As soon as you suspect a heart attack, call 911. Tell the dispatcher you may be having a heart attack. Your community may have ambulances that carry advanced cardiac life support technicians and equipment.

Get a ride. Even if you experience a cluster of subtle symptoms, such as clammy perspiration and shortness of breath, don't try to drive yourself to the hospital, advises Andreas T. J. Wielgosz, M.D., Ph.D., head of the Division of Cardiology at Ottawa General Hospital in Canada.

If it is a heart attack, your heart could develop an irregular rhythm and you could pass out behind the wheel.

Go to the front of the line. If a friend takes you to the emergency room, remember that it is important for you to get treatment as quickly as possible. The medications known as clot busters can actually stop a heart attack and allow the blood to get to your heart. Explain that you may be having a heart attack. If you're asked to wait, be assertive and make sure that everyone understands that if you are having a heart attack, you need immediate treatment, says Dr. Pashkow. Look for a triage nurse, the person who decides the order of treatment.

- Problems concentrating

- Feelings of hopelessness or helplessness

- Appetite and weight loss

- Sleep problems

- Crying for no apparent reason

The good news is that there is a lot you can do to end isolation and depression.

Get a confidante. Having just one close friend makes a difference. You need someone that you feel comfortable sharing your worries and feelings with. "Heart patients who have someone that they can confide in generally do better than those who don't," says Martin Sullivan, M.D., a cardiologist at the Duke University Center for Living in Durham, North Carolina.

A lot of people are more isolated than they realize. Ask yourself: If your car was broken down, would someone drive you to the doctor? If the answer is no, you need to work on getting friends and a possible confidante. And that takes practice. Start by getting out—get involved in a church, club, and neighborhood activities.

Make an appointment. Talk to someone in your church, a social worker, or a counselor. Talk about your feelings and worries. Even if this activity seems foreign to you, remember that you are helping your heart.

Give advice. Be part of the community, helping others as you help yourself. Do volunteer work, perhaps as a senior business consultant or in a partner program in which you work with disadvantaged young people, such as Big Brothers and Big Sisters. You will benefit your community and lower your risk of a second heart attack because you will feel part of a social network.

Join the survivors. Join a focused support group for heart attack survivors. These groups often engage in community activities. They may do fund-raising for nonprofit heart associations. Groups often sponsor educational sessions, meet with nutritionists and exercise specialists, and just discuss their problems with people who have had similar experiences, says Dr. Wielgosz.

Usually, group members also get together to discuss their heart attack experiences and their concerns for the future. Some cardiac rehabilitation programs include programs of this type. "Group sessions are very important in our program," says Dr. LaFontaine. "After an attack, patients are scared, nervous, depressed, and anxious. It helps them to interact with other people, to know that other people have the same worries and concerns. Once they get better and find that they can exercise and carry on life normally, they can bring that information back to the support group to help other people who have recently had a heart attack. It benefits everyone."

These groups also provide an important sense of community. "Studies show that people who belong to groups and have social interaction are less likely to have a second heart attack," says Dr. Pashkow.

List your questions. Next time you visit your doctor, ask questions. You will feel more in control of your fate, which helps reduce depression and isolation. You will also get used to interacting with people that you don't know very well. "Many elderly patients, especially women, don't ask questions," says Dr. Wielgosz. The more you ask, the easier it will be to talk in other settings and become involved.

Before your next appointment, write down the issues that you want to discuss with your doctor. Ask a spouse or other family member to go over it with you to help clarify the issues that are important to you. Take the list to your appointment—and talk it over with your doctor, suggests Dr. Pashkow.

Stay informed. Subscribe to one of the quality newsletters, such as *Heartline* or the *Harvard Heart Letter,* that keep heart patients up to date on research and relevant issues, says Dr. Pashkow.

Get a follow-up. Your cardiologist or cardiac rehabilitation program can help you avoid depression, says Dr. Wielgosz. A Canadian study showed that simple things make a significant difference. For instance, patients showed more improvement if a nurse made a follow-up call to check on their progress and, if necessary, referred them to a doctor.

If your program or doctor doesn't do such follow-ups, ask for it or look for an alternative program, suggests Dr. Pashkow.

Get family support. Emotional support from friends and family is critical. "People who are depressed feel isolated," says Dr. Carney. "They worry that they don't have anyone who cares for them. They often ask after a heart attack, 'Is there a future for me?' " Discuss your feelings with family members and friends. You will all benefit—you won't feel as isolated, and they will understand your needs better.

Consider purchasing a pet. A pet will provide you with crucial support and interaction. "Pets depend on you, and that gives your life some purpose and gratification that sustains you," says Dr. Wielgosz.

Researchers at the University of Montreal in Canada found that people who are depressed and angry are much more likely to die within one year of a heart attack than people who aren't. And at Brooklyn College of the City University of New York, researchers found that cardiac patients who owned pets had better survival rates than those who didn't. Pet owners were less anxious, less depressed, and less angry. Dog owners fared the best in the study, but Dr. Pashkow says that you should benefit from any pet to whom you are strongly attached.

Get a grip. Emotions play an important role in heart attack risk. Teach yourself to spot and defuse anger and hostility, emotions that could pave the way for a second heart attack. When you are feeling upset, just stop, step back, and try to analyze the emotion. Distance yourself from your feelings. Ask yourself if what is bothering you is really important, says Dr. Sullivan.

If, for instance, you get cut off in traffic, is it worth getting mad? Did the incident really slow you down? Is your anger at another driver worth an increased risk of a heart attack? With time, putting your emotions into perspective will become second nature, and you will learn to control heart-threatening feelings.

Redefine yourself. A lot of people define themselves by what they can do: their jobs, their physical activity, or their health. A heart attack can lower your self-esteem, says Dr. Sullivan. "It can take away a layer of who you are, especially if you define yourself by things you can't do right after a heart attack." Determine other ways of defining yourself. Even though you've had a heart attack, you are still just as important to family and friends, for example.

Use existing resources. If you're just recovering from a heart attack and have physical limitations, use the resources already in place in your community. Take advantage of programs that offer senior transportation or home delivery of meals—at least until you feel better.

A lot of cardiac patients don't like to feel dependent, but these organizations also help you feel like a part of the community, which speeds recovery and lowers your risk. Remember that the whole community benefits, because staying healthy is a lot less costly. "You're doing everyone a favor by taking advantage of resources and staying involved in the community," says Dr. Pashkow.

Prescription for Prevention

Get back on track for a healthy, active life by making the lifestyle changes that both help your heart recover and protect it from a second attack. If you don't, your risk of another attack soars.

Do:

- *Become a label reader in the grocery store. Choose low-fat, low-cholesterol, and low-calorie products.*

- *Increase your consumption of breads, cereals, pasta, grains, fruits, and vegetables.*

- *Choose a doctor and a cardiac rehabilitation program that provide you with encouragement and follow-up.*

- *Reduce stress. Make time for quiet reflection, contemplation, and hobbies.*

- *Get 2 to 5 hours of aerobic exercise a week.*

Don't:

- *Smoke.*

- *Let small things get you stressed out.*

- *Live in isolation. Get involved in a church, club, and neighborhood activities. Do volunteer work. Join a focused support group for heart attack survivors.*

Chapter 20

Cancer

An Eating and Exercise Plan for a Longer, Healthier Life

The fear that cancer will return dances a ceaseless jig in your mind. Sure, you're scared. Yes, you're nervous.

But never forget that you are in remission.

"Every time you go to bed think, 'I'm in remission.' Every morning when you wake up think, 'I'm in remission.' Always, always think about remission instead of recurrence. Thank God every day that you are in remission. Embrace that feeling and hang on to it as tightly as you can," says Thommye Stewart, a Houston breast cancer survivor in her seventies who has been in remission for more than 25 years.

There is plenty that you can do to increase the odds that you'll stay in remission, doctors say.

"People shouldn't just sit around waiting to die. Sure, you have a chance of recurrence. But assuming that you didn't come in with a cancer that was in an advanced stage to begin with, the chances are you're going to be cured or survive for many years," says Hugh Shingleton, M.D., the American Cancer Society's national vice president for cancer detection and treatment. "So you should keep on practicing good health habits."

Although no direct evidence exists that lifestyle changes can reduce the risk of recurrence, some doctors suspect that the same measures recommended for preventing an initial cancer—a low-fat and high-fiber diet, regular exercise, weight control, optimism, spirituality, not smoking, and avoiding excessive alcohol use and nitrites—can help fend off a return of the disease.

"These preventive steps, which are beneficial to the general public, may be of heightened importance for someone who has already had a cancer," says Wendy Schlessel Harpham, M.D., attending physician at Presbyterian Hospital of Dallas, cancer survivor, and author of *After Cancer: A Guide to Your New Life.* "All people are at risk for developing the same cancer again. Many survivors are at an increased risk for developing another type of cancer just because of the original type of cancer they had. Some treatments themselves increase the risk of developing cancer. Taking these steps to prevent cancer can reduce survivors' overall risk of future cancers."

The Odds Are with You

For certain cancers that are detected and treated early, a cure is likely, and the odds of a recurrence are small, Dr. Shingleton says.

Take breast, colon, and prostate cancer, for instance. These three cancers are some of the most common cancers among men and women over age 60 and account for about 44 percent of all cancers. For women, the risk of renewed breast cancer rises by about 1 percent each year after treatment. So after 10 years, there is about a 10 percent chance of cancer developing in the other breast, says Charles Taylor, M.D., director of medical oncology at the Arizona Cancer Center in Tucson. In the colon there is a 10 to 15 percent risk of a second new cancer occurring in the remaining bowel.

Prostate cancer seldom recurs if the tumor is confined to the prostate and the organ can be surgically removed, says Paul Engstrom, M.D., a medical oncologist and senior vice president of population science at Fox Chase Cancer Center in Philadelphia. As with all cancers, there is a small chance that some prostate cancer cells will elude detection and spread to other organs even after the prostate has been removed. But if caught early, there is less than a 1-in-10 chance that prostate cancer will revive in some other part of the body in the next five years.

On the other hand, lung cancer is difficult to detect early and cure. Patients that are cured of lung cancer are more prone to develop new cancers of the lung, throat, or mouth. That's because smoking—the number one cause of lung cancer—damages many cells in the respiratory tract and makes them more susceptible to cancer, says Dr. Engstrom. At five years the risk is about 15 percent and doubles to 30 percent within a decade.

Living with Uncertainty

Yet, even with these favorable statistics, doctors can not guarantee that your cancer will never recur. Why? Sometimes, radiation or chemotherapy doesn't destroy all the cancer cells in a person's body. These microscopic cells, which often are undetectable, begin to grow, and eventually the tumor takes hold in another spot, says Peter Greenwald, M.D., head of cancer prevention and control at the National Cancer Institute in Bethesda, Maryland.

In other cases it is possible for cells at several sites in the same organ to be damaged by carcinogens like cigarette smoke. These damaged cells can develop into cancer at different rates. So even while you're being treated for one tumor, it is possible that a second or even third cancer may be slowly evolving within the same organ, according to Dr. Greenwald.

If a cancer does recur, it is often more difficult to fight than the initial cancer, Dr. Engstrom says. That's because the remaining cancer cells usually are more resistant to treatment than those destroyed the first time around.

"Unless all of the factors, such as smoking, that may have contributed to that cancer developing in first place are reversed, the risk of it happening again is still high," Dr. Harpham says.

That is why improving your diet and getting regular exercise like walking 30 minutes a day, three times a week, are so important after cancer. These and other preventive steps bolster the immune system and increase its ability to seek out and destroy any stray cancer cells, Dr. Harpham says.

"If your immune system is in good shape and you are well nourished, I do think that helps the body keep a cancer in check," Dr. Harpham says.

Making Your Remission Last

Your battle against recurrence begins in the doctor's office, since early detection is your first line of defense.

"In a sense, follow-up is further assurance for both you and your doctor that everything is okay," Dr. Shingleton says.

Your doctor will determine the best follow-up plan for you. In general, most oncologists like to see patients every three months during the first year of remission, every four months in the second year, and then every six months until year five. After that, your doctor will probably want to examine you annually, says David Bouda, M.D., assistant professor of oncology at the University of Nebraska College of Medicine in Omaha.

Here are a few tips to make your appointments more satisfying.

Chart your progress. Keep a record of your medications, side effects, and symptoms, Dr. Shingleton says. Take it with you every time you see your oncologist. It will help you plan the next step in your recovery.

Express yourself. Before each appointment, make a list of questions that you may have about your follow-up treatment. Then ask the oncologist to discuss these concerns with you, Dr. Bouda says.

"You need to be open about your feelings. Some people never discuss anything with their doctors, so they don't have a clue that there are any concerns," Dr. Bouda says. "Your doctor isn't a mind reader. You need to talk with your physician regularly and give him a fair chance to address your concerns."

If the doctor doesn't seem interested in your problems, find another oncologist. "The doctor-patient relationship is a partnership. If your doctor isn't your partner, fire him," Dr. Bouda says.

Don't panic. Blood tests such as prostate-specific antigen (PSA), which measures cancer activity in the prostate, can provide doctors with valuable clues about the status of your remission. But don't panic if a single test is elevated. Some tests have a wide range of normal readings, while others may be prone to imprecise results, Dr. Bouda says.

"People who focus on the outcome of every test tend to be fixated on recurrence," Dr. Bouda says. "They're often paralyzed to the point that they can't enjoy life."

How I Did It: A Survivor Helps Others Cope

Thommye Stewart still cries a lot.

"Crying is a blessing," says the Houston woman. "If I couldn't cry, I couldn't have gotten through all of this."

"All of this" began in 1970 when she was diagnosed with breast cancer and underwent a radical mastectomy and radiation treatment at M. D. Anderson Cancer Center in Houston. More than a quarter-century later and now in her seventies, she's still in remission.

"The prognosis was really grim. But from the beginning I told myself, 'Thommye, you're not going to think about dying,'" Stewart says. "I've known so many people who from the minute they knew they had cancer told themselves that they were going to die. And many did. I simply didn't want to think like that. I focused on living."

Once she recovered, she became a volunteer at the cancer center, visiting new patients and running errands for families. She is still at it.

"Volunteering is healing. If you can help patients get through their trauma and their anger, that certainly helps you, too," Stewart says. "The possibility of recurrence does pop into the back of my mind every once in awhile, particularly when someone comes in with a recurrence after 20 years. But I just focus on helping others, and any fear or anxiety that I may have about my cancer coming back just fades away."

Instead, she reserves her tears for others. "I hurt when someone doesn't make it. And I cry whenever I hurt. That's when I feel angry about cancer," she says. "I didn't have those feelings for myself because I literally thought, 'Thank God, it's not my kids. I can handle anything but that.'

"I'm happy because I've had 25 years that I wouldn't have had," Stewart says. "I thank God for every day that I've had. I love every day that I'm alive, whether it's good, bad, or indifferent."

If you're like that, you may be better off not getting tested, because any fluctuation is going to drive you nuts, Dr. Bouda says.

In fact, doctors may be able to detect some forms of recurrent cancer just as well without fancy tests. Researchers, for instance, have found that doctors who used sophisticated medical testing detected breast cancer recurrence only four weeks earlier than doctors who relied solely on physical exams, Dr. Bouda says. The earlier detection by testing made no difference in overall survival rates. Ask your doctor what a test really means, Dr. Bouda suggests. How reliable is it? What does it actually measure? How concerned should you be if the test isn't normal? Is it really necessary?

"If it's a simple, specific test, it should be done. But ordering too many tests just causes unnecessary anxiety," Dr. Bouda says.

Suspend alternative treatments before your appointment. Let your doctor know if you are using any alternative treatments like homeopathy, ayurveda, or vitamin and mineral therapy, Dr. Bouda says. These treatments may interfere with traditional medicines and testing.

Saw palmetto, for instance, an herbal treatment used by some men to prevent swelling of the prostate, may decrease PSA test readings. That can mislead you and your doctor into thinking that your prostate cancer is under control, says E. David Crawford, M.D., chairman of the Division of Urology at the University of Colorado Health Sciences Center in Denver.

"If you're doing something that is off the mainstream, you probably shouldn't take any alternative therapy for at least 24 hours before or after your conventional treatment," Dr. Bouda says.

Know the warning signs. Ask your doctor to explain the most important signs and symptoms of a possible recurrence, Dr. Harpham says. If you have any concerns about a symptom, don't hesitate to phone your doctor and make an appointment.

"After surviving cancer, particularly soon afterward, it is very normal to be a bit alarmist about changes or symptoms," says Dr. Harpham. "But you owe it to yourself and your doctor to go in with your concern and get it checked out. If it turns out to be nothing, what have you lost? If it does turn out to be something, you have maximized your health."

Diet: Get Back to the Pyramid

No diet or foods have been proven to suppress the return of cancer, says Carolyn Clifford, Ph.D., chief of the diet and cancer branch at the

Six Supplements That May Subdue Recurrence

After cancer treatment, vitamin supplements, diet modifications, and lifestyle changes can reinforce your body's natural defenses and help prevent a recurrence, says Kedar N. Prasad, Ph.D., director of the Center for Vitamins and Cancer Research at the University of Colorado Health Sciences Center in Denver.

"Taking these supplements may boost your immune system so it can seek out and destroy any undetected cancer cells that remain in your body," says Dr. Prasad, author of *Vitamins in Cancer Prevention and Treatment.*

Here is the combination of oral supplements that Dr. Prasad recommends.

Beta-carotene: 15 milligrams a day.

Vitamin A: 5,000 international units a day, divided into two doses, taken once in the morning and once in the evening. Most vitamin A supplements come in a 10,000 international units dose, so quarter the tablet (equivalent to 2,500 international units) to get your 5,000 international units a day.

Vitamin C: Up to 2 grams a day, divided into at least two doses, in the form of calcium ascorbate. *Note:* Amounts of vitamin C over 1,200 milligrams a day may cause diarrhea in some people.

Vitamin E: 400 international units per day, divided into two doses, taken in the morning and evening. Each dose should contain 100 international units of alpha-tocopheryl-succinate and 100 international units of alpha-tocopherol.

B vitamins: Take a multiple vitamin containing two to five times the Daily Value for thiamin, riboflavin, and vitamins B_6 and B_{12}.

Selenium: 100 micrograms a day, divided into two doses, once in the morning and once in the evening. Levels above this should only be taken under medical supervision.

Selenium must be taken in the form of organic selenium. Inorganic selenium, such as sodium selenite, is absorbed poorly by the small intestine.

National Cancer Institute in Bethesda, Maryland. But several ongoing studies sponsored by the Institute are attempting to determine if eating a low-fat, high-fiber diet will lower recurrence rates of breast, lung, head, and neck cancer.

Although the results of these long-term studies are several years away, following the U.S. Department of Agriculture's food pyramid recommendations after you have had cancer is probably prudent.

"The feeling is, it is best to follow these guidelines to reduce the risk of recurrence as much as possible," says Christine Polisena, R.D., an oncology dietitian at the Cleveland Clinic Foundation. "For someone who has successfully gotten through cancer treatment, the recommendations I would give are to maintain your desirable body weight, watch your fat consumption, increase your fiber intake, try to eat more fruits and vegetables, and limit nitrate-cured foods and alcohol consumption."

Here are a few specifics that are especially important after cancer.

Eat more lean meat. "When some people are recovering from cancer, they'll think now is the time to become a vegetarian. But that's not necessarily true," says Cheryl Ritenbaugh, Ph.D., head of nutrition research at the Arizona Cancer Center in Tucson. "Many people lose muscle mass rapidly while fighting the disease, so getting enough lean meat and other forms of protein onto your plate is important at that point."

To help your body rebuild muscle, eat three servings—a total of 5 to 7 ounces a day—of fish, poultry, and lean meat for at least four months after your treatment ends, Dr. Ritenbaugh suggests. "You don't need to go overboard on meat. You don't need to eat a 16-ounce steak," she says.

Target 20 percent. In laboratory experiments excessive amounts of dietary fat fuels growth of certain types of tumors like prostate cancer, says William R. Fair, M.D., chief of urologic surgery and chairman of urologic oncology at Memorial Sloan-Kettering Cancer Center in New York City. Reduced dietary fat also may slow recurrence.

Try to limit yourself to 20 percent of calories from fat daily, Dr. Fair recommends. If you eat 2,000 calories a day, for instance, that means you can consume about 400 calories—44 grams—from fat. Look for total fat grams on food labels.

Stoke up on fruits and vegetables. Try eating at least five servings of

How I Did It: A Super Bowl Coach Wins the Big One

There is only one recurrence that Marv Levy would welcome in his life.

"A chance to go back to the Super Bowl and win," says Levy, the 70-plus coach of the National Football League's Buffalo Bills.

But even if he never gets that opportunity, Levy has already won the biggest challenge of his life. In 1995 he survived prostate cancer.

"I think I was doing all the right things before I got prostate cancer. I was exercising. I was eating a very low-fat, high-fiber diet. So I don't know what else I could have done to prevent it. I was just fortunate that it was detected early during an annual physical," Levy says.

He opted for surgical removal of the prostate. Like many other men, Levy feared impotence and incontinence, but neither of these two possible side effects of prostate cancer surgery affected him. After surgery, his faith in his lifestyle remained strong.

"I got back into living a healthy life very quickly after my surgery," Levy says. "I work out, I run, I lift weights at least twice a week, I eat correctly, and I make sure that I get the proper amount of rest. I think all of that helped me come back very quickly."

Still, anxiety about a recurrence does rumble through his mind every once in awhile like a blitzing linebacker.

"Those concerns exist, but I can't live in fear," he says. "One thing that helped was that I did quite a bit of studying about prostate cancer once I discovered that I had it. That was very reassuring to me because I found out about treatments and ways to live with it even if it does spread. So education always helps.

"I also talked with a lot of people who have been through similar experiences. And I found that to be very helpful."

He also advises diving back into your regular routine.

"As quickly as possible, I'd say return to as vigorous a life as you can," Levy says. "You don't have to become a workout nut. But don't make yourself an invalid mentally just because you've had cancer. Don't ever let this disease make you feel old."

fruits and vegetables like apples, oranges, carrots, and broccoli a day. These foods are loaded with antioxidants, fiber, and other cancer-preventing nutrients, says Polisena.

Fruits and vegetables are good sources of fiber, which speeds food through your body so that fewer carcinogens can be absorbed by your digestive tract, Dr. Bouda says.

Nix the nitrates. Limit or avoid nitrate-cured, salt-cured, or smoke-cured foods like ham, sausage, or bacon, Polisena says. These foods are linked to stomach cancer.

Go light on the hard stuff. Alcohol may promote recurrence of head, neck, mouth, and esophagus cancer. Limit your consumption each day to no more than one 12-ounce beer, a 4-ounce glass of wine, or one cocktail containing an ounce of liquor, Polisena says.

Look to the Future

When she was diagnosed with lymphoma in 1990, Dr. Harpham didn't know what to do about her magazine subscriptions.

"I always used to renew my magazines and medical journals for several years at a time," she says. "When I first got sick, I questioned whether it was worthwhile renewing any of them. Then when I felt a little more secure, I renewed them for a year. Now I renew them for three to five years at a time again. Instead of making me feel vulnerable, these subscriptions empower me, because I plan on being here to use them."

The lesson? Hang on to hope and cling to the future as you move into remission, she says.

Not only can that improve the quality of your life and lessen your fears of recurrence, it may boost your immune system's ability to wipe out any emerging cancers, Dr. Bouda says.

"Try to figure out some way to think positively every day, despite having had cancer," Dr. Bouda says.

Here are some suggestions.

Seek support. Cancer support groups can be breeding grounds for optimism, Dr. Bouda says. You'll probably meet many long-term survivors who can inspire you and offer lots of empowering self-help tips.

"A doctor may just tell you what the textbook says," Dr. Bouda says. "Someone at a support group meeting may tell you, 'Yeah, I tried what my doctor suggested, and it never worked. But I tried this instead, and I haven't had a problem since.'"

Most cancer treatment centers or hospitals can provide you with a list of support groups in your area.

Look to your past. You have lived for 60-plus years and probably have coped with many stressful and tragic situations before. Evaluate those experiences and try to identify what helped you survive those emotional upheavals, suggests Joan Hermann, director of social work services at Fox Chase Cancer Center in Philadelphia. Did it help to jot down your feelings? Talk to close friends? Pray? Whatever it was, it probably will help you deal with your fears now.

"Older people often handle cancer and its aftermath better than younger men and women because of their wisdom and experience," Hermann says. "An older person tends to think, 'This is how I dealt with another tragedy in my life, and I can get through this situation in the same way.' The younger person simply doesn't have that experience to fall back on."

Tame your imagination. Sometimes it is easy to imagine the worst. But if you learn to control your imagination, it can actually help calm your fears and strengthen your body's natural defenses, says Gloria Malone, Ph.D., a Phoenix psychologist in private practice who counsels many older people who have cancer.

"It's like a remote control on your television. With a little practice you can literally learn to turn off an unwanted thought," Dr. Malone says.

To do it, you might begin by imagining yourself in a very relaxed place in nature like a meadow filled with wildflowers or a lush tropical beach. See it, feel it, smell it, sense it. Practice that for a minute or two, 20 to 30 times a day, until visualizing your special place becomes almost automatic, Dr. Malone says. Then when fear or any other unwanted thought pops into your mind, imagine reaching for a remote control. Press the button and—zap—turn the unwanted thought or fear out of your sight. Take a deep breath, then press the button again and visualize yourself calm and relaxed in your special place in nature.

Treat yourself. Plan to do something special for yourself each day.

It doesn't have to be time-consuming or costly. List two dozen nurturing activities like watching a sunrise, playing with your grandchildren, or reading an inspirational book. Then pick one a day and do it, Dr. Malone says.

"Doing something nurturing for yourself each day will help you feel less angry or deprived," Dr. Malone says. "It will help you focus on the positive aspects of your life instead of negative thoughts about recurrence."

Find hope. Inspirational posters and meaningful pictures from your life can help, too.

"I have a poster in my kitchen that reads, 'Keep on hoping, keep on wishing, keep on believing.' It would be easy to say that poster is childish and silly," Dr. Harpham says. "Well, you know what? This physician and mother derives benefit from looking at that poster. It is one more thing that helps me believe that I can get well again and stay well."

Prescription for Prevention

Fear of a recurrence is a common emotion after surviving cancer. Although doctors can't guarantee that you won't get cancer again, the odds of a complete cure for many forms of this disease are getting better every day, particularly if you adopt a healthy lifestyle.

Do:

- *Focus on remission rather than recurrence. Rejoice every day that you are cancer-free.*

- *Know the warning signs of a recurrence. Like your initial cancer, early treatment of a recurrence increases your chances of recovery.*

- *Consume no more than 20 percent of daily calories from fat. If you eat 2,000 calories a day, that means you can have about 44 grams of fat daily.*

- *Eat plenty of fruits and vegetables rich in antioxidants and other cancer-suppressing nutrients. Try to eat at least five servings of foods like oranges and broccoli daily.*

Don't:

- *Get hung up on test results. Small fluctuations in a single test don't necessarily mean your cancer has returned.*

- *Take alternative treatments within 24 hours of a conventional cancer treatment or test. Some alternative medicines can interfere with more traditional treatments.*

- *Overindulge. Excessive alcohol consumption can promote head, neck, and other cancers. Limit yourself to one drink a day.*

- *Eat bacon and other nitrate-laden foods. Salt-cured, smoke-cured foods like ham or bacon might reignite cancer. If you can't completely give up these foods, limit your intake.*

Chapter 21

Stroke

Take Command and Reduce Your Risk of Another One

As he walks, his right foot slowly rises about 2 inches in the air before it mechanically plunges to the ground, as if it were attached to a puppeteer's string. Often he still says "water" when he really means something else like "hand," "chair," or "tree." But John Candido is happy.

"I feel great. I'm not sick anymore," says the former New Jersey landscaper who had a massive stroke in June 1995.

Indeed, John, who was nearly 60 when it happened, came a long way in the first year after his stroke. With the help of therapists, he regained the use of his paralyzed right arm and leg. His speech, which was once limited to "One, two, three, water," returned to complete, understandable sentences after months of rehabilitation. He recovered so well that he is a volunteer—transporting patients in wheelchairs—at the center where he was treated, the Kessler Institute for Rehabilitation in West Orange, New Jersey.

But as healthy as he seems, John still is at high risk for another stroke.

"He doesn't worry about it, but I do because I know the statistics," says Mary Jo Candido, R.N., John's wife and chapter coordinator for the Northern New Jersey Chapter of the National Stroke Association.

In fact, people over age 60 who have had a stroke are 10 times more likely to have another one. Up to one in three will have another stroke within five years of their first one.

But even if you've had a stroke, this doesn't have to be your fate.

"Changing your lifestyle now can make a dramatic difference," says Lawrence M. Brass, M.D., professor of neurology and co-director of the Yale Cerebrovascular Center at Yale University School of Medicine. "In some cases, lowering blood pressure, quitting smoking, and making other lifestyle changes can reduce your risk of subsequent stroke by more than 50 percent."

Anatomy of a Stroke

When you were going through stroke rehabilitation, you probably noticed a lot of people your age working through similar problems. There are reasons for that.

Every minute, someone in the United States has a stroke. Of those, two of every three—more than 350,000 a year—occur in people over age 65. And after age 55, the risk of stroke doubles with each passing decade you live.

Stroke becomes more common as we age, in part, because it is provoked by many of the same lifelong habits—smoking, sedentary living, high-fat eating—that trigger heart attacks. In fact, most strokes are caused by the same mechanism as a heart attack, says Arthur Ancowitz, M.D., author of *The Stroke Book* and founder of the Stroke Foundation in New York City.

These "brain attacks," or ischemic strokes, occur when a blood vessel gets blocked and blood flow to a part of the brain ceases, causing death of brain tissue. A less common type of stroke, called a hemorrhagic stroke, happens when a weakened blood vessel bursts and causes bleeding in the brain. This kind of stroke, which killed president Franklin Roosevelt, is often more debilitating than an ischemic stroke, says Michael Schneck, M.D., assistant professor of neurological sciences at Rush–Presbyterian–St. Luke's Medical Center in Chicago. Regardless of type, "most effects of stroke can improve with therapy," he says.

Even a small stroke, if it occurs in a vital part of the brain, can cause extensive damage that may rob you of speech, vision, or movement, Dr. Schneck says.

But at least one-third of all strokes are mild, meaning the person may have little or no disability. Another third of stroke survivors are completely debilitated, requiring special care. The rest are somewhere in between—such as having extreme weakness in one or more limbs. Those with moderate effects are often functionally independent in their daily activities, although they may or may not be able to return to work. But no matter how severe the initial damage, most stroke survivors do get better, says Richard C. Senelick, M.D., neurologist, medical director of HealthSouth Rehabilitation Institute of San Antonio, Texas, and co-author of *Living with Stroke*.

Some early improvement probably occurs as swelling surrounding the damaged area of the brain slowly diminishes in the first few weeks after the stroke, says Carlos Kase, M.D., professor of neurology at Boston University School of Medicine. It is also possible that in the months following the stroke other parts of the brain take over some of the functions of the damaged area, he says.

Still, it may take up to a year before a survivor regains many of the capabilities that he had prior to the stroke, Dr. Schneck says. "The first six months of rehabilitation are the hardest. Don't let yourself give up."

Preventing Another One

Now that you are better, you certainly don't want it to happen again. Depending on the type of stroke you had, your doctor may prescribe an anticoagulant drug like anisindione (Miradon) or antiplatelet drugs like ticlopidine (Ticlid) or aspirin.

Your doctor also might recommend a surgery, called a carotid endarterectomy, to unclog your carotid arteries. A surgeon makes a 3-inch incision in your neck and cleans plaque out of one or both of the carotid arteries, two major arteries that supply blood to the brain. Although surgery can't reverse the damage already done by stroke, says Dr. Ancowitz, this procedure can help prevent a recurrent or even an initial attack in those at high risk. Among people who have had a previous stroke, this surgery reduces the risk of recurrence in the following two years from 27 percent to 8 percent, says Richard Libman, M.D., assistant professor of neurology at the Albert Einstein College of Medicine of Yeshiva University in New York City.

But even if you take drugs or have surgery, it is still important to take command of your own health after a stroke.

Some risk factors for stroke are out of your control. Among these are family history of stroke, age, gender (men are slightly more prone to

Seek Help for These Warning Signs

Strokes can fool you. The warning signs of a recurrent stroke, such as blurred vision, dizziness, and gait unsteadiness, can be subtle, says Michael Schneck, M.D., assistant professor of neurological sciences at Rush-Presbyterian–St. Luke's Medical Center in Chicago.

A symptom like numbness in the hands will last only a few minutes, for instance, then suddenly disappear. But don't be deceived.

"If there is even the slightest chance that you're having symptoms of a stroke, don't wait to see your doctor. All that does is delay treatment. Go to a hospital emergency room immediately, then have someone notify your doctor of the situation," says Richard Libman, M.D., assistant professor of neurology at Albert Einstein College of Medicine of Yeshiva University in New York City.

Since a stroke can impair your judgment and ability to communicate, it's also important that people in your life be aware of a stroke's warning signs, says Harold P. Adams, Jr., M.D., director of the Division of Cerebrovascular Diseases at the University of Iowa in Iowa City.

It's also important to remember that a stroke can occur in any area of the brain, affecting different parts of the body. So a subsequent stroke can have completely different warning signs than your first one.

Here are some of the key warning signs of any impending stroke.
- Sudden weakness or numbness of the face, arm, or leg
- Sudden dimness or loss of vision, particularly in one eye
- Double vision
- Any sudden unexplained drowsiness, nausea, or vomiting
- Sudden difficulty speaking, finding words, or understanding speech
- Sudden severe headache with no known cause
- Unexplained dizziness, unsteadiness, or sudden falls, especially with any of these other symptoms
- Difficulty swallowing
- Memory loss
- Loss of consciousness

strokes than women), and race (African-Americans are almost twice as likely to have a stroke than Whites).

But many others, such as high blood pressure, high cholesterol levels, diabetes, a smoking habit, overweight, a sedentary lifestyle, and excessive alcohol consumption can and should be tamed.

"If a person has a stroke and doesn't stop smoking or change his diet or get his blood pressure under control, then his chances of having a second stroke in the next year are overwhelming," Dr. Ancowitz says. "Without those changes, all the ingredients that caused stroke number one will still be there to provoke stroke number two."

Here's a look at how you can dampen your chances of a recurrent stroke.

Banish High Blood Pressure

"Uncontrolled high blood pressure is a major cause of stroke. Treatment is crucial," says Sidney C. Smith, Jr., M.D., professor and chief of the Division of Cardiology at the University of North Carolina at Chapel Hill and past president of the American Heart Association.

In fact, after a four-year study of 662 men and women in their sixties and seventies who had strokes, researchers at Allegheny University in Philadelphia concluded that those people who didn't correct high blood pressure were substantially more likely to have a recurrent stroke, says Milton Alter, M.D., Ph.D., clinical professor of neurology at Allegheny University Hospitals, a neuroepidemiologist, and co-author of the study.

That's because high blood pressure—a reading consistently more than 140/90 millimeters of mercury (mmHg)—strains your arteries, especially in the brain. This makes them more susceptible to clotting or rupture, Dr. Ancowitz says.

There are many ways to combat soaring blood pressure.

Shed pounds. If you lose excess weight, you'll be less likely to have high blood pressure, Dr. Ancowitz says.

Curtail cocktails. Limiting your daily consumption of alcohol to no more than two 12-ounce beers, two 4-ounce glasses of wine, or two cocktails containing 1 ounce of alcohol also can slash your chances of having a stroke, Dr. Ancowitz says.

429

Stay physically active. "Exercise is extremely important after you've had a stroke for many reasons. Not only will it help lower blood pressure and protect against the development of cardiovascular disease, but it will help you maintain muscle tone that is so vital during rehabilitation," Dr. Ancowitz says.

Regular exercise dilates blood vessels so that blood pressure falls and stays down when you're not exercising. Sweating also may coax sodium out of your bloodstream and help lower blood pressure, Dr. Ancowitz says. Plus, developing muscle strength through exercise will make daily tasks that much easier to perform.

Ask your doctor or physical therapist about the types of exercise that are best for you. But in general, try to get some type of moderately intense aerobic exercise for at least 30 minutes daily, Dr. Ancowitz suggests.

"If you can still walk, do that. If you can't walk, then try upper-body exercises like swinging your arms over your head. Just do as much as you can," Dr. Ancowitz says.

Stoke up on calcium. If you're not getting enough calcium in your diet, not only will you be at greater risk of osteoporosis but also you may be more likely to have high blood pressure. "Individuals that fail to meet the Daily Value for calcium are more likely to develop hypertension," says David McCarron, M.D., professor of medicine and head of the Division of Hypertension at Oregon Health Sciences University in Portland.

Edith Howard Hogan, R.D., a spokesperson for the American Dietetic Association in Washington, D.C., recommends consuming 1,500 milligrams of calcium daily. A 1-ounce slice of Swiss cheese, about the size of a domino, has 270 milligrams of calcium and only 7 grams of fat. A cup of low-fat yogurt, an 8-ounce glass of skim milk, or canned sardines or salmon packed with bones are also good sources. If you think that you're not getting enough calcium from your diet alone, ask your doctor about taking a supplement to boost your intake, says Hogan.

Dash for the herbs. Instead of reaching for the salt, which can raise blood pressure, add a touch of herbs and spices like ginger, oregano, garlic, or onion powder to your foods, Dr. Ancowitz suggests. Not only will that add aroma and zest to your meal but also it will cut down on your salt consumption and may lower your risk of a recurrent stroke.

You can save money by looking for these products in unusual places, Hogan says. Some drugstores, for example, sell spices for about half the price that you would find in a grocery store.

Try the dilution solution. In many cases, you can do a lot to shave the sodium content of a favorite food or ingredient, Hogan says. If, for example, you buy a sodium-rich spaghetti sauce, try adding a can of no-sodium-added stewed tomatoes to the mixture. That will dilute the sodium in the sauce without affecting the flavor.

Be wary of salt substitutes. Many salt substitutes contain potassium in the form of potassium chloride, which can help lower blood pressure in healthy people. But some men and women over age 60 who have weakened kidneys may not be able to rapidly excrete potassium from their bodies, says Thomas Pickering, M.D., professor of medicine at New York Hospital–Cornell Medical Center in New York City and author of *Good News about High Blood Pressure.* Also, excessive amounts of potassium in the blood can cause abnormal heart rhythms. Before using a salt substitute, check with your doctor, he suggests.

Snuff Those Puffs

Days after John Candido's stroke, his wife found him digging through her purse looking for something.

"He was still in the hospital, he couldn't walk and could barely talk, and here he was rummaging around for a cigarette," recalls Mary Jo Candido. "I said, 'Are you crazy? That's the worst thing you could do to yourself.'"

In fact, smoking elevates blood pressure, speeds up the narrowing of artery walls, and forces the heart to work harder. Overall, smoking at least doubles your chances of having another stroke.

"If you want to increase your risk of a recurrent stroke and take the chance of being further debilitated, then you should continue to smoke,"

Make "I Can" Your Motto

If you've had a stroke, it's easy to give in. If you're a caregiver, it's easy to overprotect.

Resist these temptations.

People who have had strokes often can do much more than many caregivers suspect, says Michael Schneck, M.D., assistant professor of neurological sciences at Rush-Presbyterian–St. Luke's Medical Center in Chicago.

"Whenever possible, I advise caregivers to err on the side of independence," Dr. Schneck says. "Let the person who has had the stroke do as much as they want to, and then some. Don't let the survivor be an invalid."

With adaptive equipment and techniques, many people who have had strokes can master skills like driving, gardening, woodworking, and other activities, says Caryn Abel, a recreation therapist at the Kessler Institute for Rehabilitation in West Orange, New Jersey. If you have a

---

Dr. Libman says. "Smoking is the most modifiable risk factor for stroke. You have complete control over whether you do it."

Although John Candido did smoke for a brief time after he returned home from the rehabilitation hospital, he eventually snuffed out his 40-year habit cold turkey.

Of course, there are many ways to quit. Deep breathing, for instance, helps many people learn to relax without cigarettes and can help you resist cravings, experts say.

Long, deep breaths mimic the sensation of smoking and can be reassuring and satisfying to someone who is trying to quit, says Mitchell Nides, Ph.D., a psychologist specializing in smoking cessation at the University of California, Los Angeles. "Deep breathing may be one of the best ways cope with an urge to smoke," he says.

Try the following deep-breathing exercise whenever you feel an urge to smoke.

hobby or vocation that you would like to try, first clear it with your doctor, then ask your recreation therapist how you might do it, Abel suggests.

It is also important that the stroke survivor be allowed to reassume a role within the family, says Wayne Sotile, Ph.D., director of psychological services for the Wake Forest University Cardiac Rehabilitation Program in Winston-Salem, North Carolina, and author of *Heart Illness and Intimacy*.

"If the person with a stroke becomes a spectator instead of a participant in life, that can be devastating emotionally," Dr. Sotile says. "Allow the stroke survivor to be as much of a person as he can."

So if the stroke survivor loves to cook, for example, but no longer has use of his arms, he can still be helpful in the kitchen by sharing his expertise with others, Dr. Sotile suggests. That will relieve depression and boost self-esteem.

Take a deep, slow breath through your nose or through pursed lips as if you were smoking a cigarette. But instead of smoke, feel the fresh air fill your lungs. Hold it in for a count of three. Then exhale slowly, letting all of the air out of your lungs. As you exhale, feel the muscles in your neck and shoulders relax. Repeat this exercise two or three times, Dr. Nides says.

Sex: Love Conquers All

Intimacy hasn't been forgotten at Jim and Cathy Kalal's home in Harlan, Iowa.

"We're keeping on pace with the national record for sex in a month by a stroke survivor," Jim Kalal says, laughing. "I'm holding up my end."

Jim, a retired public utility administrator in his sixties, survived a paralyzing stroke in 1982.

(continued on page 436)

Caregivers: You Deserve a Break Today

Caregiving is a grind that can wear even the best of us down.

In fact, up to half of all long-term caregivers will seek help for a stress-related disorder. Often, the wearing routine of this ceaseless job creates more stress for the caregiver than the illness itself does for the person who is ill, says Wayne Sotile, Ph.D., director of psychological services for the Wake Forest University Cardiac Rehabilitation Program in Winston-Salem, North Carolina, and author of *Heart Illness and Intimacy*.

"It's important for caregivers to realize that this isn't a sprint. It's a marathon, so you have to pace yourself," Dr. Sotile says. "The best gift you can give to people that you care for is taking time to care for yourself both mentally and physically."

Here are some ways to lessen the strain of caregiving.

Reach out for help. Don't be afraid to ask family members, friends, and neighbors to take some of the load off your shoulders, suggests Pam Erickson, R.N., private care manager for Eldercare Advisors in Denver. Make a list of people willing to care for your loved one when you need a break. Call upon those who have said, "If there's anything I can do, just ask." Even if the respite person will just cook a meal, do laundry, or do other chores for you once a week, accept it. It will ease your burden and allow you to have more quality time for yourself. If friends or family aren't available, consider home health care or nursing services listed in the Yellow Pages. Rates range from $10 to $18 an hour.

Get away from it all. Take 30 minutes daily to do something that you enjoy, like gardening or reading. At least once a week, get outside the home, Dr. Sotile says. Go to a movie, walk around a park, or play bridge with friends for a couple of hours.

Not only will these activities boost your morale but also, when you come home, you'll probably have new experiences and stories to share with your less-mobile loved one, Dr. Sotile says.

Vent your feelings. At times every caregiver feels frustrated, angry, guilty, lonely, and overworked. Form a telephone network of caregivers who are facing similar problems so that you can share your ups and downs, Dr. Sotile suggests. The National Stroke Association, 96 Inverness Drive East, Suite I, Englewood, CO 80112 (phone number 1-800-STROKES), can provide a list of stroke support groups in your area with interested members.

If you're having a particularly bad day, don't try to hide it from the person you're caring for, Dr. Sotile says.

"Holding in your feelings and letting interpersonal tension accumulate isn't healthy for either you or the stroke survivor," Dr. Sotile says. "Sometimes you need to proclaim to the person you're caring for, 'I really need your help, love, and care today as much as you need mine.'"

Set limits. People who have had strokes have mood swings, frustrations, and bad days, too. But that doesn't mean they have a right to take it out on you.

"Ask yourself how you would react to this behavior if the stroke had not occurred," Dr. Sotile says. "If your loved one came home from work and started calling you names, you probably wouldn't tolerate it. So take off those kid gloves. Say, 'Listen, I love you, I care about you, and I know you're scared. But you can't treat me like this and get away with it. It's important to me that I am respected and loved. We can't let a stroke ruin what we have built between us.' You simply can't let yourself be violated, or else you're going to end up resentful, and that doesn't help anyone in this situation."

If mood swings and other emotional outbursts persist for more than six months for either the patient or anyone in a caregiving position, seek counseling, Dr. Sotile says. The emotional effects of dealing with serious illness can be far-reaching, he says, so it is important for each family member to examine his feelings and seek help if needed.

How I Did It: Iowa Man Leads an Electrifying Life

Jim Kalal has a message for everyone who has had a stroke: Life goes on.

"A stroke isn't the end of the world. You just change your routine, switch to another track, and proceed onward. You can still have the same enjoyment of life. I used to love golf. But since my stroke, I've found lots of other things to do," says Kalal, a retired public utility administrator in Harlan, Iowa.

Now in his sixties, Kalal has lived with complete paralysis of his left arm and leg since his stroke in December 1982. He can stand and walk with the aid of a leg brace.

"I was at least 30 pounds overweight, I had high cholesterol, my blood pressure was running high, I drank more than I should, and I was working in a high-pressure job," he says. "But for some reason, I didn't think it would happen to me."

After rehabilitation, he went back to work but made little effort to change his lifestyle. His job overseeing the water, electrical, and natural gas needs of 2,500 customers continued to wear him down. His daily routine still included two or three drinks after work. In addition, he and his wife, Cathy, continued eating a high-fat diet that included

"I don't think you should ever give intimacy up because of a disability. You find what is the best way for you to fulfill your intimacy with each other. We have managed to do that. We're probably as sexually active as some of the younger couples in our neighborhood," says Cathy Kalal, R.N.

"I don't see Jim's disability," she adds. "I don't look at him like I'm longing for something that isn't there. He is who he is, and I am who I am."

Many stroke survivors and their spouses fear that sexual activity will trigger another stroke. In reality, although blood pressure and heart rate do increase during sex, the increase probably isn't enough to be concerned about, according Roger Crenshaw, M.D., a psychiatrist and sex

lots of fried foods. In January 1991, he had a massive heart attack that forced him to retire.

But a lesson was learned. Now he adheres to a low-fat diet, walks as much as possible, limits himself to one beer a day, and lives at a slower pace.

"I think one of the things that saved me from another stroke is that I got away from the pressures. That's very important. I'm just more relaxed. I'm not living my life full speed ahead anymore."

But he remains active. He uses a power mower to cut the grass on the couple's 4-acre lot, enjoys building doll furniture and wooden storage trunks for his grandchildren, and serves on his community's cemetery board.

"I don't understand people who sit around and feel sad about what life has dealt them," he says. "I just don't have any room for that in my life."

Still, there are times when anxiety does overwhelm him.

"It's unrealistic to believe that a fear of recurrence isn't going to be in the back of your mind occasionally," Kalal says. "I just do everything that I can, including prayer, to prevent a stroke from happening again."

therapist in private practice in San Diego.

"The sexual part of the brain doesn't dissolve during a stroke," Dr. Crenshaw says. "Just because there has been a muscular difficulty doesn't mean that the person can't desire and enjoy sexual activity."

In fact, intimacy of all kinds, including hugging and kissing, can boost self-esteem and relieve depression, says Dr. Senelick. The better your primary intimate relationship is after a stroke, he says, the better your odds are that you'll have a more complete recovery.

"It's a huge boost to your self-esteem if your partner still finds you attractive," says Domeena Renshaw, M.D., director of the Sexual Dysfunction Clinic at Loyola University of Chicago Stritch School of Medicine.

---

10 Empowering Ways You Can Help Your Caregiver

Jim Kalal, a retired public utility administrator in Harlan, Iowa, wrote these 10 commitments after his paralyzing stroke in 1982. They have helped him maintain an understanding and fulfilling relationship with his wife and caregiver, Cathy. Originally published by the National Stroke Association, the commitments are as follows.

1. Don't ask my caregiver for anything that I can do for myself.

2. Make sure that I thank my caregiver each time she provides assistance to me.

3. Make sure that when my caregiver suggests we go out to eat, shopping, and so forth, I make every effort to go.

4. I will do my best not to complain about my stroke or handicap and my limitations.

5. I will try my utmost, on my own, to improve my skills, so as to improve the quality of my life and my caregiver's quality of life.

6. Encourage my caregiver to do things on her own, always giving my caregiver some space.

7. I will try to never feel sorry for myself, and I will do my best to keep my sense of humor.

8. I enjoy telling my caregiver that she looks nice, and to me she is always attractive.

9. I will not live in the past but live for today and the future, learning to live with my new lifestyle, my handicap.

10. I tell my caregiver I love her, because I do.

"And yes, it's still possible to be a very good lover even if you've had a stroke."

Ask your doctor if and when you can resume sexual relations, Dr.

Crenshaw recommends. Like all aspects of stroke rehabilitation, regaining intimacy may require some adaptation and experimentation. Here are some suggestions.

Take it slow. After you and your partner decide to resume sexual relations, put intercourse out of your mind for a couple of weeks. Instead, focus on the other pleasures of intimacy like kissing, touching, and hugging, suggests Dr. Renshaw, author of *Seven Weeks to Better Sex.* Gradually building up to renewed sexual relations will boost your self-esteem and self-confidence, reduce performance anxiety, and foster feelings of mutual trust.

"Love play that avoids the genitals can strengthen the relationship between a couple in this situation," she says. "It lets the person who had the stroke know that his partner really loves him in many ways. And that ultimately makes sex much easier."

Play it again, Sam. Setting the right mood is important, particularly after a life-changing event like a stroke, Dr. Renshaw says. Take time to reminisce about past romantic moments in your relationship. Play a favorite love song on the stereo. Take a moment to gaze at a full moon together and realize that the romance you had before the stroke can continue.

Stay in sight. Many people who have strokes lose vision in one eye. Either ask your spouse to move so that you can see him or her or tilt your head to the side so that your partner remains in your line of sight when you're making love, Dr. Renshaw says.

Go with your strength. Lie on the side of your body that is weaker so that your strong hand is free to caress your spouse's body. This position will also allow you to thrust by using your strong leg to push off against the foot of the bed or a wall, Dr. Renshaw says.

Keep laughing. Sex at any age or with any physical problem is better if you don't take it so seriously. Have fun, be frivolous, use your imagination, Dr. Renshaw says. Remember that you're not at a stockholders meeting—you're with someone you love. Enjoy it.

Check out your drugs. If you have difficulty getting or maintaining arousal, ask your doctor about it. Some medications prescribed for high blood pressure or depression, for instance, can interfere with your sexual abilities, Dr. Renshaw says. But under no circumstances should you dis-

Hormone Replacement May Stop Stroke Recurrence

For women, estrogen may bolster the fight against stroke and its recurrence.

Preliminary data show that postmenopausal women who take the hormone appear to have a 50 to 70 percent lower risk of heart attacks than women who don't. They also may be less susceptible to strokes, says Lawrence M. Brass, M.D., professor of neurology and co-director of the Yale Cerebrovascular Center at Yale University School of Medicine.

That's important because women account for more than half of all strokes and 60 percent of stroke-related deaths.

"We don't have conclusive evidence that estrogen does lower stroke risk. But there are more than 400 known effects of estrogen in the body, many of which could contribute to a better outcome for this disease," Dr. Brass says.

Estrogen may diminish the chances of a stroke or a recurrence by lowering blood cholesterol levels, slowing atherosclerosis, dilating blood vessels, or preventing blot clots, Dr. Brass says.

The Women's Estrogen for Stroke Trial, a study being conducted by Yale University researchers of 652 postmenopausal women who use the hormone, may unravel some of the mystery in the near future, Dr. Brass says. If estrogen is proven to reduce stroke risk among women, it also may have the same preventive effects for men, he says.

If you've had a stroke, it is worthwhile to ask your doctor about taking estrogen to reduce your risk of recurrence, Dr. Brass suggests.

continue taking a drug without your doctor's consent.

Give yourself time. After six months, if you're not back into the same sexual routine that you were in prior to your stroke, consider seeing a sex therapist who has experience in dealing with stroke survivors and their families, Dr. Crenshaw says.

"It usually isn't protracted therapy—just six to eight sessions that will help the couple deal with their specific concerns," Dr. Crenshaw says.

Rehabilitation Is a Lifetime Job

Although rehabilitation probably won't directly lower your risk of a subsequent stroke, it can vastly improve the quality of your life and help keep you more active.

Dr. Senelick says that exercise, along with other lifestyle changes like quitting smoking, can lessen your risk factors—such as hypertension, diabetes, or obesity—as well as reduce your chances of having another stroke.

That's why it is important to keep the muscles in the affected area of your body well toned even after rehabilitation ends, says Matthew Lee, M.D., medical director of the Rusk Institute of Rehabilitation Medicine at New York University Medical Center in New York City.

"If you don't do the exercises recommended for you, if you don't maintain what flexibility you've gained during rehabilitation, you're going to lose it. Your movements are going to get tighter and tighter, and eventually you may not be able to put a shirt or pair of pants on again. What's going to be affected is your quality of life," says Dr. Lee, co-author of *Recovering at Home after a Stroke*.

In addition to walking, strength training, or any other regular exercise you can get, the daily arm and leg toning regimen on the following pages is suggested by Regina Kelly, a physical therapist at Kessler Institute for Rehabilitation in West Orange, New Jersey. If you have recently had a stroke, be sure to check with your doctor before starting any exercise program.

Do one set (10 repetitions) of each exercise. Then rest for 1 minute, or until you feel able to continue, and do two more sets of 10 with rest periods in between. Switch sides where appropriate and then repeat the cycle.

Wear comfortable, loose-fitting clothing and do these exercises slowly and smoothly. Count out loud during your workout, says Kelly. Saying numbers aloud will require you to breathe normally, while helping to keep track of your reps.

UPPER-BODY EXERCISES

MAKING FISTS
Curl your fingers, beginning at the tips, and make a fist. Uncurl your fingers, completely straightening and spreading them. You can work both hands at once or alternate sides.

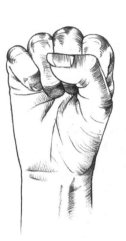

WRIST FLEXIONS
To strengthen your wrist, sit in a chair and rest the forearm of your left hand on a table placed beside you, with your wrist extending over the edge, palm down. Bending at the wrist, raise the hand up and down, leaving your forearm on the table. Do three sets, rest, then turn your palm up and repeat. Switch arms.

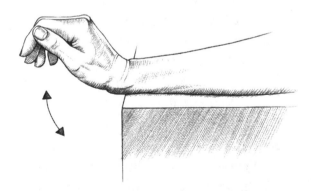

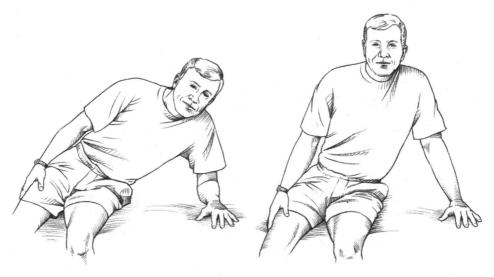

SITTING PUSH-UPS

To strengthen your triceps muscle, sit on a firm surface like the edge of a bed and lean to one side. Support your weight with your bent elbow and forearm. Now push up so that your weight is on your hand and your arm is straight. Slowly lower yourself again and repeat for three sets. Switch sides.

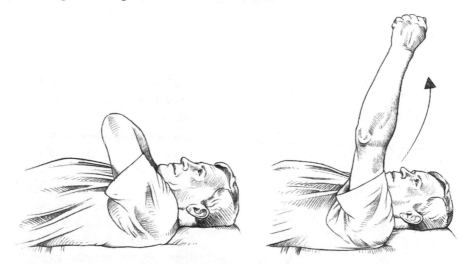

ELBOW EXTENSIONS

Lie on your back on a firm bed. Touch your left hand to the opposite shoulder. Your elbow should be pointing toward the ceiling. Raise your hand slowly toward the ceiling until your arm is straight. Then lower your hand to the starting position. Do three sets with rest periods in between. Repeat with your other arm.

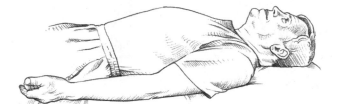

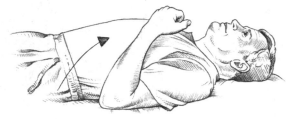

BICEPS CURLS

This exercise can be done lying down, sitting, or standing. Begin with your arms straight and at your sides. Bend your left elbow, bringing your left hand toward your left shoulder. Straighten your arm and repeat for three sets. Rest, then switch sides.

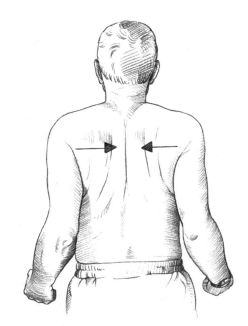

SHOULDER SQUEEZES

To improve your posture and strengthen your back muscles, stand or sit straight and tall. Tuck your chin in and relax your arms. Pull your shoulders back and squeeze your shoulder blades together. Try to get your elbows as close together as possible behind your back. If you're sitting, you can bend your elbows slightly as you draw your arms back. Otherwise, try to keep your arms straight. Relax and repeat for three sets.

LOWER-BODY EXERCISES

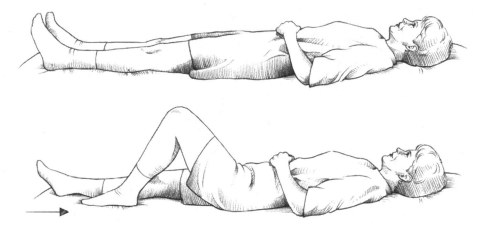

HEEL SLIDES

On a firm bed, lie on your back with your legs straight. Bend your left leg at the hip and knee, sliding your heel up toward your buttocks. Your knee should eventually point toward the ceiling. Hold for a count of five, then return to the starting position. Do three sets with rest periods in between. Repeat with your other leg.

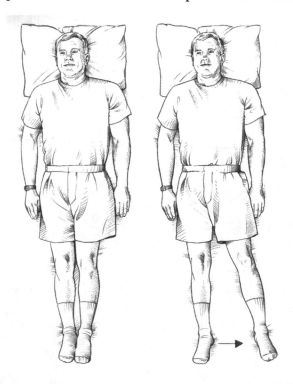

LEG SLIDES

Lying on your back with your legs straight, slide your left leg out to the side. Keep the leg straight and toes pointed up. Don't lift the leg, just slide it. (As you get stronger, you can try lifting your leg up slightly as you swing it out.) Return to starting position and repeat. Do three sets with each leg.

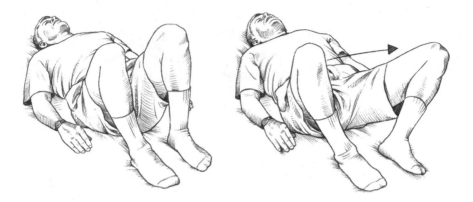

MORE LEG WORK

Lie on your back on a firm bed with knees bent and feet flat. Keeping your knees bent, slowly lower your left knee out to the side as far as possible. Return to starting position. Repeat for three sets. Rest, then switch legs.

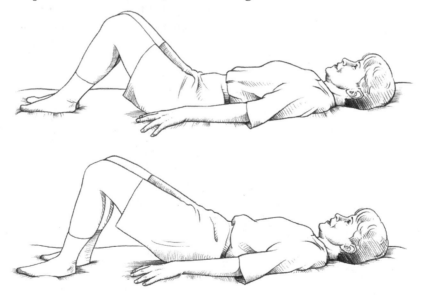

BOTTOM LIFTS

To strengthen your buttocks, lie on your back on a firm bed with your legs together and your knees bent and pointing toward the ceiling. Your feet should be flat on the bed. Using your arms for leverage, if necessary, lift your bottom as high as possible. Don't forget to breathe regularly. Slowly lower, then repeat for three sets.

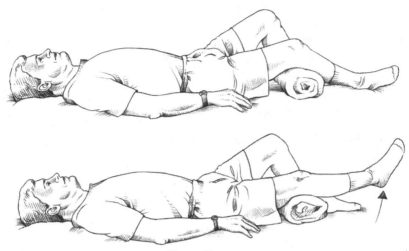

KNEE EXTENSIONS
Lie on your back with a pillow or large towel rolled under your knees. Slowly lift one foot up a couple of inches. The back of your knee should remain on the pillow and your leg should become as straight as possible. Slowly lower and repeat for three sets. Rest, then switch legs.

Prescription for Prevention

With therapy, many people can regain use of the arms, legs, and speech after a stroke. Strokes are often provoked by many of the same lifelong habits— smoking, sedentary living, high-fat eating—that trigger heart attacks. But modifications in lifestyle can diminish your chances of having a recurrence.

Do:

- *Exercise. Walking and other activities will help lower blood pressure, a major risk factor for stroke.*

- *Season foods with herbs instead of salt. Excess sodium can drive up blood pressure in some people who are salt-sensitive.*

- *Quit smoking. Lighting up doubles your chances of having another stroke.*

- *Continue practicing the exercises your physical therapist or doctor has recommended for you.*

Don't:

- *Drink too much alcohol. In excess, alcohol increases your risk of stroke. Limit yourself to no more than two drinks a day.*

- *Reach for salt substitutes. Many are made with potassium chloride, which can cause irregular heart rhythms in some people over age 60.*

- *Shy away from intimacy. Sex can boost your self-esteem. It is unlikely to cause a stroke.*

- *Give up.*

Index

<u>Underscored</u> page references indicate boxed text. **Boldface** page references indicate illustrations. *Italic* page references indicate tables.

449

<u>Underscored</u> page references indicate boxed text. **Boldface** page references indicate illustrations. *Italic* page references indicate tables.

Underscored page references indicate boxed text. **Boldface** page references indicate illustrations. *Italic* page references indicate tables.

Underscored page references indicate boxed text. **Boldface** page references indicate illustrations. *Italic* page references indicate tables.

Underscored page references indicate boxed text. **Boldface** page references indicate illustrations. *Italic* page references indicate tables.

Cruciferous vegetables. *See also specific cruciferous vegetables*
for preventing cancer, 70, 71, 72, 74
Cucumbers, health benefits of, 109
Currants, health benefits of, 110
Curry, health benefits of, <u>128</u>
Cyclic hormone therapy, 379

D

Daily Value, 87
DDT, cancer from, 320, 329, 330
Deep-breathing exercise, for smoking cessation, 432–33
Deli foods, low-fat, 33
Depression
exercise, to elevate mood in, <u>218</u>–<u>219</u>
heart attack recurrence from, 405, 408–11
heart disease risk from, 253, 349–50
Desserts, portion size, 42
Diabetes
disease risk from, 350–53
exercise for controlling, <u>219</u>, <u>224</u>
metabolism and, 399
screening, 313–14
Dining out, low-fat eating when, 39–43
Doctor, choosing, <u>398</u>
Double shoulder rolls exercise, 197
Doughnuts, fat in, 33–34
Drinking alcohol. *See also* Alcoholic beverages
cancer recurrence and, 421
deciding on merits of, <u>295</u>
health benefits of, 293–98, 357
smoking cessation and, 277

stroke recurrence and, 429
supplements needed with, <u>162</u>
to stimulate appetite, <u>209</u>, 210

E

Eating habits, for weight control, 200–201, 203–11
Eggs, substitutes for, 36
Elbow extensions, as poststroke exercise, 443
Elbow rolls exercise, 197
Electrocardiogram (EKG), 314
Emotions
heart attack risk and, 410
overeating and, <u>188</u>–<u>89</u>
positive, good health from, 248–70
Endometrial cancer
hormone replacement therapy and, 375
overweight and, 185, 186
Energy, from hormone replacement therapy, <u>376</u>–<u>77</u>
Environmental hazards
air pollution, 320, 327–29
asbestos, <u>332</u>–<u>33</u>
health risks from, 319–37
cancer, 320–21, 322, 324–25, <u>328</u>, <u>332</u>, 335
heart attack, 320, 327–29
occupational, <u>324</u>–<u>25</u>
passive smoking, 323–25, 327
pesticides, 321, 329–30, 332–33, 335
radon, 321, 335–37
Esophageal cancer, overweight and, 185, 186
Estrogen
dietary fat and, 15

Underscored page references indicate boxed text. **Boldface** page references indicate illustrations. *Italic* page references indicate tables.

functions of, <u>374</u>, <u>376–77</u>
phytoestrogens, health benefits of, 73–74, 75, 79
for stroke prevention, <u>440</u>
Estrogen replacement therapy. *See* Hormone replacement therapy
Evaporated skim milk, in cooking, 27, 36
Exercise(s) <u>224</u> 227
aerobic, for heart attack recovery, 397, 400–401
benefits of, 213–14, <u>218–19</u>, 224–25
calisthenics, 233, **234**, **235**
cooldown, <u>220</u>, <u>221</u>, 227–28
danger signs from, <u>222</u>
deep-breathing, for smoking cessation, 432–33
doctor's approval of, <u>216</u>, 225–26
guidelines for starting, 225–30, <u>241</u>, <u>242</u>, <u>244</u>, 245, <u>246</u>
immune system and, 223
perceived exertion rate of, <u>232</u>
for preventing
atherosclerosis, 346
cancer, 223
heart attack recurrence, 397–403
heart disease, 214–15
high blood pressure, 215–17, 355
stroke recurrence, 430
preventing injury from, <u>220–21</u>
rating exertion level of, <u>232</u>
relaxation, 190–91
shoes for, 240–43
sticking with, <u>400</u>, 401, 403

strength-training, 195–96, 217–23, 237, **237–40**, 397
stretching, <u>228</u>, **229**, 383–84
after stroke, 441, **442–47**
supplements needed with, <u>162</u>
two-phase program of, 213–14
walking as, 226, 227, 230–31
warm-up, <u>220</u>, <u>221</u>, 226, <u>228</u>, **229**
for weight control, 194–96, **197–99**, 199–200
Eyelids, skin cancer on, <u>366</u>
Eye round roast, as healthy meat, <u>92</u>

F
Faith, positive feelings and, <u>260–61</u>
Fat, body
distribution of, <u>184</u>
health risks from, 179–80
Fat, dietary, 6–8, <u>7</u>, 8–9, *See also specific types*
cholesterol from, 356–57
counting grams of, <u>13</u>, 20
cutting grams of, *22–23*
functions of, 6
health risks from, 4–6, 10–11
percentage of saturated and unsaturated fat in, 7
recommended percentage of calories from, 10, 20, 419
Fecal occult-blood test, for colon and rectal cancer screening, 312–13
Fiber, 45–61
adding, to diet, <u>76</u>
calcium absorption and, 172
for cancer prevention, 19, 45, 47, 48, 421

Underscored page references indicate boxed text. **Boldface** page references indicate illustrations. *Italic* page references indicate tables.

Fiber *(continued)*
   food sources of, 88, 89–90, 91, 92,
      93, 94, 95, 96, 97, 99, 102,
      103, 104, 106, 109, 110, 114,
      116, 117, 118, 119, 120, 121,
      125, 127, <u>128</u>, 129, 131, 134,
      137, 138, 140, 141, 143, 148,
      149, 153, 154
   gas from, 25, <u>46</u>
   health benefits of, 45, 47
   insoluble
      for cancer prevention, 47–48
      sources of, 49, 52–53
   for lowering
      blood pressure, 395
      cholesterol, 357, 394
   soluble
      getting 10 grams per day of, <u>58</u>
      health benefits of, 53–55, 58
      increasing intake of, 59–60
      for lowering cholesterol, 53–55,
         <u>59</u>, 60
      sources of, 53, *56–57*, <u>58</u>
      supplements, 58
   for weight control, 205
Fibrinogen, heart disease and, <u>340</u>,
      348
Figs, health benefits of, 110
Fish. *See also specific types*
   for low-fat eating, 33
   poaching, 35
Flatulence, from high-fiber foods, 25,
      <u>46</u>
Flavonoids
   adding, to diet, 83–84
   food sources of, 89, 96, 98, 99, 100,
      113, 114, 118, 120, 122, 150
   for preventing

cancer, 82–83
      heart disease and stroke, 83, 114
   in wine, 297–98
Flaxseed, health benefits of, 79–80
Flounder, health benefits of, 111
Fluke, health benefits of, 111
Folate, food sources of, 90, 91, 93, 94,
      95, 96, 99, 100–101, 102,
      103, 104, 106, 107, 108, 119,
      121, 126, 127, 128, 129, 132,
      133, 135, 136, 137, 138–39,
      140, 144, 147, 148, 151, 154,
      156, 157
Folic acid supplements, 166
Footwear, athletic, 240–43
Free radicals, phytochemicals and,
      66–67
French fries, low-fat alternative to, 35
Frozen foods
   as high-fat, high-sodium foods,
      35–36
   low-fat homemade, 37
Fruit ices, as snack, <u>113</u>
Fruits. *See also specific fruits*
   for low-fat eating, 35
   pesticides on, <u>331</u>
   for preventing
      cancer, 62, 63, <u>64</u>, 66, 419, 421
      heart disease, 66
   serving size of, 87
Frying, alternatives to, 35, <u>40–41</u>

G

Garlic
   deodorized, 70
   health benefits of, 67, 68, 69, 111–12
Garlic powder, 68, 69, 70
Gas, from high-fiber foods, 25, <u>46</u>

<u>Underscored</u> page references indicate boxed text. **Boldface** page references
indicate illustrations. *Italic* page references indicate tables.

Underscored page references indicate boxed text. **Boldface** page references
indicate illustrations. *Italic* page references indicate tables.

<u>Underscored</u> page references indicate boxed text. **Boldface** page references indicate illustrations. *Italic* page references indicate tables.

Underscored page references indicate boxed text. **Boldface** page references indicate illustrations. _Italic_ page references indicate tables.

Underscored page references indicate boxed text. **Boldface** page references indicate illustrations. *Italic* page references indicate tables.

Underscored page references indicate boxed text. **Boldface** page references indicate illustrations. *Italic* page references indicate tables.

Underscored page references indicate boxed text. **Boldface** page references
indicate illustrations. *Italic* page references indicate tables.

Underscored page references indicate boxed text. **Boldface** page references indicate illustrations. _Italic_ page references indicate tables.

Prostate cancer *(continued)*
   preventing, with
      exercise, 223
      low-fat eating, 15–17
   recurrence rate of, 413
   screening for, 315–16
Prostate-specific antigen (PSA) test,
      for prostate cancer
      screening, 315, 415, 417
Prunes
   as fat substitute, 26
   health benefits of, 139–40
PSA test, for prostate cancer
      screening, 315, 415, 417
Psyllium, in fiber supplements, 60
Puddings, evaporated skim milk in
      low fat, 36
Pumpkins, health benefits of, 140–41
Push-ups
   bent-knee, **234**
   sitting, as poststroke exercise,
      443

R

Radishes, health benefits of, 141
Radon, 325–27
   lung cancer from, 321, 335
Radon detectors, 336
Raisins, health benefits of, 141
Raspberries, health benefits of, 142
Recipes
   chili, <u>50</u>
   spaghetti sauce, <u>51</u>
Rectal cancer, screening for, 312–13
Rectal examination, for prostate
      cancer screening, 315
Reflux, gastric, cancer risk from,
   186

Rehabilitation
   after heart attack, 401–3, 404–5, 409
   after stroke, 441, **442–47**
Relaxation
   for coping with grief, 263, 265
   for weight control, 190–91
Resistance training. *See also* Strength-
      training exercise; Weight-
      lifting
   exercises
   for weight control, 195–96
Respiratory infections, heart disease
      and, 348–49
Restaurant dining, low-fat eating in,
      39–43
Rhubarb, health benefits of, 142
Riboflavin
   food sources of, 88, 91, 104, 105, 125,
      129, 133, 138, 140, 141, 144,
      149, 151, 152, 153, 156, 157
   supplements, 166
Rice, health benefits of, 143
Roasting foods, in low-fat cooking, <u>41</u>
Rutabagas, health benefits of, 143

S

Salad dressings, served on the side,
      41–42
Salads, high-fat additions to, 42
Salmon, health benefits of, 144
Salt
   high blood pressure from, 355, 395,
      430
   substitutes for, 430–31
Sardines, health benefits of, 144–45
Saturated fats, <u>8</u>
   cancer risk from, 5–6
   cholesterol from, 356

<u>Underscored</u> page references indicate boxed text. **Boldface** page references
indicate illustrations. *Italic* page references indicate tables.

Underscored page references indicate boxed text. **Boldface** page references
indicate illustrations. *Italic* page references indicate tables.

Underscored page references indicate boxed text. **Boldface** page references
indicate illustrations. *Italic* page references indicate tables.

Underscored page references indicate boxed text. **Boldface** page references indicate illustrations. *Italic* page references indicate tables.

Underscored page references indicate boxed text. **Boldface** page references indicate illustrations. *Italic* page references indicate tables.

Underscored page references indicate boxed text. **Boldface** page references indicate illustrations. *Italic* page references indicate tables.